Private Practices

Private Practices

Harry Stack Sullivan, the Science of Homosexuality, and American Liberalism

NAOKO WAKE

RUTGERS UNIVERSITY PRESS

NEW BRUNSWICK, NEW JERSEY, AND LONDON

LIBRARY OF CONGRESS CATALOGING-IN-PUBLICATION DATA

Wake, Naoko.
  Private practices : Harry Stack Sullivan, the science of homosexuality, and
American liberalism / Naoko Wake.
     p. ; cm.
  Updated version of author's doctoral thesis—Indiana University, 2005.
  Includes bibliographical references and index.
  ISBN 978–0–8135–4958–3 (hardcover : alk. paper)
  I. Sullivan, Harry Stack, 1892–1949. 2. Gay psychiatrists—United States—Biography
3. Homosexuality—United States—History—20th century. I. Title.
  [DNLM: I. Sullivan, Harry Stack, 1892–1949. 2. Psychiatry—United States—
Biography. 3. Psychiatry—history—United States. 4. History, 20th Century—
United States. 5. Homosexuality, Male—history—United States. 6. Homosexuality,
Male—psychology—United States. 7. Politics—United States. WZ 100 S949w 2011]
  RC440.84.W35 2011
  616.890092—dc22
  [B]   2010021011

A British Cataloging-in-Publication record for this book is available from the
British Library.

Visit our Web site: http://rutgerspress.rutgers.edu

Manufactured in the United States of America

For my partner, Steve, and my parents

CONTENTS

Acknowledgments ix

Abbreviations xiii

Introduction 1

1 A Man, a Doctor, and His Patients 13

2 Illness Within a Hospital and Without 51

3 Life History for Science and Subjectivity 85

4 Homosexuality: The Stepchild of Interwar Liberalism 121

5 The Military, Psychiatry, and "Unfit" Soldiers 157

6 "One-Man" Liberalism Goes to the World 187

Notes 219

Index 257

ACKNOWLEDGMENTS

My journey to this book began when in 1995 at a college bookstore in Kyoto, Japan, I picked up a work titled *Schizophrenia as a Human Process*, one of Harry Stack Sullivan's posthumous publications translated into Japanese. The chapters were filled with patient records and testimonies of their illnesses from an American psychiatric hospital called Sheppard and Enoch Pratt Hospital, or Sheppard-Pratt. For reasons I both did and did not know, I found the records unforgettable. Three years later, I was on my way to the hospital archives, taking my first trip to the United States—and my first international trip of any sort—anxious to find out if these records still existed and what I might find. At Sheppard-Pratt, everyone warmly welcomed me, thanks to Lawrence Breslau, a psychiatrist who had worked at the facility. He and his wife, Erica, exemplifying American hospitality, showed me around Baltimore and made sure that I did not get lost in the huge hospital. The manager of its medical records department, Janet Fry, helped me dig up clinical records from the 1920s in a dimly lit basement storage room that she called a dungeon. Just as I will not forget the excitement of discovering the precious, if dusty, records, I will not forget the lunch she treated me to at the hospital's cafeteria on the last day of my stay, during which we—a middle-aged American woman and a Japanese graduate student who could not speak fluent English—did not really know how to talk to each other. But we gave it our best shot anyway.

I have been fortunate in receiving generous support from institutions that are key locations for my research. At the Washington School of Psychiatry in Washington D.C., Carolyn A. Morrisey and Barbara Wayne were a great resource. From the William Alanson White Institute in New York City, I received not only openhanded assistance in my archival work, but also the best intellectual engagement that a historian of medicine can hope for from medical professionals. A special thank you goes to Mark J. Blechner, Jay Kwawer, and Sondra Wilk. Beyond these institutions, Stewart E. Perry and Michael S. Allen stood out both as avid believers in the value of intellectual inquiry and as distinctive personalities who helped define what I was up to. Without the Sullivan-related sources to which they generously offered me access, this book would have been impossible. I am grateful to the late Joanne Finley, whose history of affiliation with the Washington School of Psychiatry and Sheppard-Pratt inspired my thinking about history in both personal and professional ways. She also became one of my dearest friends, and her energy, honesty, and charm will forever stay in my memory.

In my present academic life, I thank Elizabeth Simmons, dean of Lyman Briggs College at Michigan State University, whose support for my research has come to occupy an important place in my scholarship. A warm thank you, too, to the historians of science at Briggs—Richard Bellon, Georgina Montgomery, Mark Waddell, and John Waller—whose minds, collegiality, and friendship have kept me writing. I also thank other colleagues at Lyman Briggs, Sharon DeGraw, Daniel Dougherty, and Chris Ganshoff in particular, who took time to offer their thoughts on my research, despite disciplinary boundaries that could have prevented it. And I am happy to acknowledge colleagues Aaron McCright, Robert Pennock, and Robert Shelton, who have inspired me with their passion for life and work in academia.

James H. Capshew saw my dissertation through to completion at Indiana University, Bloomington and has continued to be a warm supporter of my academic life. Peter Hegarty and Jack Drescher have never failed to urge me to think, as the saying goes, outside the box. Their work on gender roles, sexual identity, and science has shaped scientific and political frameworks against which I measure my historical thinking. Gerald N. Grob, who first became familiar with my work as an outside reader of my dissertation chapters, has come to know it even more as a reviewer for Rutgers University Press. I have benefited enormously from his crisp, thoughtful suggestions. Elizabeth Lunbeck's insights into my work, which she offered to me particularly when I was working on Chapters 3 and 6, have been sharp, original, and invaluable.

I have benefited from two editors at Rutgers University Press, each of whom brought different virtues to this monograph. I appreciate Doreen Valentine's cogent editorship of style, rooted in her interest in issues of gender, health, and illness. Peter Mickulas has instilled this book's production process with energy and stability. My hope is that our collaboration, his first with an author at Rutgers, was as positive an experience for him as it was for me.

I say a special thank you to my parents, Shigemi and Hirotsugu Wake. While I grappled with this book, their lives went through significant changes, including my father's retirement. I wish I were closer to them in their process of readjustment—I was far away across the ocean, working on this thing called a book manuscript. But they are very happy about its publication, and about the great gratification they knew that I took in it. I am fortunate to have such sincere, loving parents.

Steven M. Stowe is everywhere in this book, as much as he is in my life. There is no single word that he did not read more than ten times; there is perhaps no single sentence that remained unchanged after he went over it. If there is anything as powerful as such intellectual rigor and generosity, it is his quiet, and yet abiding, love for me. I was often not sure if this book was going to be finished; but his daily presence has shown me that there are some things that we can learn to trust in our lives.

ABBREVIATIONS

APA	American Psychiatric Association
ASS	American Sociological Society
CACSS	Civilian Advisory Committee on Selective Service
IPC	International Preparatory Commission for the International Congress on Mental Health
NCMH	National Committee for Mental Hygiene
WFMH	World Federation for Mental Health

Private Practices

Introduction

Homosexuality in the twenty-first-century United States is highly politicized. As the issue of same-sex marriage enters courtrooms or appears on ballots, often with a brusque *no* as an outcome, supporters of such unions express their dismay and anger at the denial of equal rights for sexual minorities. On another, related front, the military's "Don't Ask, Don't Tell" policy has been one of the most contested issues in the United States today, stirring up the one-century-old discussion about the "damage" that sexual minorities might do to the army's morale, as well as the question of what qualities Americans hope to see in men and women serving the nation. As much as in 1993, when the policy was implemented, these discussions remind us of angst and frustration that is still in need of relief and resolution. But these ongoing debates are also an indication of the long distance toward equality that sexual minorities have traveled. Notwithstanding the steep road that lies before sexual minorities and their allies, the fact that their concerns have made their way to the states' highest courts, popular elections, the U.S. Congress, and the armed forces indicates significant progress toward a fuller recognition of people with "different" sexuality. The issue of homosexuality, as well as that of sexual minorities more generally, is "in play" in American public life.[1] No matter what stance we take, the issue is something that must be openly confronted and that must be checked against our belief in justice, fairness, and equality.

Homosexual men and women had to come a considerable historical distance before their lives assumed this public dimension. Far from being plain and straight, their road to equality was circuitous and full of detours leading only to dead ends. Despite the flourishing of urban gay culture and the rise of progressive views about homosexuality among liberal intellectuals during the 1920s and 1930s, the following decades witnessed extreme

1

hostility against gays and lesbians in many aspects of U.S. public life. American mass media's fascination with "mannish" women and "effeminate" men who dressed, acted, and made life and career choices outside traditional gender boundaries in the earlier decades of the twentieth century became overshadowed by some of the most rampant government-led antihomosexual campaigns in the nation's history by midcentury. Although sexually "free" men and women of the 1920s explored sexual relationships for pleasure, gratification, and happiness outside marriage, the United States in the 1950s became emblematic of strict gender roles, domestication of sexuality, and conformity.[2] Certainly, the economic hardships of the 1930s and Americans' increasing desire to reaffirm traditional gender relationships set the stage for the conservatism of the 1940s and 1950s.[3] National mobilization during World War II made it seem natural that individual differences be tamed and controlled for the greater good. The atmosphere of fear and anxiety, as well as Americans' desire to protect family values during the Cold War, made homosexuality an easy scapegoat.[4] Many scientific experts seemed to justify the marginalization of sexual minorities. Indeed, the gradual, often painfully slow growth of liberalism on the issue of homosexuality in American science—psychiatry, psychology, and the social sciences in particular—in the first half of the twentieth century suggests that intellectual liberalism took a long time to mature before affecting (or being affected by) the public's awareness. Often, the most tenacious conservatism was embedded in scientists' "sympathetic" approach to homosexuality. Thus, before—and in some cases, even after—homosexuality was no longer defined as illness by physicians, many "therapeutic" procedures were administered to homosexual men and women in hospitals and clinics throughout the nation, to "cure" them so they would become heterosexuals.[5] It is no wonder, then, that gays and lesbians experienced setbacks. Researchers of human sexuality did not focus on what most of their subjects needed: an acceptance of who they were.

In this uncertain journey before the politicization of homosexuality, a gap between "public" and "private" views of homosexuality among certain U.S. liberal scientists was a significant factor. Of course, again, the Great Depression, the war, and the fight against communism created an atmosphere favoring conservatism over liberalism: these national challenges made the modern United States' struggle with fear and prejudice difficult. But this is not the whole story. This picture of the battle between liberalism and conservatism does not tell us how liberals—including a number who were sexual minorities—themselves responded and contributed to setbacks in the history of homosexuality. As much as ideological disagreements between liberals and conservatives raised barriers to equality for sexual minorities, certain assumptions and practices among liberal scientists circumscribed their reform impulses from within.[6] Many scientists developed accepting approaches to homosexuality in private, while expressing more compromised views in public. In published writings, lecture notes, and the proceedings of meetings and conferences—"public" documents created with an intention to be shared by a professional or lay audience—the scientific approach to homosexuality seems tentative at best, hostile at worst. In contrast, scientists' opinions expressed in more "private" documents— personal letters, memoirs, and transcripts of one-on-one clinical sessions between a doctor and a patient—often seem uncompromisingly supportive of the normalization of homosexuality.[7] To be sure, scientists of homosexuality did not necessarily see this gap as a flaw. Many regarded the distinction between public and private as a promising means for promoting the eventual acceptance of homosexuality. The separation of the private from the public was as plausible an approach to reform as today's activism seems to us twenty-first-century observers. But their stance did not result in what we see as mainstream political activism today; rather, their effort ended up feeding the homophobic public policies of the 1940s and 1950s.

The life and work of gay psychiatrist Harry Stack Sullivan (1892–1949), the central figure of this book, offer a way into this troubled history of the making of the gap between public and private liberalism in the science of homosexuality. Sullivan is well known for his "interpersonal theory," which defined mental illness in general, and homosexuality in particular, in nonbiological, less stigmatizing sociocultural terms. Moreover, he worked with leading anthropologists and sociologists—Edward Sapir, John Dollard, Charles S. Johnson, Lawrence K. Frank, Ruth Fulton Benedict, and Margaret Mead, among others—to pursue broad, cross-disciplinary social reform.[8] Mirroring the era's high spirit for social betterment and fairness, their hope was to create an overarching, multidimensional, and rational agenda—a liberal agenda—to understand and benefit the socially marginalized, such as mentally ill and homosexual individuals. Because medical and social scientists were the leading scientific authorities examining human sexuality in general, their willingness to recognize homosexuality as a legitimate subject of science could, and to a certain extent did, encourage a better acceptance of homosexuality. Their disciplinary views overlapped in exciting ways. Just as psychiatrists considered homosexuality a meaningful stage of personality development, the social scientific literature of the 1920s and 1930s conveyed intellectuals' fascination with non-Western societies' accepting attitudes toward homosexuality. Because of its potential to reveal Americans' unique characteristics during a time of increasing exposure to social and cultural "others," homosexuality became a much discussed subject. When cultural relativism began to question all things familiar in the medical and social sciences—including the universality of "normal" sexuality—"abnormal" sexuality seemed to illuminate a truth, rather than an exception, about modernity. For, as many scientists of the era agreed, modernity was about the recognition that ambiguity, rather than clear-cut categories, was where all understanding begins. Moreover, the rising interest in homosexuality corresponded with the making of the "life history" method in the medical and social sciences, which urged scientists to go beyond objective mass analysis to reach out to subjective, individual experiences.[9] Implicit in this approach was an attempt to create a place for a modern self—a fluid, unpredictable, and unfamiliar self amid shifting gender roles and sexual relationships—in a coherent narrative of science. Not surprisingly, a range of descriptions of homosexuality appeared in life histories collected in the 1920s and 1930s. Homosexuality in these decades represented a unique locus of scientific inquiry, a liberal current that pushed for individuality and particularity against the mainstream, which tended to suppress these qualities under the assumed regularity and uniformity of nature.[10]

However, the rise of homosexuality as a scientific subject did not mean that scientists who were sexual minorities themselves were able to come out of the closet and assert an equal treatment of homosexual individuals; instead, it meant that these scientists artfully separated what they argued in public from who they were in private. For instance, Sullivan and his colleagues continued to describe heterosexuality and homosexuality in dualistic terms—"healthy versus sick," "virile versus effeminate," and "mature versus immature"—in their published writings. Following the precepts of Sigmund Freud, these psychiatrists did not think of homosexuality itself as an illness unless it caused a person distress, a belief that was in sharp contrast with the mainstream medical notion that sexual "perversion" constituted a clinical entity. Nevertheless, their position most often expressed in public was that, given the prevailing homophobia, homosexual persons tended to be mentally and socially unstable, constituting a risk group that often required medical attention.[11] Anthropological reports of cultures open to homosexuality did not create an intellectual tide of better acceptance of sexual minorities in the United States, either. Although these reports certainly illuminated "primitive" societies' nonstigmatizing attitudes toward homosexuality, anthropologists did not assume that it was immediately applicable to the "civilized" United States. Thus, anthropologist Ruth Benedict's view that American bias against sexual minorities was locally and arbitrarily constructed did not develop into a concerted effort to eradicate homophobia in the United States. She did not engage in a study of homosexuality outside the country herself, nor did she synthesize other researchers' observations to argue for the destigmatization of homosexuality at home. This approach constrained their liberal reform's impact, as it allowed scientists to continue to portray homosexuality as either a mental or a social "problem," at least in public. Scientists of homosexuality did not see equality between the "problem" population and those who examined and tried to find solutions for it. Neither did they make an evenhanded comparison between "primitive" and "civilized" societies.

This limitation becomes more complicated if we look at what Sullivan and other liberal scientists did or said in private. They had a distinct sense of what constituted appropriate public debate and what should remain in private, creating different forms of liberalism in different spheres. It is clear that Sullivan was willing to take more risks and adopt a more radical approach to homosexuality in his clinical practice. That is, Sullivan as a gay psychiatrist pursued a fuller depathologization of homosexuality in his treatment of psychiatrically disturbed homosexual men, even as he defined them as "immature" individuals in his published writings. Benedict's unpublished writings suggest a similar gap between her positive acceptance of homosexuality as revealed in private and the more restrained views that she expressed in public. Her published writings were silent about her more critical ideas about sexual relationships confined to marriage and reproduction, which she expressed passionately, and often lightheartedly, in private.

This was not only because of their concern that critiquing American homophobia in public might do damage to their reputation. Because the subject was still in an uncharted area in science, these scientists had to figure out logic and language that best served their purpose of destigmatization. They wondered, for example, if it would be better to discuss homosexuality as a purely sexual matter, or if the subject should be related to other pressing issues, such as racism and gender inequality. Should homosexuality be dealt with in its own right, or should it be seen as part of the broader social problem of intolerance? These scientists' ultimate practice to embed their critique of homophobia in that of racism and sexism had a significant impact on their colleagues, friends, families, and patients. The issues of racism and sexism, compared with that of homosexuality, were less apt to raise for scientists the troubling matter of their own subjectivity, underscoring a belief in scientific communities that the subjectivity of scientists should not be part of science. To destigmatize, scientists assumed, you could not be part of the stigmatized population. By literally embodying two distinctively different views—living closeted lives as sexual minorities while publishing theories of the sexually "immature"—these intellectuals contributed to a scientific culture in which a careful separation of the public from the private was an accepted norm.

Because of the relative lack of sources about scientists' private views, as well as the vexed place that subjectivity (sexual subjectivity in particular) occupies in the history of science, this culture has often escaped historical scrutiny.[12] Indeed, in the scholarship of Sullivan, Benedict, and Mead, silence and ambiguity about their sexualities—not to mention the connection between their subjective experiences and their scientific ideas—have been most conspicuous. Some of this concealment has been the result of the scientists' desire to protect their privacy, extended over time by their partners, families, and friends. For instance, James Inscoe, Sullivan's lifelong partner, reported that he had burned Sullivan's personal letters soon after Sullivan died in 1949, to protect his deceased partner's reputation. Inscoe believed that Sullivan had "experienced hostility from a great many people" throughout his life; hence he must be defended against "nasty rumor" that might rise out of releasing any aspects of his personal life.[13] Similarly, Ruth Benedict's former lover Margaret Mead did not disclose intimate expressions they had exchanged in their correspondence throughout their adult lives when she published *An Anthropologist at Work*, a biography of Benedict, in 1959.[14] The biography included their letters, but they were framed as an example of Benedict's mentoring of her student Mead. Thus it remained hidden that Benedict's letter to Mead almost invariably began with "Margaret darling," "Darling," or "Dearest Margaret," and ended with lines such as "I love you, darling, always. Take care of yourself. And love me, dear, too" and "Be happy, darling. I love you."[15] Also undisclosed was that Mead responded with similar, ardent language. Only in 2000, a century after Mead's birth, did the personal, more avid original letters become open to researchers.

The lack of acknowledgment of scientists' sexualities also has elements of a barely disguised homophobia, as well as feelings of embarrassment and inappropriateness about discussing sexual matters, apparent among some scholars who wrote about the scientists. Sullivan's biographers, for example, have avoided discussing his homosexuality, for reasons ranging from fear of doing "harm [to] families" involved, "irrelevancy," "silliness," and "uselessness" of the subject, to a belief that his sexual life "was [not] very important" in understanding his professional accomplishments.[16] Benedict's sexual life does not seem to occupy a legitimate place in the scholarship of her career as one of the United States' intellectual giants, either. Just as Benedict herself refrained from publicly claiming rights for homosexual individuals, her life as a sexual minority has been conflated with—and in some cases, made secondary to—her life as a woman and a feminist.[17] The tension between the subjective life histories of scientists and the history of (supposedly) objective science has not been easily dissoluble.

A range of private texts that have not been previously examined, most notably Sullivan's clinical records and the letters and memoirs of his associates in the medical and social sciences, shed light on the underappreciated, crucial characteristics of interwar liberalism on the issue of homosexuality. These sources present a history of science edging out of the closet, revealing a kind of scientific practice—a practice that raises questions about shifting relationships between the "normal" and "abnormal," subjectivity and science, and sexuality and modernity—that has been largely invisible in the scholarship. But this is not to suggest that private practices occurred in some preexisting, static place where the scientists hid anything that was potentially embarrassing or threatening—anything that needed to be closeted because of social oppression. Instead, defining and redefining what needed to be private, why, and how, were the central concerns of these scientists. Many of the people we encounter in this book were famous and powerful individuals. As scientific experts and authorities, they had relatively generous room to negotiate what to say about homosexuality. In this sense, their relationship to their sexualities was different from that of their research subjects. Unlike their homosexual "patients" or their informants in "primitive" societies, who rarely made an immediate input regarding their sexualities in historical documents, scientists of homosexuality had a large measure of control over what facts and interpretations went into what kind of records. It is virtually impossible to understand the subjectivity of sexual minorities in Native American societies during the 1920s and 1930s based on anthropological observations of the subject; there is no first-person voice in these scientific studies.[18] In contrast, scientists were consistently the subject—"I"—of all the sentences they wrote, either explicitly or implicitly. Thus, although their homosexuality constituted a certain risk to their professional status, it could—and often did—turn into a strength for them as individuals. Their words and practices offer unmistakable signs of how they made strategic choices as well as inadvertent decisions. In some cases, scientists attempted to keep open the interactions between public and private aspects of scientific practice; for instance, Sullivan obliquely criticized homophobia at an academic conference, using insights arising from his far more straightforward one-on-one discussions with his patients in clinical settings. Other times scientists chose to keep their private views completely invisible. Some psychiatrists who privately supported the better acceptance of sexual minorities wrote dismissively about them in their published works. Both Benedict and Mead preferred to be "Mrs." in public, perhaps in part to shield off possible doubt about their sexualities. The unintended result of this shifting process was an ultimately unbridgeable distance between the public and private in science.

There were, of course, more than self-protective reasons for scientists' choice to keep the private apart from the public. For one, in clinical settings, private liberalism offered comfort, acceptance, and adjustment to mentally disturbed homosexual individuals. Keeping certain practices secret made the most of therapies, as well as protecting doctors from being criticized as too unconventional or as "queers" getting personal satisfaction out of their work. Oftentimes this secrecy supported the belief that members of the protected, "therapeutic" community were the most "civilized" and "sophisticated" in sexual matters. This heightened pride may have empowered people within the private circle, both doctors and patients, and in particular individuals whose homosexuality had no place in their public life. Some were encouraged to adjust to mainstream, heterosexual society by being "tolerant" of people who could not think beyond traditional sexual norms. Others felt proud to be part of the community in which intellectuals upheld homosexual experiences as key to a better understanding of mental illness. To the members of this community, homosexuality was not purely a medical matter, but a site at which their emotional lives, intellectual curiosity, and social critique encountered and deepened each other. Their exploration of homosexuality comprised not only science taking shape in person-to-person interactions, but also clinical relationships shaped by the surrounding cultural and personal imagination. In this unique, relatively safe environment, at least some of the people involved began to envision a society that tolerated a variety of sexual acts, desires, and wishes.[19] By the same token, however, their sense of pride and hope hindered their ability to counter homophobia in public debate. Rooted in a protected setting, the critiques and aspirations shared by the members of this community were not easily translated into broadly understandable, appealing language and ideas. Thus the gap between public and private revealed its striking consequences during World War II, as psychiatrists, including Sullivan, created a Selective Service policy discriminating against homosexual individuals. By keeping their critique of homophobia private in the 1920s and 1930s, U.S. scientists were unprepared to create egalitarian public policies at the dawn of the war. The texture of conservatism in the politics of sexuality among liberal scientists, as well as the more intransigent conservatism among politicians during the economic recession and the war, shaped the climate of unabashed discrimination against homosexual men and women.

Contradictory as it may seem, the restriction of homophile scientific practices to the private arena occurred partly because of liberal scientists' belief in the potential for social change. In their minds, what worked in a small-scale environment might be, at some later point, applied to the public sphere. Psychiatrists in the 1920s and 1930s embraced this hope particularly because of the impact of Freudian psychoanalysis, which valued careful examinations of patients' life histories, and also because of the rise of the mental hygiene movement, which created a number of clinics and counseling rooms suitable for individualized treatment.[20] These changes allowed psychiatrists to believe that mental health care would soon become accessible to all in local communities. The increased accessibility would encourage communities to be more accepting of mental illness, they believed, which in turn would help create a better therapeutic environment for the sick. This belief in the connection between clinics and communities discouraged psychiatrists from questioning the existing distance between their private and public approaches to homosexuality. Psychiatrists did not publicly criticize homophobia as such, because it seemed more reasonable, as well as safer, to suggest the critique between the lines. This was, to a certain degree, a coerced choice forced by a homophobic society, but not one without hope that, at some time in the future, the implicit critique would yield desirable consequences. Just as small outposts of psychiatric care would help improve an entire community's mental health, a homophile climate that "sophisticated" individuals created in their small circle would eventually work against homophobia in the public. This optimism made it difficult for psychiatrists to problematize the existing gap between published writings and person-to-person interactions. Homophile doctors and patients were persuaded that their practice in a small group would influence the rest of the society in the long run, if not now. Thus they did not see an immediate need to invent rhetoric and other means that would translate private liberalism into public discourse.

This approach revealed its limitations in domestic policies of discrimination against homosexuality. But the impact of the gap between public and private liberalism went beyond national boundaries, as the United States tried to establish a new identity as a global power after World War II. Making an impressive leap from theoretical to political argument, the biased language that liberal scientists had used to discuss homosexuality—it was "immature"—in their publications in the 1920s and 1930s began to be used to describe non-Western countries, so as to claim U.S. leadership in the postwar world. In this assertion of international hegemony, the conceptual and metaphorical link between psychosexual "immaturity," imbalanced masculinity and femininity, and cultural "otherness" functioned as a scientific assumption that needed no questioning. The United States' working for the betterment of "immature" countries provided an image of assistance rather than imposition, driving liberal scientists' attention away from the authoritarian dimension implicit in programs in the United Nations Educational, Scientific and Cultural Organization (UNESCO) and the World Federation for Mental Health (WFMH). At this point, it was clear that a more daring liberalism occupied no place in public policies, whether national or international. The intellectuals' aspiration to extend the most liberal agenda from private to public reached a certain dead end.

The next generation of Americans would choose a different approach to ensuring the rights of sexual minorities. Political activism, as it developed in the second half of the twentieth century, was based on the failure of the tactics that the preceding decades had embraced. Thus the liberal scientists from the 1920s to the 1940s were not "predecessors" of the current civil rights movement for sexual minorities. Rather, these were the people whose drive for destigmatization was, despite their best hopes and intentions, largely lost. Harry Stack Sullivan's life offers the most remarkable illumination of this loss; when he started his career as a psychiatrist in the 1920s, his approach to homosexuality was full of unique, inspiring, and great possibilities. By the late 1940s, however, his work was no longer linked to the interests or aspirations of sexual minorities. Although he did not talk about his feelings about this change, Sullivan toward the end of his life was a deeply unhappy person. This unhappiness may be seen as his era's intellectual and cultural limitations, as much as it was a poignant aspect of his biography. It was these limitations—not merely the general conservatism of the 1940s and 1950s—that shaped our determination to pursue political justice for sexual minorities.

A word about key concepts and terms used in this book is useful here. This study examines the "science of homosexuality"—a range of scientific approaches to homosexuality, if not an established field of inquiry with a specialized body of knowledge—that flourished in the 1920s and 1930s. The scientists who were involved in the science of homosexuality were primarily people who were intellectually connected to Sullivan, although they also included scientists who were not in his immediate group but had important things to say about the issues to which Sullivan's associates were drawn. This resulted in the inclusion of people who do not necessarily belong to science's hall of fame, and only passing attention to better-known scientists who wrote about homosexuality, most notably Katherine Bemont Davis, Robert Latou Dickinson, George W. Henry, and Alfred C. Kinsey. Besides the difference in the specific focus of their interests, what separates this study's main figures from these notable scientists is their self-conscious effort to create interdisciplinary scholarship, grounded in close and continual collaborations with scientists from different fields. The science of homosexuality as it is defined in this book always aspired to be—and most of the time, was—interdisciplinary, and this offers a unique path into the history of science as it grappled with the changing meaning of subjectivity, sexuality, gender, culture, and modernity. Thus interdisciplinarity is a primary—if not exclusive—source of guidance for the scope of this book.

In discussing particular individuals' sexualities, it is imperative to confront head-on anachronism and stigma. Most of the time, I use *homosexuality*, not *gayness* and *lesbianism*, to refer to sexuality that was marked as different from the "normal" and thus became a subject of scientific interest. This is because *homosexuality* was the term that scientists themselves used. Although *gay* and *lesbian* were used in emerging communities of sexual minorities during this time, these terms did not enter the language of the scientists examined in this book. This created something of a problem for my writing, especially when it seemed useful to acknowledge a person's sexuality as homosexuality because the person had done so. But *a homosexual scientist*—as opposed to *a gay scientist*—sounds hopelessly rigid and in many cases derogatory in our contemporary vocabulary. Thus sometimes I use *gay* or *lesbian* as an adjective to describe a person, although I do so only when sources indicate that the person's sexual identity would comport with what we would call "gay" or "lesbian" today. That is, that this person had a sense of being a minority because his or her sexuality was socially marked as "abnormal"; at the same time, this person had some sense of belonging to the emerging community and culture of sexual minorities. Alternately, then, such a person is referred to as a *sexual minority*, even though this does not mean that the sense of being a minority included political awareness as it began to in the second half of the twentieth century. The lack of organized effort to better the status of sexual minorities was a definitive characteristic of interwar liberal science.[21]

Interestingly, *queer*, in addition to *homosexual*, are terms that scientists used, and thus they seem appropriate adjectives to describe the sexual identities of some of the scientists discussed in this book. Indeed, these scientists thought that sexual minorities could offer special insights into mainstream culture because of their minority status, and thus *queer* might seem somewhat similar to usage today. But again, language changes over time. *Queer* carries specific meanings in today's usage that were not present in the 1920s and 1930s, particularly when the term addresses a desire to go beyond the categories of lesbian, gay, bisexual, and transgender. These categories can imply that it is acceptable to divide people based on their sexuality, and many would say that such a view itself needs to be questioned by using the term *queer*—a term that does not usually imply any specific gender and sexual identities but highlights a critical stance to normalcy.[22] Given this, it is more appropriate to use the word *queer* with an explanation of specific meanings associated with it in the past than to apply it generally to my discussion of scientists' sexual identities. There was such a thing as a "sexual identity" in the 1920s and 1930s; however, it did not involve a critique of sexual categories themselves in the same way as the term *queer* in today's usage does.

The charged nature of sexual terms shapes sexual matters we choose to—or choose not to—discuss, as much as it influenced scientific discourse in the past. When I began to make inquiries in the late 1990s about Sullivan's romantic and sexual relationships, I encountered a considerable amount of elusiveness and a quick change of topic by many people with whom I talked—perhaps more than I would if I were to make the same inquiries today. This elusiveness not only posed a challenge to this nonnative English speaker ("Perhaps I just missed something," I often thought), but also caused a strong desire on my part to figure out the nature of that challenge. Of course, I was puzzled and frustrated, and sometimes it seemed easy to conclude that I was not getting information about Sullivan's homosexuality because it did not exist. But then, I realized that my frustration was what many other scholars must have experienced. Thus I set out to know what people were trying to convey by being ambiguous and incomplete in their sentences, and why. I wanted to see my experience in historical context, not just as a matter of miscommunication; I wanted to believe that we can talk about sexuality cross-culturally. This curiosity and desire have been one of the driving forces of the discussion that follows.

1

A Man, a Doctor, and His Patients

When Harry Stack Sullivan came to Sheppard and Enoch Pratt Hospital, a psychoanalytically oriented mental hospital in Towson, Maryland, in late 1922, he doubtless did not know how much he would become fascinated in the coming years with a condition called schizophrenia. Nor did he know that he would become so intensively and deeply involved in issues of homosexuality through his interaction with patients with schizophrenia. He was a thirty-year-old physician with some experience in general medicine, but he did not have much familiarity with the fields of psychiatry and psychoanalysis. He did not have—as far as we know from the existing records—a clear sense of how his own sexuality would become an important part of his public and private lives, either. By the end of his time at Sheppard-Pratt in 1930, however, he would be living with a man who was to become his lifelong partner, James Inscoe. He would also become a famous figure in psychiatry and psychoanalysis, a star in the treatment of schizophrenia, one of the most serious and difficult illnesses a person's "self" can suffer from.[1]

Unusually rich clinical records at Sheppard-Pratt illuminate this crucial time in Sullivan's life and career. In particular, his interaction with patients who had homosexual concerns reveals how his clinical practice helped shape his own identity as a gay psychiatrist during the decade in which modern and traditional views of homosexuality coexisted and competed. As a scientist, he became an expert in the definition of schizophrenia as a socially and culturally constructed illness of the modern United States, a development that would eventually pull him out of the medical clinic to a broader intellectual community and to collaborations with sociologists, cultural anthropologists, political scientists, and social psychologists. As a person, he became a determined sympathizer with homosexual men whom he considered to be uniquely oppressed by sociocultural "inhibitions." He frequently encountered evidence of moralistic teachings against sexual "sin," internalized by patients, as he talked to those who were diagnosed with schizophrenia. He responded to this personally, because, for him, it was more than a medical condition that needed attention.

Thus Sullivan faced issues of homosexuality both scientifically and subjectively—sometimes reluctantly, other times with determination. His interactions with patients occurred in a protected environment within hospital walls, making a clean line between the scientific and subjective almost impossible. As such, the clinical setting at Sheppard-Pratt was where Sullivan began to create his particular form of liberalism, which drew upon his values as both a man and a scientist. He did not forge his liberalism in a seamless cooperation with patients; some of his patients decidedly resisted the doctor's ideas and suggestions. On the other hand, there were moments when a patient's concerns and the doctor's interests seemed to come together or, at least, recognize each other. Sheppard-Pratt's clinical files, then, are not only records of medical science in practice; they are also records of encounters between a doctor's and patients' subjectivities, different ways in which their life histories intersected and shaped each other.

Through agreement and disagreement, competition and negotiation, and mutual recognition and rejection with his patients, Sullivan formulated a liberal "treatment" of schizophrenia (and implicitly, of homosexual conflicts), at the center of which was physical contact between male attendants and male patients that included touching, holding, and kissing.[2] This was not a treatment he introduced based on a well-worked-out theory; rather, it was a practice that emerged piecemeal out of doctor-patient interactions, which were fluid and open to a range of possibilities. The intended goal of this treatment was to make patients feel comfortable with their sexuality and understand the nature of their mental problems. Most of Sullivan's colleagues found this approach inconceivable as therapy, and it led to his being ostracized by staff. Moreover, Sullivan's life with James Inscoe provoked troubling gossip. The development of the former's private liberalism was intimately tied to his personal life as a homosexual man, and the fact that his colleagues at Sheppard-Pratt responded to this tie with firm rejection suggests the contested place of subjectivity in 1920s science. As Sullivan encountered these responses of the public, he began to restrict certain aspects of his liberalism to "private" spheres. The confidentiality involved in his controversial approach certainly helped both the doctor and his patients to talk frankly about their feelings, but it also made it difficult for Sullivan to encourage more sympathetic, or at least less homophobic, attitudes outside his clinic. At the same time, the accountability of his homophile practice became difficult to measure, because the practice itself—and his freedom to make any professional decisions he wanted—was insulated from public

scrutiny. His decision to keep aspects of his liberalism private had significant if unforeseen consequences for any expression of public liberalism.

A Place to Come, a Place to Go:
Sheppard-Pratt in the 1920s

Sheppard-Pratt in the 1920s was a desirable place to be for a young doctor
interested in mental illness. It was one of the few mental hospitals in the
nation associated with a research department based in a university, in this
case Johns Hopkins University and its clinical research outfit, the Henry
Phipps Clinic. Since its opening in 1891, the hospital's financial base (a $2.2
million endowment from local merchants Moses Sheppard and Enoch Pratt)
had been stable, making it feasible to admit a certain number of patients
who were considered useful subjects of research but who were unable to
pay the hospital's standard fee. Moreover, the hospital's focus was on acute
cases at the beginning of the illness, considered curable by intensive therapies. This reflected an emerging paradigm of the 1910s and 1920s, called the
"new psychiatry," which was shifting the focus of mental health care from
large state institutions to small-scale mental hospitals and clinics.[3] Unlike
traditional mental hospitals where much of physicians' work consisted of
the care of chronic patients, new outposts of mental health care, such as
Boston Psychopathic Hospital, McLean Hospital, Chestnut Lodge Hospital,
and Sheppard-Pratt, encouraged doctors to spend time with patients, so as
to better understand the personal, familial, and social causes of their illness
and the course of its progression.[4] At Sheppard-Pratt, the relatively small
number of beds (250) and of patients per doctor (25) were crucial in this
individualized treatment.[5] Most patients admitted in the 1920s underwent
examinations of their life histories (under headings such as "birth and early
development," "sexual development and function," and "occupation") and
of their past and present illnesses. In addition, attendants carried out frequent clinical observations of patients' conditions (both physical and mental, ranging from daily to weekly), occupational therapies, and recreational
activities. In some cases, the hospital employed social workers who reported
on patients' conditions during a parole or after discharge, illustrating that
the hospital's medical interest literally extended beyond its walls.

The hospital's doctors regarded patients as subjects of both research
and treatment, transferring them to a state mental hospital or a sanitarium
for long-term care when it was determined that a patient's prognosis was
poor. After Ross McClure Chapman, an exponent of psychoanalysis, was
appointed as medical superintendent in 1920, this trend became more
powerful. Building on Sigmund Freud's theory of psychoanalysis, doctors
at Sheppard-Pratt inquired about patients' childhood memories, sexual

experiences, and dreams, to understand the underlying causes of their patients' illnesses. Along with the routine examinations and therapies, these in-depth, analytical interviews in both group and individual formats made up the main segment of treatment. Physicians in these interviews tried to obtain as much information as possible; thus it was crucial that all patients at Sheppard-Pratt were inpatients, with whom doctors expected to spend a considerable length of time. This approach did not necessarily reflect doctors' formal training in psychoanalysis, however. While some, such as Ives Hendrick, Lewis B. Hill, and William V. Silverberg, had completed or were completing training in either Europe or the United States, others were acquainted with psychoanalysis only through their reading and clinical experiences, not through training in a recognized program. Ross M. Chapman, George E. Partridge, and Sullivan belonged to this latter cohort. Before 1935, there were no guidelines for the number of hours that analysts had to spend in training, and it was not unusual for physicians who were inclined to use an analytic approach to do so without a certificate. Psychoanalysis in the 1920s was broadly defined and did not demand a strict adherence to Freudian theories and techniques.[6] The doctors were aware of both the research component of their practice and the potential for their research to find preventive measures of illness. Such interest in prevention, as seen in their focus on early and acute cases, clearly reflected the hospital's aspiration to be an agent of public health.

In a piecemeal but convincing way, clinical records at Sheppard-Pratt illuminate a fascinating variety of men and women whose lives intersected with the mental hospital. Patients came to Sheppard-Pratt from different places and for different reasons.[7] Most of them were from the middle class, although the economic conditions of about 15 percent of the patients admitted between 1923 and 1928 were described as either "marginal" or "dependent." About 90 percent of the patients were from "urban" districts and the rest from "rural" areas. This does not necessarily mean that most of the patients had grown up in and were familiar with an urban environment. The 1920s is a time when emerging urban posts drew people from small towns and villages. Some Sheppard-Pratt patients were sons and daughters of farmers who had come to a city to pursue educational or job opportunities, which rural life could not offer. Thus a number of "urban" patients were, in fact, newcomers to cities who were trying to figure out changing ways of life and living. The majority of patients were from Maryland, but a significant minority came from eastern and midwestern states such as New Jersey, New York, Connecticut, Maine, Delaware, Pennsylvania, Ohio, Michigan, Illinois, and Missouri, as well as from Washington D.C., and also from southern states such as Virginia, West Virginia, North and South Carolina, Tennessee, Georgia, Alabama, Mississippi, Louisiana, Texas, and Florida. This suggests both the hospital's good reputation and the relative lack of clinics that offered treatment that patients and families deemed desirable.

The Sheppard-Pratt patients in the 1920s were somewhat diverse in their ethnic and religious backgrounds as well. First-generation immigrants, mostly Jews from Russia and Germany, made up 6.7 percent of the patients. Among the patients whose religion was specified, 11.8 percent were Catholic and 12.3 percent Jewish; ethnic diversity would have been greater if second-generation immigrants (who were not consistently recorded as such) were included in the statistics. Other patients were Protestants of various denominations, among them Presbyterian, Episcopalian, Baptist, Methodist, Lutheran, Friend, Congregation, and Christian Science. Many were raised by churchgoing parents and still belonged to churches, while a number described feeling less active than they should be as church members. This was something that the hospital's doctors were interested in finding out, apparently because they considered religious inhibitions to be related to patients' illness, both pathogenically and symptomatically.

People of all ages came to the hospital, from their teens to their eighties, but Sullivan and his research team were most interested in males from the midteens to the early thirties. The hospital accepted about equal numbers of male and female patients, although men, particularly those diagnosed with schizophrenia, seemed to enjoy slightly more opportunities for in-depth interviews with doctors than did women. This might be because of some doctors' belief that psychoanalysis required a certain degree of intellectual sophistication and self-awareness, which male doctors often failed to recognize in disturbed female patients. As for Sullivan, he did not seem either skilled or interested in treating female patients. In his comments during interviews with them he was often tense, frustrated, and disagreeable, more frequently so than when he was with male patients.[8] Sullivan's gift as a psychiatric interviewer shined when he talked to young men with sexual concerns, not with their female counterparts.

Patients' experience of coming to Sheppard-Pratt varied. Some were brought to the hospital by concerned parents, siblings, aunts, or uncles. Most signed for voluntary admission, but they often did not believe the hospitalization necessary. In particular, the first hospitalization seemed to hit patients hard as a misguided, unfair, and embarrassing event. Many desired an early "parole," even what doctors considered a premature discharge. But leaving the hospital would not entail a normal life back home. When discharged, as patients often speculated, they would never be as good as they used to be. The stigma of having been at a mental hospital was certainly felt strongly.[9] But these negative feelings do not convey the whole picture. Some patients thought that something had been wrong with them, and they came to the hospital willingly. Several had relatives who had been treated at Sheppard-Pratt and felt that they, too, could benefit from a stay there. Others, in particular those who had been to a psychiatric hospital before, thought that Sheppard-Pratt was a place to come to when things were not going well. One of these patients, at the end of his second hospitalization, said that if he "had another attack [he] would want to come back here."[10] Some had their favorite doctors, and they expected to get the doctors' help when needed. These are patients who had a way of "using" the hospital for their benefit, even though it might not have meant that they did not experience the downside of being hospitalized. In more extreme cases, patients wanted to stay in the hospital for long periods, without an apparent desire to get well. Although it is easy to see this as a sign of illness (and indeed, these patients often had serious symptoms), it is also possible to see them as individuals who had finally found a place to be. The hospital offered companions (other inpatients), activities, and recreational opportunities, and not a few patients expressed their appreciation of them. For some, friends and social occasions were something that they could enjoy only within hospital walls. When they were transferred to a state hospital, their worry was not about being unable to go back home, but about being separated from the comfortable, familiar environment of Sheppard-Pratt.[11]

The clinical records refute a simplistic image of doctors as guardians of social order and public health.[12] Neither do they present physicians as benevolent protectors of the mentally sick.[13] To be sure, some doctors made what might seem to us to be judgmental comments, especially when patients resisted revealing their feelings. (To a patient who seemed to be evasive, one doctor said: "Be quiet, I am tired of hearing you talk."[14]) Although subtle, a bias against female patients (and not infrequently, male patients with limited education, too), engendered by the view that they were not smart enough to benefit from analysis, was present. But in many ways, doctors were more willing to shed critical light on social and cultural ills than to dissect a person's sickness as a clinical entity. Such interest in societal, not individual, causes of mental problems came up most strikingly when doctors discussed sexual matters with young men. In particular, men who had a concern about their homosexual experiences, both real and imagined, compelled doctors to reconsider assumed differences between health and illness, the normal and abnormal, and the personal and social. As these male patients' discussions of homosexual experiences and desires became a central theme in therapy, doctors and patients at Sheppard-Pratt created perhaps one of the most striking forms of social critique to take shape in modern medical practice in the United States. In particular, Sullivan's increasing awareness as a homosexual psychiatrist made him an outstanding figure in the making of this social critique, an adamant critic of traditional definitions of manliness and male sexuality.

Although rich in their contents, these clinical records have certain limits as a source of information. For one, there is much information that is missing. Oftentimes, a doctor made a reference to a meeting he had had with a patient, but the record, for whatever reason, is not to be found in the file. The hospital made it standard practice to type up any doctor-patient exchanges made during meetings since 1926; thus some of these records must have been created but are missing. Moreover, as might be expected, there are frequent disparities in what was recorded. For instance, a patient's mother would relate the patient's sexual experience, while the patient's wife would tell an entirely different story. The patient would have yet another version of it. Doctors were aware of this and would write a note about it. One such note from 1929 reads, "The reminder of the history [of the patient that his mother had given] is absolutely unreliable, and is placed in the folder merely for the purpose of comparison."[15] The doctors—those who created the clinical records—were attentive to different, conflicting stories that people might bring.

The doctors were not equally attentive to the gap between patients' claims and medical interpretations, showing that doctors did not see the possibility that their ideas might be influenced by their subjectivity as well. One patient from 1928, for instance, admitted that he had had a habit of masturbation and that it had been continuing after marriage. A doctor noted that the patient "admits his practice without any show of shame, and states that he has a perfect right to do it during his wife's menstrual periods." A few pages later, however, the doctor recorded his own view of the issue, which does not seem to reflect the patient's attitude: "Masturbation is playing a large part in his [thought] content at this time, and it is believed that he has a great amount of self accusatory ideas in relation to it."[16] Unlike contradictions in informants' stories, the apparent discrepancy between the patient's attitude and the doctor's interpretation invariably remained unacknowledged. The doctors had established ideas about illness, and these ideas exercised conclusive power in virtually every case. Even when the doctors expressed their uncertainty about diagnoses and prognoses—which was not unusual, given the complex nature of mental problems in general and the changing terminology of the era in particular—clinical records had to be marked with recognizable signposts, and it was doctors who decided what medical signals should be placed on what conditions. Thus patients' words recorded in their files must be read with caution, because they appeared only after being processed through medical reasoning.[17]

The standard clinical file had eight parts: an admission note, a family history, a personal history, a record of a physical examination, a record of a mental examination, clinical observations, one or more conference reports, and a discharge note.[18] Conference reports are particularly dense because they recorded conversations between a team of doctors (usually six or seven of them) and a patient, which were an in-depth examination of a patient's life experiences. Usually two or three typists were present to transcribe a conference. This careful recording of doctor-patient conversation started early in 1926, soon after Sullivan became the director of clinical research. Earlier, in 1922 and 1923, conference reports were brief summaries and did not include records of words exchanged between doctors and patients. In 1924 and 1925, doctor-patient conversations were included in conference reports, but they were minimal. This suggests that conferences were short or that doctors did not think the documentation of conversations particularly important. It is likely that Sullivan encouraged the expansion of a conference and its verbatim documentation following the model of the new psychiatry.[19] This was also connected to the increasing interest in life history as a method of scientific inquiry in the medical and social sciences in the 1920s and 1930s.

The primary purpose of the conference was to settle on a diagnosis and a prognosis, so that doctors could agree on a treatment plan for a patient.[20] Another important purpose after Sullivan became the director of clinical research was to decide whether a patient was a useful subject for his intensive treatment. When he found patients suitable, Sullivan initiated a series of special interviews with them. Most selected patients were young men with homosexual conflicts and a diagnosis of schizophrenia. Their files include transcriptions of special interviews in addition to the standard eight parts. These verbatim transcriptions show how Sullivan's scientific reasoning and his subjectivity were joined as he talked with patients with minimum formality. The interviews usually occurred in Sullivan's office, where there were just a few others (one or two other doctors and stenographers) or, sometimes, nobody other than Sullivan, a patient, and a stenographer. There were no prearranged questions; thus doctors and patients could say whatever their conversation suggested. Unlike the conferences, these special interviews allowed the doctor's subjectivity to come into play almost as much as patients'.

As Sullivan began to have more special interviews, he became less concerned with regular hospital activities. In 1926, his first full year as director of clinical research, he attended 247 staff conferences. In 1927, the number decreased to 87. In contrast, he had fourteen special interviews with seven patients in 1926, and the number increased to thirty-four with thirteen patients in 1927.[21] The following pages focus on the patients with whom Sullivan had one or more special interviews, as well as those who did not have such an interview but attracted Sullivan's interest, judging from the length and depth of the conference reports. This selection resulted in the in-depth examination of 62 patient files out of the total 1,696.[22] Twenty-two out of the 62 files included a record of special interviews, while 40 had an unusually elaborate record of staff conferences. The analysis of the 62 files illuminates the doctor-patient interactions concerning homosexual experiences and feelings. Issues other than those of homosexuality, which also came up in the doctor-patient conversations, will be examined in the following chapter. This focus on the patients whose records are more extensive than those of others allows us to look at the kind of patients that the hospital was particularly interested in. Because of the written nature of the records and the hospital's reliance on interviews, Sheppard-Pratt clinical records do not shed much light on those who were unwilling or unable to talk.[23] But among a few exceptions to this rule are the patients who had difficulty in talking but appeared to have homosexual conflicts at the root of their illnesses. To these patients, the Sheppard-Pratt doctors in general, and Sullivan in particular, paid special attention. These patients' files include unusually long records of interviews during which the patients said virtually nothing. But the hospital recorded the interviews anyway, suggesting that homosexuality was an important issue that overrode a patient's reluctance to communicate. Without being fully aware, Sheppard-Pratt doctors were discovering homosexuality as a fascinating subject of science, bringing up a host of questions about sexuality, gender, illness, and culture. Ultimately, the subject allowed them to see themselves in a setting larger than a clinic.

Homosexual Matters

As one might imagine from a comment made by Arthur Linton, a former Sheppard-Pratt attendant who worked with Sullivan in 1928 and 1929, that "all of Sullivan's patients were young male homosexuals whom he personally picked from the general hospital population," one of the issues Sullivan talked about most intensively during interviews was homosexuality.[24] Some patients were aware of this. Discussing his homosexual desire and his inability to accept it, a patient told Sullivan: "If someone would only tell me where I was at and what path to follow I would be the happiest person in the world. . . . [One doctor] said if anybody could help me it was you. . . . Please tell me, Dr. Sullivan." That Sullivan specialized in patients with homosexual conflicts, however, does not mean that other doctors did not collaborate with him. Indeed, some colleagues seemed to share his emerging critique of homophobia, although to a more limited degree. This collaboration was therapeutically desirable because interactions with patients occurred not only on a one-on-one basis but also in a group. It was crucial, then, that a team of doctors were at least willing to go along with Sullivan's critical attitude toward homophobia, so as to offer consistent treatment.

The homosexual experiences of Sheppard-Pratt patients were in no way uniform. For instance, many admitted having had mutual masturbation with their brothers or male school friends when young. Entries such as "[the patient] and his brother three years younger slept in the same bed until the patient was sixteen and they practiced mutual masturbation for a period of about one year"[25] are not uncommon in patient files, even among those that are not included in the selected sixty-two files. But the patients' response to such experiences varied significantly. To be sure, most patients considered mutual masturbation bad and felt guilty about it even as young children. But some considered it embarrassing because it was a form of masturbation, not because it occurred with a person of the same sex. One patient related that, when he was a child, he slept with his younger brother and that they had engaged in mutual masturbation. After he was given a separate room, the patient began to masturbate alone. When he became an adolescent and began to develop pimples, he became self-conscious around girls because he believed that "they knew his habit by the pimples on his face."[26] Thus, for this patient, mutual masturbation was the beginning of a troubling habit of masturbation, not of homosexuality. This was not the case with another patient, who as a teenager masturbated with his school-mate. He said that he had felt "disgusting" about it, but then he began to pursue homosexual encounters at "Central Park and elsewhere" in New York City. On one such occasion, he went to a man's apartment, permitting him "intercourse per anal" in exchange for cash. In this case, the mutual masturbation was presented as an early episode in the patient's history of homosexual relationships.

Homosexual experiences in youth often involved exploitation by older persons. One patient recalled his older brother "going into my rear" when they were sleeping in the same bed. The patient "couldn't understand it." He related, "I said I wanted a separate bed," and claimed that mutual mastur-bation with the brother, as well as anal sex with him, was "revolting." This was, the patient said, because he did not want to "think of [himself] as the sexual object of a man." While the patient apparently was disgusted by same-sex sexual contacts, he also acknowledged the possibility that the brother had been the sexual object of an older man "against his will." A series of same-sex acts of sexual abuse, not simply the brother's homosexual advance, seems to have been at the core of the problem.[27] In the case of another patient, the abuser was the patient's father. Sullivan made a presentation of the father's imposition on the patient during a staff conference, conveying his frustration with the father and his protectiveness toward the patient: "The father is . . . a man struggling most clumsily against an homosexual interest in his son, the patient. . . . The father's conflict result[ed] in . . . [an] indefinite number of atrocious, destructive performances upon the patient:

1) repeatedly submerging the boy in a full bath tub to compel admissions of actual or fancied peccadillos . . . [and] 7) a frank if abortive homosexual assault on the boy one night when they were both somnolent." Sullivan and other doctors were worried about the patient's defensive response to these "performances": the patient might repress his homosexual desire because homosexuality had been associated with the father's offensive behavior. Such repression, in Sullivan's belief, was unhealthy, an obstacle that needed to be removed in treatment. Thus, when the patient noted that he liked to dance, Sullivan said that, to dance, the patient would "have to have nice girls to go around with," as if to suggest that this could present a problem for the patient. The patient agreed that he would need girls, but then Sullivan asked if the patient "would prefer to dance with a nice boy." The patient's answer was negative, but the drift of Sullivan's questions suggests he did not believe it.[28] These cases make it clear that Sullivan searched for homosexual content, especially those of a traumatizing nature, regardless of what a patient was willing to admit.

For many men it was not easy to admit homosexual experiences. Homophobia apparently had found its way into the minds of many patients, and some were not shy about expressing it straightforwardly. A patient who had confessed his sense of guilt over masturbation and a relationship with a prostitute, but nothing of a homosexual nature, still noted that he did not want Sullivan "to have the idea that [when] all doors were closed . . . I was a cock sucker." Moreover, the patient believed that there were many "such people [cock suckers]" on one of the hospital wards. He was afraid that he might be sent to the ward if Sullivan suspected any homosexual content in the patient's thinking. The patient "certainly didn't want to be put in any worse class than [he] was in," suggesting his belief that, among various sexual "deviations," homosexuality seemed the worst.[29] Others seemed to suffer from less explicit, but equally troubling, homophobia. One patient, for instance, told doctors that he had had "many homosexual . . . experiences" and that he had a constant "craving . . . [in] my throat [for fellatio]." Indeed, he believed "he was really a woman, and wishe[d] an operation to remove his genital." But then he backed off, saying, "I am a man myself. . . . I can't love any man." He was "undecided" about what he wanted, "just thinking [that] the only way I can be is homosexual . . . I can't be any other way—the way I want to be."[30] Thus he understood that his gender and sexual identities were not conventional, but at the same time, he did not want to be unconventional.

One sexual act that proved troubling to many patients was fellatio, which helps us understand the moral and gendered implication of how patients experienced homosexuality. It was considered a behavior that signified homosexuality, but patients' descriptions of their fear were so vivid that it seemed as if fellatio was a form of unconventionality in its own right. One such description, recorded by one of Sheppard-Pratt doctors, reads as follows: "When the patients on the ward are discussing homosexuality, as they frequently do, he [the patient] says, 'It slides in and takes hold of me.' He feels a sensation in his mouth, and his mouth waters. He associates cussing and homosexual. Cussing is low, and so is the other. . . . He says, when he cusses he opens his mouth and grits his teeth, and therefore there must be some connection."[31] What is striking in this statement is how this patient's homosexual interest was powerfully represented by fellatio. A strong, alarming sensation that fellatio provokes reminded him of cussing, which was considered an undesirable act. Thus the homosexuality is undesirable, too. For him, what seems most upsetting was the immediate physicality of fellatio more than homosexuality as an abstract idea.

Another patient was also afraid of fellatio, but in a different way. This is the patient who had rejected his brother's attempt at anal sex and mentioned an older man who might have sexually abused the brother. Further describing this older man, the patient said that he had studied the man's "motion of his lips." The man is a "fairy," the patient concluded. As the patient's story goes, he further learned to "judge a person . . . that is one [a fairy]" when he met "a young gentleman [who] once seemed to force my mouth." This incident left "a deep impression," and since then, the patient has been able to detect "feminine ways, sucking of lips—pulling the tongue out" as evidence of homosexuality. Unlike the other patient, he did not seem to suffer from an internalized sensation of fellatio. But again, fellatio, and "fairies—people who use their mouths," represented to him what was fearful about homosexuality.[32] Such was the case regardless of some indication that the patient's brother and the other men in his story were not "fairies." Given the feminine attributes of fairies, femininity—and the succumbing of masculinity to it—was what ignited in this patient the worst fear of homosexuality.

Sullivan was aware of the uncanny effect of fellatio. During a one-on-one interview with another patient, he argued that fellatio could "expose an area of weakness to another person." He did not mention the gendered nature of such weakness, while he surely thought that fellatio should not cause weakness in anyone. In the same interview, he said that he had "had a theory for a long time that fellatio was avoided by a large number of people . . . for the effect that it would have on their prestige."[33] If there were no fear of disgrace, there would be no stigmatization of fellatio. Thus Sullivan encouraged the patient to see the sexual act as something that just "is," not something entangled with social preconceptions.

Sullivan and his colleagues at Sheppard-Pratt certainly dealt with a number of stories related to homoeroticism, ranging from same-sex mutual masturbation, molestation, and fellatio, to cruising and the selling of sex.

The doctors called all of them "homosexual content," making no clear distinction between sexual desire and sexual action. Nor did they draw a clear borderline between homosexuality and homophobia. In the Sheppard-Pratt clinical setting, someone who was fearful of homosexuality was deemed to have a conflict with homosexual content as much as others who had a substantial history of homosexual experiences. Further, the doctors did not seem much interested in labeling certain patients as homosexual. They took note of patients who had a long record of exclusively homosexual relationships—they would say, for instance, that a patient's relationships had been "essentially homosexual"—but the doctors did not distinguish these patients from those who admitted heterosexual and homosexual experiences.[34] For instance, the patient mentioned earlier, the one who had practiced mutual masturbation with his brother, did not have any other homosexual experience. His current worry was about his habit of masturbation and sexual intercourse he had had with a prostitute. These experiences made him feel that he was "sexually excessive." As his habit of masturbation continued, he came to believe that he was "no good sexually," unable to get an erection because of the exhaustion after masturbation. Sullivan carried out a long interview with the patient during a staff conference and told him that in that case he must have "thought [he] had lost [his] manhood." Clearly, Sullivan considered both homosexual content and masturbation part of a larger story of men's fear and failure. Homosexual experience was one of the things that could undercut manhood, not necessarily a reason to put a patient into a special category of sexuality. Thus, this patient was no different from others who had had a number of homosexual experiences *and* suffered from the sense of lost manhood. Neither received a sexuality-specific label at any point during their stay at the hospital. The science of homosexuality, as it was taking shape at Sheppard-Pratt, did not see homosexuality as a clear-cut entity. The Sheppard-Pratt doctors' broad, flexible use of homosexual content was a way for them to focus on the social and cultural factors of mental illness, instead of seeing a homosexual experience as a problem by itself.

Amid this heightened interest in the sociocultural origin of illness, Sullivan began to develop his view that the sense of failed manhood, or failed "virility," in modern society was one of the main causes of mental illness, particularly schizophrenia.[35] Cultural changes exposed the youth to a number of sexual opportunities (petting, dancing, and drinking are common topics of patients' histories), while traditional morals made them feel terrible about even the faintest sign of their sexual desire. Sexual dreams could make them upset, even if they did not include homosexual content. Mutual masturbation, both homosexual and heterosexual, and homosexual relationships, both in experience and imagination, could cause a deep sense of losing self. These dangerous experiences and feelings were not uncommon, because unmarried men did not have many other ways to deal with their sexual desire. As Sullivan claimed during a special interview with a schizophrenic patient, it was still a common belief that "it is wrong to deal with a real [woman] unless you marry her." This is the situation that confronts all people, not just those who are mentally ill. Thus Sullivan went on to argue, "One thing [you can do in this situation] is to get sick . . . and live in another world; another one heads toward men . . . ; and the other is to abuse yourself." Indeed, the patient to whom Sullivan was talking had had all of them—masturbation, homosexual relationship, and then mental illness, in that order.[36] Freud's belief in a causal relationship between sexual repression and neurosis was applied to a psychosis here, with a focus on specific sexual experiences that caused the illness. Sullivan seldom discussed the Freudian idea of repression in his clinical practice, although it would have been a crucial concept for examining sexual conflicts were he an orthodox Freudian. Sullivan's approach was more oriented to acts and experiences than to theories and interpretations. He tried to get facts, or at least get patients to talk about what they considered to be facts, so that they could have something concrete in front of them to work with. In Sullivan's view, such immediacy and direct connection to patients' real-life situations were highly effective. Within a few years this approach was precisely what would bring medical doctors together with social scientists who were interested in an individual's life history.

Sullivan's careful attention to specifics stood out in his examination of the sociocultural context of illness, in both his published articles and his clinical practice. A 1925 article illuminates his critique of the modern United States as trapped in old-fashioned attitudes toward sex. In this era of transformation, Sullivan argued, it was difficult for youths to find a role model in adults. Apparently using Sheppard-Pratt patients as his source, Sullivan claimed that what dominates a family was not children's respect for parents, but "an attitude of . . . concealed jealousy and hatred" between a husband and a wife. In particular, when the wife is "[sexually] cold and struggle[s] to hold him [the husband] to it [the marriage]," she can propel the husband into extramarital affairs. There are abundant sexual opportunities and increasing social tolerance for them in cities, offering a hotbed for infidelity. Once an affair happens, however, the husband can feel that he must raise his child in a way "so [that] he won't be like his father." This deprives the husband of his confidence as a father. The wife, too, could suffer from the gap between the reality and her ideal of a good mother: the wife can then feel forced to be a "boss," because she believes it is necessary to play the fatherly role that she feels is not appropriately played by the betraying husband. But because of traditional social expectations for women, she would also be prohibited from becoming a fatherlike, dominant figure. At this point, it is almost certain that a "disaster to the offspring" would follow. One such "disastrous" consequence is the boy's attempt to avoid all things sexual, because of what he sees as their inevitable consequence: a dysfunctional marriage, just like his parents'. But soon, the child would find it impossible to eliminate his sexual desire, and either masturbation or a homosexual contact would follow. Both of them require, as Sullivan put it ironically, "an infinity of rationalizations . . . in our so advanced society," meaning that it is in fact unconscionable for many.[37] They would ruin the boy's budding sense of manhood, leading him to a mental breakdown. While Sullivan used a boy as a prototype, and suggested that women, rather than men, were the beginning of marital problems (by being "cold"), he still considered "Mrs. Grundy"—outdated social expectations for both men and women—as the ultimate problem behind illness.[38]

The life history of one Sheppard-Pratt patient further highlights the conflict between the changing reality for youths and the stagnant morality of the older generation. This patient was a medical officer in the Naval Reserve during World War I. When on a ship, he served on "the Board of Officers who tried a fellow officer for sodomy"; during the trial, he became "argumentative, and fought against the Board" to defend the accused. Whether or not the patient believed this was related to his "sexual experiences with boys of the same age" during his adolescence was not clear. He ran into further problems when he returned to civilian life, because he "worried tremendously" about what might go wrong in his medical practice. He was employed in his father's hardware store, where he worked until he came to Sheppard-Pratt in 1928. A few years before his hospitalization he had become religious, as reported by his brother. The patient's psychosis emerged in church. One day during a sermon he became restless, and when the congregation was singing a hymn, "without warning, [he] jumped up . . . in the pew, and broke out in a loud argument about . . . prohibition, and berated the churches for their non-Christian attitude in attempting to prohibit something that was authorized by Christ." He went on to discuss sexual matters, saying that "dogs [were] having intercourse" and "if they did it, there was no reason why . . . people couldn't." He also talked about "the colored people, and said there was no reason why the black and white people should not mix. . . . There was no more harm in a black man raping a white woman than a white man having intercourse with a black woman." Not surprisingly, "the church, by this time, was completely upset, and several members of the congregation went to him, and removed him quickly from the building," as a Sheppard-Pratt doctor recorded somberly.[39] Here again, society's (in this case, the religious community's) refusal to acknowledge sexual matters and the resulting tension in modern life seemed to be the main points of conflict. The hospital doctors were certainly aware of this, as shown in their frequent comments about a patient's or a patient family's religious background. Regarding another patient who "became greatly interested in religion [and] is overwhelmed with ideas of sin and guilt," one doctor noted that the patient "impresses one as a man who . . . [is under a considerable] amount of confusion and perplexity." The doctor also pointed out that the patient had "a very limited education and a total lack of knowledge of mental things," suggesting how the doctors considered outdated social norms, religious teaching in particular, to be damaging to mental health.[40]

Of two high-risk behaviors that highlighted the conflict between social expectations and real-life experiences, masturbation was considered more common and less harmful to patients' self-esteem than a homosexual experience. The latter was considered likely to lead to a long-term, possibly untreatable illness such as schizophrenia. One patient, whom Sheppard-Pratt doctors did not consider psychotic, had a history of "misbehaviors," including homosexual attempts with young boys. Sullivan's view of the patient was that, although he was not currently psychotic, "he [would] have a very excellent chance of becoming schizophrenic."[41] In contrast, discussing another patient, whose history of illness fitted well into Sullivan's "loss of manhood" story, Sullivan nonetheless argued that he would not give a diagnosis of schizophrenia to the patient. This was because the patient "[had] made heterosexual adjustments in numbers," suggesting that a lack of homosexual content indicates a lack of schizophrenia. The patient was diagnosed instead with a psychopathic personality, a term that Sheppard-Pratt doctors used for a wide range of problems, including those similar to schizophrenia but lacking symptomatic severity.[42] Instead of being labeled as "homosexual," then, patients whose histories included substantial homosexual content could have been called "schizophrenic." Indeed, some patients Sullivan diagnosed as schizophrenic seemed to lack typical symptoms of the illness, such as hallucinations, delusions, and catatonia, which Sheppard-Pratt doctors used as evidence of schizophrenia. What these patients exhibited instead was a concern about homosexuality. Of course, psychiatric diagnosis was (and is) a delicate matter, and it is impossible to argue that all patients with any indication of homosexual content were diagnosed with schizophrenia. The clinical files are not a complete record of doctor-patient interaction, and it is possible that patients whose records do not indicate signs of schizophrenia showed some unrecorded behaviors suggestive of the disease. But still, it is hard to miss Sullivan's belief in the connection between homosexual content and schizophrenia. The belief comes through his comments over and over again.

Why did Sullivan see a connection between homosexuality and schizophrenia, and what does this tell us about the science of homosexuality at

Sheppard-Pratt? Some psychiatrists of the time believed that these conditions shared behavioral characteristics.[43] Patients in so-called acute panic—those who exhibited episodes of excitement, rapid and incomprehensible speech, an unusual degree of perspiration, the feeling of being followed, rumored about, or persecuted, all of which were deemed to be the beginning of certain types of schizophrenia—often related "homosexual content" in their recent past. This is not surprising, given the prevailing homophobia of the time. Homosexual men could actually be an easy target of rumor and accusation, resulting in, at least for some men, an exhibition of panic and paranoia. Since such an exhibition was considered one of the indications of schizophrenia, it was not entirely surprising that doctors suspected some ties between a homosexual experience and a schizophrenic breakdown. Homosexuality and schizophrenia also shared ambiguity in definition. The term *homosexual content*, as it was used at Sheppard-Pratt, could mean a range of things, from a self-conscious, homosexual act to unconscious homophobia. The definition of schizophrenia was just as broad. For example, during a staff conference with an Italian-born Catholic patient, Sullivan and his colleague Dr. Martin discussed problems of definition and diagnosis:

SULLIVAN: Do you imagine the diagnosis of schizophrenia is made too frequently among the foreign born?

MARTIN: That is my opinion. When we find ourselves with something strange we are inclined to label it as schizophrenia when it may be due to difference in race. I have in my mind Osmena [sic] and certain Jews, then these Italians. I would like to see what the Italians call manic depressive and what they call schizophrenia.

SULLIVAN: I think doctor Martin has raised an important question. . . . If we make a diagnosis of schizophrenia because we . . . do not understand him, we are making a serious diagnosis on very poor grounds.[44]

Here, the doctors seized upon the possibility that some patients might be diagnosed with schizophrenia because of their ethnicity. It also seems possible that the doctors did not understand the nature of some patients' illness and hence put them in a black box named *schizophrenia*. Given the fact that sexual experiences and the ease with which people talked about them varied significantly between cultures, it is not unlikely that the definition of schizophrenia had a considerable overlap with that of homosexual content.

The connection Sullivan recognized was more than symptomatic similarity or diagnostic ambiguity. Both homosexuality and schizophrenia were fascinating conditions, which, Sullivan believed, revealed the core of a person's self. In an article published in 1924, he discussed his view of schizophrenia as follows:

[In schizophrenic dissociation of a personality,] the regressive process goes deeper in the mental structures; and the function appearing in [thought] content and behavior become lower and lower in the scale of psychologic [sic] ontogenesis. Thus it is here that we see that really marvelous demonstration (by regression) of the intra-uterine mind— the prenatal attitudes, sometimes with . . . uterine environment (tightly enwrapping blanket, darkness, wetness, etc.). Here we see the unmistakable evidence of prenatal experience.[45]

This description of the illness assumes that schizophrenic patients' personalities derive from their childhood, or even from their status before birth. This is apparently intriguing to Sullivan, as seen in his repeated reference to the "prenatal" status. It was "really marvelous" for him, because such a phenomenon gave him a rare opportunity to see what he believed to be the beginnings of a person's self. Such a developmental view of schizophrenia was not uncommon among psychiatrists of the 1920s, in particular those who were influenced by psychoanalytic thought.[46] However, Sullivan was unique in his strong belief that a regression to the prenatal status was a hopeful sign for recovery, because it might offer a patient a chance to do the process of growing up all over again. The fundamental nature of the illness and its presumed openness for treatment were what intrigued Sullivan.

Sullivan saw a formative stage of a person's self in homosexuality, too. In a 1927 paper, he argued that a person's interaction with society and competition with peers carried "everyone through the incest and the homosexual stages to heterosexual adjustments," suggesting his developmental approach to human sexuality. To be sure, unlike schizophrenia, which belongs to the prenatal stage, incestuous and homosexual behaviors belong to more advanced stages of a person's development, infancy and adolescence, respectively. Moreover, unlike schizophrenia, both autoeroticism and homoeroticism can result in an established, satisfying pattern of adjustment. As long as these patterns are gratifying, and as long as people whose sexual adjustment relied on these patterns developed "a friendly attitude toward behavior, interests, and sexual motivations which they know to be contrary to the prevailing social ideals," they would be free of mental disorder. But these conditions were difficult to satisfy. If a homosexual person did not have enough awareness of the "contrary" nature of his or her sexuality, even a single episode of homosexual contact could cause a schizophrenic breakdown.[47] Some might not act on their homosexual desires, but would still develop a so-called homosexual panic because the mere presence of such desire could shake a person's sense of security. This is unfortunate, Sullivan argued, particularly because the homosexual mode of adjustment came right before the heterosexual stage, in his theory of human psychosexual development.

If there were no social prohibition of same-sex intimacy, people would grow healthily into "mature" sexuality. But given the current prevalence of homophobia, homosexual experience was inevitably an episode that preceded and even produced the illness.

The crucial place that homosexuality occupied in the pathology of schizophrenia and, more important, the association of homosexual and schizophrenic conditions with the early stages of psychosexual development, contributed to Sullivan's and other doctors' fascination with both. For reeducation and readjustment of sick individuals to normal, healthy life in a community was an important tenet of the "new psychiatry" in general, and of the sociocultural approach to illness at Sheppard-Pratt in particular. The hospital's doctors, including Sullivan, were eager to offer more than just comfort to troubled minds. They wanted to treat and cure illness, and they reached a conclusion that the redoing of a person's mental growth is one of the most reasonable ways to undo the old-fashioned training that patients had received. They asked questions that spoke to this point: What do you make of your parents' sexual incompatibility, when the only teaching you hear about sex is that it should not be talked or even thought about? What about your homosexual feeling, when your culture tells you that it means that you have failed not only in your adjustment, but also in your manliness and maturity? The doctors' answer was that going back to an early stage of personality development was the most thorough way to help people who had been tormented by the disparity between ideal and reality. It was precisely the primal nature of schizophrenia and homosexuality that made them key to retrieving sanity in modern society. When society was moving away from traditional patterns of sexual behavior and, at the same time, exhibiting its tenacious attachment to these patterns, a complete reeducation of personality seemed plausible and necessary.

Doctors' broad definition of "homosexual content" thus was a double-edged sword. On the one hand, such broadness allowed them to avoid an instant, uncritical association between homosexual feelings or experiences and a mental disorder. In sharp contrast to the mainstream theory of homosexuality, Sheppard-Pratt physicians' approach to homosexual content was much less stigmatizing. At the same time, the flexible—even loose—use of the term promoted the sense that what was observed in a clinical setting was applicable to the general public. To be sure, Sheppard-Pratt doctors encountered a range of sexual issues through their patients. What they did not see frequently was well-adjusted homosexual men and women who had accepted and appreciated their sexualities. As Sullivan's article on auto-eroticism and homoeroticism suggested, he was aware that there were such people. But in this article and elsewhere in his published writing, Sullivan nonetheless emphasized mental instability in such individuals. Discussing

the social unacceptability of homosexuality, for instance, he pointed out
how "the homosexual love object all too frequently fails to 'stay put,'" causing homosexual men "one disappointment after another." Also, "when the
love objects recant the covenant of friendship to enter the sacrament of
wedlock, so much the greater is the shock" to those who stayed in exclusive
homosexuality.[48] These warnings implied that even healthy homosexual men
were at risk: homosexual men, both inside and outside a mental hospital,
constituted a risk group. Although homosexuality itself was not an illness,
a homosexual experience could be traumatic and thus a social pathogen
because of the stigma associated with it. In this way, the science of homosexuality at Sheppard-Pratt was part of the era's expansion of the psychiatric
domain—the expansion of the field that shifted its focus from the care of
serious illness to the treatment of mild disturbance, discomfort, and maladjustment in everyday life.[49]

While Sullivan promoted such expansion of psychiatric authority in his
writing, he encountered a far more complex reality in the clinical setting,
creating a sharp contrast between his published works and his clinical interactions. Some of his patients refused to be placed in the risk group, while
others questioned Sullivan's sincerity in claiming the need for homosexual
men to "grow up" to become heterosexuals. No patients seemed to know
that Sullivan was living with a male partner; nonetheless, some sensed a
gap between Sullivan's unconventionality as a person and his conventional
advice as a doctor. As he talked with these particularly perceptive patients,
he began to create a clinical approach that was detached from those
described in his published articles, or even from collaboration with his colleagues at Sheppard-Pratt.

The Private Liberalism in the Making

"Why not talk about yourself? . . . You are not exactly in public here," Sullivan told a patient during a special interview in 1927. The patient resisted,
saying that he "[felt he was] in public because [of] these gentlemen," referring to attendants taking notes. This exchange illuminates a few emblematic qualities of Sullivan's special interview with patients. For one, Sullivan
considered it a unique occasion during which both doctor and patient
could discuss things in an unguarded manner. He was more than willing to
impress a patient with the fact that the doctor is a regular person with his
own emotions and limitations. Thus, in response to this patient's protest,
Sullivan explained: "I very rarely talk without having notes taken—I hear a
great many things in a day and can't keep everything straight, you know."
Further, when the patient complained that he had not been benefiting from
the interview and hence they should "call it quit [sic]," Sullivan persisted:

"No. I can't. Merely because a thing is difficult, I can't quit. . . . You are able to concern yourself about Masons and all that [the patient believed that Masons persecuted him], whereas I have to concern myself about you." This put the patient and the doctor on an equal ground in a single stroke, while the comment also illuminated Sullivan's frustration with the patient's unwillingness to open up, which was, ultimately, an expression of his serious interest in the patient's well-being.[50] Even if the interview did not go well, Sullivan would be staying in the room, and he would not let go of the patient, either. Such was the demeanor Sullivan projected in the special interviews.

It is not surprising, then, that he and some of his patients created something more than a formal medical relationship—it was a personal and private environment in which a doctor and patients who shared a concern about their own homosexual feelings and experiences could forge a bond and a critique of homophobia. In a 1926 interview, for instance, we can see one of the earliest examples of an in-depth discussion of homosexuality, which no doubt called for considerable confidence in the relationship on the part of both the doctor and the patient. In spite of the presence of two other doctors, who remained silent after a few exchanges at the beginning of the interview, Sullivan and the patient freely discussed the latter's feelings for another male patient.

PATIENT: Well—about this fellow *** over here—I began to love him and it was discontinued because I was removed from that ward.
SULLIVAN: Had your love for him been permitted . . . what would have been its end?
PATIENT: Wouldn't have been an end.
SULLIVAN: Would have gone on forever, increasing?
PATIENT: Wouldn't have amounted to anything.
SULLIVAN: What was lovable about him?
PATIENT: Just a mere fact of his being alive—that's all.[51]

Sullivan and the patient conversed with the apparent assumption that they could talk about love between men without fear or embarrassment. Given the medical consensus of the time that homosexuality constituted an illness, it is not difficult to assume that the doctor and patients had to travel a long distance to share such an assumption in a clinical setting. Although Sheppard-Pratt doctors obviously did not adhere to the stigmatizing view of homosexuality and encouraged patients to discuss homosexual experiences, the patient still could have been afraid that his confession of his current attraction to the person of the same sex would be seen as an unquestionable sign of illness. The doctor, too, could have been worried that he would be seen as too understanding of the patient's homosexual feelings. But none of these concerns seemed to affect this exchange, suggesting a firm mutual trust that that all was being done to explore the patient's illness, and nothing would go outside the room to do harm. This allowed them to further explore the patient's "love" toward ***.

PATIENT: Sometimes when he was hollering and crying—and whining—I would hold him and he would go right to sleep. Maybe if you Doctors try some of that instead of so many orders and theories.

SULLIVAN: It might be misunderstood.

PATIENT: Yes—I know you are handicapped. And these orders of attendants—they knock people around—if the attendants had more intellectual powers and the doctors more manual powers I think it would be possible.

SULLIVAN: In your own case would it have helped? Shortly after you came here if someone tried to be physically affectionate to you, would that have helped?

PATIENT: Physically affectionate? There is no such thing as physical affection.

SULLIVAN: Well, pardon my ignorance. If one of them had held you, caressed you, or something of that kind?

PATIENT: If one of them had shown that he wanted to . . . I didn't want any actual holding or caressing—no.

SULLIVAN: Why not?

PATIENT: I just wouldn't—I don't know.

SULLIVAN: What is the difference between you and ***? It worked with ***. But you say you wouldn't care for any physical demonstration of that sort.

PATIENT: It would seem unnatural to me.

SULLIVAN: But it seemed . . . natural when you did it to him?

PATIENT: Because he had a trust.

SULLIVAN: Which you lack?

PATIENT: Yes.[52]

Evidently, Sullivan was intrigued by the patient's suggestion that doctors held patients to comfort them. He was aware of its risk, but wanted to know more about what the patient thought of the doctors' use of "manual powers." The patient backed off when it came to the application of "manual powers" to himself. Particularly, the words "physical affection" seemed to bother him. Sullivan's following comment, whether sarcastic or not, is illuminating, because by asking the patient to excuse his "ignorance," he seemed to express his respect for the patient. By describing "physical affection" with different expressions such as "holding," "caressing," and "physical demonstration of that sort," Sullivan showed his willingness to use language that sounded acceptable to the patient. What followed further highlights Sullivan's eagerness to learn from the patient.

SULLIVAN: If he had been suspicious it would have been bad business for us to hold him and fondle him?

PATIENT: Yes—but you could have found some way to remove his suspicion.

SULLIVAN: Would you mind telling me what would be the best way?. . . . What means would you recommend for me to overcome the suspiciousness?

PATIENT: . . . Your kindly and sympathetic attitude would be something.

SULLIVAN: Would it work with you?

PATIENT: Yes—it would work with me.

SULLIVAN: Here is a case in which you can be kindly to a patient and we cannot; because [we are] . . . restrained from doing that.

PATIENT: Well—your being here is—it rests on your reputation. Does it not?

SULLIVAN: If you are asking personally—it does not. Continue.

PATIENT: It does not? . . . I feel certain that it does . . .

SULLIVAN: If you failed [to get well] you will expect the social organization, to wit; your loved ones, to punish us—would you not?

PATIENT: No—no—no. If you do what you thought was right—why, that's all a man can do. I don't think that you can do what you don't think was right here.

SULLIVAN: Explain. You have said [earlier] that you don't think that I could do what I thought was right here. Now explain that to me, if you will.

PATIENT: . . . If you thought that holding any one was right . . . of course, you could do that, but something more than that I don't think that you would do it. . . . In that case about *** . . . I think you would be embarrassed to hold him . . .

SULLIVAN: Would you be embarrassed to permit me to do them?

PATIENT: I might—I don't know.

SULLIVAN: And what would bring about my embarrassment and your possible embarrassment?

PATIENT: Your fear to do something foolish.

SULLIVAN: . . . May I ask what that means? . . . I suppose it connects with some experience of yours . . .

PATIENT: I have been afraid to wear a beard.

SULLIVAN: Foolish, then, would be something that opened one to the disdain or criticism of others.

PATIENT: Yes,—exactly . . .

SULLIVAN: Suppose then, that it was done secretly?

PATIENT: That would be alright.

SULLIVAN: . . . The rub is not what other people may think of our doing, but what you think of it, isn't it?

PATIENT: Yes—that's what concerns you and me.

SULLIVAN: So why need we drag in these people who prohibit our methods?

PATIENT: I think—that—that situation exists between you and me.
SULLIVAN: And that's all there is to it, isn't it—just what you think?
PATIENT: Exactly.[53]

In response to the patient's earlier reference to "trust," Sullivan asked
how he might eradicate the patient's suspicion. Then they discussed the
professional "restraint" imposed on staff, the "reputation" that doctors have
to keep up, and the "social organization" that would accuse them if they
failed. Clearly, both the patient and the doctor were aware of the unconventionality of using physical contact between doctors and patients as a form of
treatment. The patient offered a fresh insight when he said that doing what
one thinks right is "all a man can do," suggesting that despite all the risks
of physical contact, what mattered most was that doctors did their best with
sympathy and sincerity. Sullivan agreed, claiming that their focus should be
on "you" and "me"; what needs to be accomplished was a feeling of security
in an actual relationship, not what seemed appropriate in abstract medical
and social standards.

Considering that this interview occurred in October 1926, it is likely
that it captured one of the moments of Sullivan's stepping into the use of
physical contact in his clinical practice. As Arthur Linton recalled of the late
1920s, "The patients could hug, embrace, and kiss the attendants without
feeling rejected, odd, embarrassed or humiliated."[54] Contact was restricted
to attendants and patients. Bernard Robbins, a doctor at Sheppard-Pratt in
the 1920s, confirmed this when he said that the practice "was left entirely
to . . . aides."[55] The reason for this distinction is unknown, although it is
possible that Sullivan could not get doctors to cooperate. Attendants, on the
other hand, could be trained (and indeed, were trained) to do what Sullivan
considered to be effective. At any rate, the contact was meant to encourage
patients' acceptance of their own homosexuality, rather than recovery from
sexual "anomalies," as one of the most respected psychiatric textbooks used
in the 1920s suggested.[56]

This interview illuminates two striking features of Sullivan's treatment.
First, it is not clear who is suggesting the use of physical contact as a means
of treatment. Sullivan can be seen as guiding the discussion to where he
wanted; he might even be seen as seducing the patient when he asked how
the patient would feel if he permitted the doctor to hold him. Nevertheless,
the patient seems assertive—he is not just listening to doctor, as he actively,
often decisively, made suggestions. Second, Sullivan was eager to get the
patient's input about ways to facilitate the physical contact. His willingness to listen to patients is affirmed in his published articles, but not in the
context of physical contact between male doctors and male patients. We see
in the interview, though nowhere in his published writing, that he was well

aware of the method's unconventionality, and suggested its application in secrecy, so that doctors and patients did not have to be concerned about outside critiques. Sullivan was not bringing an established method into his interview with a patient. The doctor-patient relationship itself was in the process of becoming, something that the interviewer and the interviewee were creating together through their careful effort to figure out what they wanted from each other, and how.

The following exchange with the same patient suggests another important feature of Sullivan's clinical practice that he did not mention in his published writings: that it carried subjective as well as scientific meanings for him, and that these meanings, combined, shaped his critique of sexual morals and standards.

SULLIVAN: What do you suppose you would do if somebody held you?

PATIENT: It all—depends who—and when—and how.

SULLIVAN: You feel you would enjoy the experience don't you?

PATIENT: No—I feel—I wouldn't enjoy the experience . . .

SULLIVAN: . . . Explain why life is too short for you to try experiments in secret, in receiving the affectionate attention of some of your fellow-men.

PATIENT: Well—just not interesting—that's all.

SULLIVAN: And yet it seems to me that that was what you recommended— that we should do that towards patients, including yourself.

PATIENT: No—I don't remember that.

SULLIVAN: Do you have any recommendations to make in that particular?

PATIENT: Well—yes, I would recommend that you go along some highroad [sic] and find a way to make your living and then if there were any men to help—help them. As a side line—not as a business.

SULLIVAN: Then you would perhaps suggest that as a preliminary we destroy the existing social system?

PATIENT: Yes. I would recommend that—I would fight for it. That I would live for and die for.

SULLIVAN: Do you think that life might be a little too short to accomplish this?

PATIENT: Yes—I do. Therefore—I am going to get what I can out of it.

SULLIVAN: Now so much for you. But we continue to be in relationship of the staff to the patient. While you feel you can't overthrow the social system and reduce everything to a delightful primitive state, what would you recommend we do in the meanwhile, between the staff and the patient?

PATIENT: . . . I wouldn't let any man I couldn't trust sleep with me—would you.

SULLIVAN: I have let men I didn't trust sleep with me—yes.

PATIENT: I mean if you were a woman.

SULLIVAN: I can't imagine it? . . . In this true marriage—when the social system is gone—will that be determined by transcendental means or what?
What will determine your being a true husband and her a true wife?[57]

Now their topic is the place of affection between men in the "existing
social system," or lack thereof. While this broadened the scope of their discussion—affection between male doctors and male patients should serve as a "preliminary" means of changing homophobic society, it also steered them into
talking about their personal beliefs. Sullivan's comments in particular indicate
that he had doubts about marriage. Further, he suggests that he prefers what
he called a "primitive state" of human relations, which was not bound to current social norms and institutions. Thus he would suggest a vision of a therapeutic colony or community where people who did not make heterosexual
adjustments were encouraged to construct homosexual relationships without
being stigmatized. Given this vision, it seems unlikely that Sullivan regretted
his experience of sleeping with a man he did not trust. He seemed to think
that there might be something constructive about sex detached from conventional love and trust, and wished to offer its benefit in a therapeutic setting.
Moreover, he was comfortable enough with this patient to talk about personal
experiences of his that he considered relevant to therapeutic practices. Indeed,
with any of his chosen patients, he was not at all hesitant in uncovering a close
connection between his scientific practice and subjective self.

Sometimes, Sullivan's openness went so far as to explore a patient's
knowledge of homosexual communities. Here is another patient in his twenties, whose interview with Sullivan occurred in February 1927. This time, no
other doctors were present, but Sullivan noted that the patient had been
"under . . . close supervision" by another doctor and that this doctor had
"talked with me [Sullivan] at great length" about the patient's situation.
The doctor, George E. Partridge, one of the two present at the 1926 interview
we have examined, seemed to collaborate with Sullivan in the treatment of
patients who had had homosexual experiences or desires. In this interview,
the patient made it clear that he recognized a homosexual tendency in himself. Sullivan asked if the patient thought the tendency was common among
people of his age, and the patient replied that he believed the tendency "exists
in quite a number of people." Then the patient mentioned a friend who was
"associated with a group of people [in] Washington—artists of talent and better class," and claimed that "among them homosexuality seems to offer quite
a good deal of food for jest." In response, Sullivan asked:

Have you seen any of the homosexual society's members go mad?
PATIENT: Can't say that I have . . .
SULLIVAN: I think there is a large number of the more cultured who are
frankly homosexual. . . . I have received exceedingly few of them as

patients in many years past. I have received a great number of people who are terribly concerned lest they are homosexual. . . . If one says, "To hell with everything, I am going to perform fellatio," the chances are all his training which is directed against immoral practices . . . will come in conflict with his impulses. . . .

PATIENT: Do you mean that a person who had no mental tension and no concern about it—that he could masturbate as often as he cared without injuring himself?

SULLIVAN: I think if one had . . . no notion of the evil of masturbation, he perhaps would do himself a wee bit of good.

PATIENT: What is the hope in my case?

SULLIVAN: To some extent that is determined by your early training and by the weakness . . . in your self-esteem. To a larger extent it is determined by the actual desire you have to get into life, rather than sitting off in a corner and thinking. . . . I think it would have been very unfortunate for you to marry the first one you came in contact with. I do believe you will gain experience which will probably diminish your interest in homosexual fantasies. . . . I . . . regard you in need of some sexual experience before you . . . select a satisfactory wife. I don't advise you to go looking for it, but if it comes your way, take it.[58]

This exchange shows that Sullivan considered a person's concern about "immoral" homosexual practices, defined as such by heterosexual norms, not homosexuality itself, to be a cause of illness. While this illuminates his critique of the social origin of mental illness, his comment also suggests upper limits he cautiously tried to place on such a critique. Not unlike in some of his articles of the 1920s, Sullivan in this exchange seemed to assume that homosexuality was one of the stages of psychosexual development, out of which people should eventually grow. Sullivan even suggested that homosexual tendencies could facilitate a person's sexual development. Thus if the patient "gain[ed] experience" with women, he should be able to rid himself of preoccupation with "homosexual fantasies." But unlike published articles, the patient was there to raise a question about such an assumption. The patient was aware of homosexual men who seemed artistic, talented, and refined. Sullivan agreed, calling them "the more cultured." How, then, could he call them immature, just because they were homosexual?

The patient recognized this inconsistency and brought it up in their next interview. This time, Sullivan believed that the patient was concealing his thoughts, and he tried out what he called "an experiment" to get the patient to talk.

SULLIVAN: Let us try an experiment and now let us be very candid—will you tell me something about myself. We are trying a practical test.

PATIENT: Well, your manner has seemed to be rather affected . . . especially your enunciation and manner of treating patients. . . . I have often wondered why it is [that] you have never married. . . . And then I tried to . . . find some association between your choice of work and the reasons you have never married—your professional manner didn't seem affected but I had an intuition that it was the result of some effort anyway. And you seem to be under some strain—that is about all, I think.

SULLIVAN: All? My goodness! Now you are trying a test as a literary person.

PATIENT: I should have to look at you. I should have to see all of your face.

SULLIVAN: Do I have to keep my eyes open?

PATIENT: No—seeing all your face enables me to form opinions and theories.

SULLIVAN: Do so, please. I wish to hear them.

PATIENT: Well, you are not averse to beating around the bush a little and evading the real truth of things just for the purpose of getting a person's mind easy. In other words, certain things which you advocate you don't really believe in yourself sincerely—but by that I mean sex questions.

SULLIVAN: Do go on.

PATIENT: I am just trying to formulate facts. You seem to be trying to get away from yourself more than you realize and I have often wondered just why a person takes up this sort of work. . . . I know attendants at an insane asylum take up that certain sort of work for certain reasons—and I was wondering if psychiatrists in an institution take up that work for the same reasons.

SULLIVAN: Do tell your reason why attendants do take it up.

PATIENT: To a great extent they take it up . . . because of their homosexual traits. . . . They take it up . . . because they feel a certain affinity for the patient. . . . A man is interested in a certain thing and there is a reason for it.

SULLIVAN: You see you are continuing a description of me.

PATIENT: You look on things in a sort of callous way. . . . You . . . gave me the impression that marriage was an excellent thing yet I knew you had never married. . . . I know that attendants have traits along that line—homosexual traits and they usually come to this sort of work—a great many of them, not all—because they are afraid of being outside of such a place. It gives them a chance to really be a patient without being one actually. May also give them a feeling of superiority where none exists.

SULLIVAN: . . . Will you smoke one of these? . . . Have you any idea that my thoughts would be any good to anyone but me—those that I don't let people know?

PATIENT: No, I don't suppose so.

SULLIVAN: Do you feel cheated because I don't say everything I think?

PATIENT: No—I merely noticed that.

SULLIVAN: Do you think I have been sincere with anything to you.

PATIENT: Yes, I think you have been sincere about everything, but I couldn't help but wonder whether they were not, well somewhat of an insincerity of your remarks about masturbation and sex—I thought possibly you were, might say taking the best road out of the difficulties which I was in or thought I was in.

SULLIVAN: If to avoid argument you should be interested in your characterization of me—do you remember it well? Because if you don't, I will be glad to give you a copy of it. It would be . . . more illuminating than anything else you have said.[59]

The patient confronted Sullivan by asking the reason for his bachelorhood if he really believed in heterosexual marriage. The patient sounded almost certain that Sullivan was not open about his homosexuality, even though Sullivan intended to conceal it from patients. Sullivan, as the patient assumed, had taken up his line of profession because he shared "homosexual traits" with patients and thus felt close to them. These pointed observations forced Sullivan to give up a clean line between his personal and professional beliefs, which he had maintained with some "effort" and "strain." Sullivan's response to these observations was forthright; he admitted more than once that what the patient has been talking about was, indeed, a description of Sullivan. As if overwhelmed by its accuracy, Sullivan became silent at one point. This silence was indicated as " . . ." in the transcript, and it seems as if he needed a break from the intense talk when he offered a cigarette to the patient. To be sure, Sullivan hoped to keep his personal and professional lives separate. Such separation would protect him from all the precarious complexity of being a gay psychiatrist. And yet, as he immersed himself in one-on-one interviews, he realized that there were times when this boundary had to be crossed. Faced with the patient's demand that the doctor abandon his "callous" manner, Sullivan had to disclose his "sincere" feeling that homosexuality was not a stage that he expected to leave behind. Indeed, homosexuality was a state of being in which he might stay for a long time, because it was most natural and intimate to him. Sullivan was not able to recommend conventionality as a doctor while he led an unconventional life as a person.

It was with this realization that he began to shape a unique form of private liberalism on questions of homosexuality, which was not open to public critique and hence did not call for a strict separation of personal beliefs from scientific observations. In this separate sphere, Sullivan and his patients were able to shape a critique of heterosexism that defined homosexuality either as a high-risk sexuality or as a passing phase in psychosexual development. Only in secrecy would they be able to pursue the unconventional method involving physical affection and emotional closeness among doctors, attendants, and patients. As the patient insisted, what bound them all together was their belief that the acceptance, not elimination, of homosexuality constituted treatment. As Arthur Linton claimed, most attendants with whom Sullivan worked were "'gay' or were latent homosexual." This suggests that such a bond was no secret among those who were involved.[60] Within this small group of insiders, a distinction between normal and abnormal sexualities came into question. In this "between you and me" circumstance, the doctor could ask gripping questions such as, "Do you think of sex relations between men with any approval at all—with any approval at all . . . ?" and "You feel in no kind of society it [homosexual relationship] would be . . . permissible?"[61] Given the pathologization of homosexuality at the time, these questions were a challenge from within against the medical establishment's authority to determine what constituted health and illness. Moreover, this was an emerging expression of identity for sexual minorities, who began to see heteronormativity, not their own sexuality, as the ultimate problem.

But their practice had to be kept hidden from outsiders. One important sign of Sullivan's effort to protect his method from outside critique was the lack of records of special interviews in 1928 and 1929. Twenty patient files from 1926 and 1927 included records of special interviews, while only two patient files from 1928 and 1929 contained them.[62] This is a crucial change, because it suggests that Sullivan's approach was shaped in front of others in earlier years (there were usually a few doctors present at the interviews we have examined), while it became more secretive (and thus its record was not included in clinical files) in later years. Most certainly, Sullivan continued special interviews in 1928 and 1929, along with the careful recording of them. Indeed, he had his own ward—"Sullivan's Ward" with six beds—in these years, and thus it is reasonable to assume that he had more one-on-one interviews in later years than in 1926 and 1927. But these interviews took place in his office, and no one kept track of when and how they occurred. As a director of clinical research, Sullivan perhaps did not find it so difficult to keep a transcript of a special interview out of a patient's official file. Indeed, William W. Elgin, an intern who worked on Sullivan's Ward in 1928, recalled that Sullivan was "always very reluctant to write the usual progress notes in the patient's charts, even though he kept copious notes for his own use. . . . He carried his personal recording apparatus to take down all of his spoken words."[63] Thus no others had a chance to look at records that could have included references to Sullivan's method.

Some conference reports from 1928 and 1929 suggest the omission of certain details as well. For example, one case presentation by Sullivan during a staff conference reads as follows:

[The patient] was seen . . . on August 23. . . . From that time to this, we have had quite a few interviews. . . . The father in this picture is characterized by his inability to actually deal with the sort of problems that his son needed his help on. For instance, one day, they were sitting in the library, and the patient was engaged in fantasy of a sexual nature, and the father rather startled him by turning to him and saying, "***, what are you thinking about?" . . . The boy then said he was thinking of . . . homosexual intercourse. The father was . . . embarrassed and said, " . . . I'll talk to you about that soon." Nothing has been said about from that date to this. . . . He engaged in . . . some feeble attempts at homosexuality when he was around thirteen. . . . His homosexual venture was the cause of . . . self-condemnation. . . . Throughout my work with him, we have both felt it important to deal with the sexual aspects of life.[64]

We cannot know any further details about the special interviews Sullivan had with the patient "for quite a few times," because there is no transcript in the patient's file. Nor was there any in-depth discussion of the patient's concern over "his homosexual venture" during the staff conference. Sullivan used to have such a discussion at least with some patients in 1926–1927 during a staff conference, but not in 1928–1929. What is left in the 1928–1929 files is a mere glimpse of what might have been rich and intense special interviews, a skeletal outline of Sullivan's "work with [his patients]" who had homosexual concerns.

The same applies to another patient from 1928, diagnosed with schizophrenia, whose file included one record of a special interview. During a conference, the patient referred to his fear of another male patient and "sex fears," which he apparently discussed with Sullivan. But the recorded one-on-one interview barely touched on these fears, an omission suggesting, perhaps, that there were other unrecorded or unfiled special interviews. These interviews may have mentioned physical contact between patients and attendants, and thus would have been too controversial to be included in the patient's files. This is of course speculation, as we lack explicit sources. But in 1926 and 1927, records of Sullivan's conversations about the possibility of physical contact between patients and attendants were filed, perhaps because such contact had not yet been put into practice. Although we cannot know for sure, it seems likely that later, when such practice became part of Sullivan's Ward, records that referred to it, if any, were perceived as too controversial to be placed in official files.

Sullivan's published articles, too, indicate his attempt to shield his clinical practice from public scrutiny. For one, his theoretical writing did not discuss a patient's acceptance of his homosexuality as a main focus of treatment, while it continued to uphold the developmental model of human sexuality. Furthermore, discussing what he called "the oral erotic" type of homosexuality, his 1929 article claimed that such was "the direct outcome of personality deviations that . . . have their nucleus in abnormal attitudes and belief cultivated in the parent-child relationship." While he suggested that not all homosexuals fitted into this oral erotic type (whom Sullivan defined as those who prefer fellatio as a sexual outlet) and the division between different "types" of homosexuality was not always distinct, he nonetheless asserted that this particular type would "encounter particular difficulty in evolving into the heterosexual phase of personality" unless a "thoroughgoing and extensive reorganization of the personality" occurred. Thus, unlike his comments in the clinical setting, which suggested that oral sex should not hurt a person's self-esteem, his published writing defined it as high-risk behavior that needed a therapeutic intervention. Moreover, unlike his clinical practice that dealt with a broad range of patients without putting them into different categories, his writing maintained a distinction between different kinds of homosexual men—the oral, anal, and urethral (genital). Among them, the oral type belonged to the most immature stage of personality adjustment and was thought to prefer feminine sexual behavior. Sullivan's public writing began to feature such categorical thinking, just as his private practice resisted and refuted these views. This disparity was not a result of his professional calculation; it was not the case that Sullivan did one thing in the clinical setting and another in his publications in order to gain from both. He was living this gap between the public and private in his personal life as well, no doubt with painstaking effort. His personal experience as a homosexual man was tightly bound up with his professional work, and in this way, Sullivan was much like many scientists of sexuality of the time whose subjectivity occupied an uneasy place in their scientific practice.

Public and Private Lives

Sullivan's relationship with his partner almost certainly shaped the striking division between the public and private during these years. Little direct evidence of their relationship survives, however, and there have been conflicting stories. But what we know illuminates Sullivan's struggle to understand the place of sexuality and subjectivity in his life and career. Sullivan began to live with a young man named James Inscoe sometime in 1928, just around the time when he began to create his own ward for young male schizophrenic patients with homosexual conflicts. James, or Jimmie, as he seems to have preferred being called, was seventeen, Harry thirty-six, and the partnership continued until Sullivan's death twenty-one years later. It is not clear how their relationship began, and this, along with the aura of secrecy with which they surrounded their partnership throughout their lives, has caused much speculation and dispute in the scholarship on Sullivan. Their first encounter, whatever the circumstances actually might have been, has produced three different stories among Sullivan's associates and biographers. These stories have appeared and reappeared in the literature on Sullivan, although none of them have addressed Inscoe's own account of the encounter.

The first two stories are found in Helen Swick Perry's 1982 study of Sullivan, the foremost biography of the psychiatrist: the first assumed that Jimmie had been Sullivan's patient at Sheppard-Pratt. The second, which does not necessarily contradict the first, related that Jimmie had been found standing in a schizophrenic catatonia in front of the office of Ernest E. Hadley, Sullivan's friend and fellow psychiatrist.[65] These episodes became well accepted over time among Sullivan's colleagues in the medical and social sciences. Indeed, Perry's main sources of information were her 1968 interview with Agnes Hadley, Ernest's wife, and another interview in 1972 with Jean Sapir, the wife of the anthropologist Edward Sapir, with whom Sullivan became a close collaborator in the 1920s and 1930s.[66] What these two stories have in common is Sullivan's role as the doctor-savior of a needy Inscoe without recognizing their relationship as partners who lived together. The third story was published by clinical psychologist Michael Stuart Allen in 1995. Allen interviewed Perry in 1987 for his research on Sullivan, and Perry told him that she understood Jimmie had been a male hustler before coming to live with Sullivan. This suggests a sexual angle—that they were a prostitute and a customer, at least up to a certain point, although Perry made no such revelation in her biography.[67]

We do not have a way of determining which (or whether) one of these stories is more accurate than another. Nor do we have Sullivan's own account of his encounter with Inscoe. But Inscoe's account, which he revealed to his friend and Sullivan's former student Ralph M. Crowley between 1971 and 1976 in a series of personal correspondences, offers yet another story.[68] According to Jimmie's account, he and Harry first met through a friend of Jimmie's aunt who was "socially prominent in the embassy's circle." Then they met "a number of times" in the office of Ernest E. Hadley. Jimmie explained that the reason for these meetings was "to get acquainted," saying nothing more. After a while, Jimmie went to see Harry "in his home surroundings" with Jimmie's aunt's friend. The friend "spent the night and I spent two days there [at Harry's home] at that time." Soon, they agreed to live together, though Jimmie does not explain why. Instead, he describes how they went to see his parents to obtain their permission:

He (Sullivan) and I went to see my mother and father for permission to come and live with him. Told them: he had not been in good health but was on the mend now, that he wanted someone in the house . . . who could run the household, and later on to take over office duties. My mother hemmed and hawed until my father finally asserted himself (which . . . he rarely ever did and said to my mother "why don't you give the boy a chance? Let him go.") My mother said nothing further. And that was that. This took only about a half-hour. I put what belongings I had in a small shopping bag and . . . caught a bus . . . for Baltimore. On the bus I felt kind of low but was glad to get away from home. . . . The first person Harry introduced me to was Clara Thompson and we became friends until she died. The second were the Chapmans who instantly accepted me without question.[69]

This account suggests a few things about Jimmie, Harry, and their relationship. First, it indicates that whatever circumstances Jimmie himself might have been in before coming to live with Harry, it was something Jimmie did not want to expand upon even more than twenty years after Harry's death. Given the fact that Inscoe, Hadley, and Sullivan met a number of times at Hadley's office, it could be that Jimmie had some mental problem that drew the psychiatrists' attention. But Jimmie did not indicate anything along these lines in his letter to Crowley. This could be because he did not want to reveal that he had had a mental problem, or because he did not want to talk about any relationship between himself and Sullivan that existed before they began to live together. It could be that Jimmie wanted to keep this to himself, until he wrote a full-scale memoir of Sullivan, a project Jimmie thought about off and on but did not act on. In any case, it is Sullivan, not Inscoe, who appears needy here. Indeed, Jimmie's description makes it clear that the "official" explanation for their cohabitation, which Jimmie and Harry decided to offer to Jimmie's parents (or Jimmie decided to tell Crowley), was that Sullivan wanted a helper around his house and office. This was something that made Jimmie's departure seem as if it were for a job, a decent position, given Jimmie's family's desperate financial situation (despite the rich aunt with prominent friends, Jimmie's parents were in financial crisis in 1928). Harry was an older, established man with money, who could help Jimmie obtain independence from his family. No wonder, then, that Jimmie told Crowley that he was "fortunate" to have "some knowledge of cooking which [I] learned from my paternal grandmother" and "some typing and shorthand and filing" skills he had learned in junior high school. These skills helped him to do the job Sullivan required of Jimmie and at the same time offered a credible title for himself: a doctor's housekeeper and secretary.[70]

And yet Jimmie's own words seem to counter such a neat designation. First, his departure from his family was not simply to take up a job, but clearly something that stirred everyone's emotions. The letter indicates that Jimmie's independence (or lack thereof) had been a cause of disagreement between his parents; when he was given permission to go, Jimmie seemed more surprised than relieved, saying "that was that"—and it took Harry *only* thirty minutes to make it happen. When Jimmie let Harry talk to his parents, then, Jimmie was putting more than just a job at stake. It was about his own future, something yet to be discovered. With only a small bag full of belongings, Jimmie was ready to seize this opportunity to begin something new. No wonder, then, that Jimmie was nervous when he met with Harry's friends and colleagues for the first time. More than forty years later, Jimmie seems eager to recall the first few people he had met as Sullivan's cohabitant. Clearly, it came with a great relief that these people were willing to accept him. With Clara Thompson, Jimmie created a close, long-lasting friendship, and Ross M. Chapman—the superintendent of Sheppard-Pratt who allowed Sullivan to establish his own ward—accepted Jimmie, in Jimmie's words, "without question, instantly." These memories illuminate how Jimmie thought that there might be a question about the nature of their relationship and was greatly relieved when there was not. This clearly seems a partner's nervousness, not a servant's or secretary's. Jimmie's account, then, raises questions about the established stories that highlighted a preexisting doctor-patient relationship between Harry and Jimmie. Moreover, the existing clinical records at Sheppard-Pratt did not include one for James Inscoe, and Jimmie himself noted that he "was only on the grounds of SEP [Sheppard and Enoch Pratt Hospital] twice in my life briefly," apparently referring to occasions after he began to live with Sullivan.[71] Nevertheless, Jimmie's mental instability became a repeated story because it fitted into Sullivan's role as a doctor. Indeed, this is the image that Sullivan himself tried to maintain, as he claimed the therapeutic value of plain, light labor and told his friends that he took Jimmie in to help his recovery.[72] But it was not clear just what problem Jimmie had to recover from. In a way, it did not matter, because not only the partners, but also possibly their friends, wanted them to adopt an appearance that did not invite uncomfortable questions about their relationship. Thus Harry and Jimmie's partnership relied on a public silence. Sullivan's associates were more than willing to live within the boundaries of what counted as public and private, as Sullivan doubtless intended.

In addition to positing Jimmie's preexisting patienthood, published accounts of Sullivan have emphasized their relationship as a father and a son; Jimmie was Sullivan's "foster son"; or he was an "adopted son, whom Sullivan took in as a vagrant at age fifteen while at Sheppard Pratt."[73] These accounts have persisted despite the lack of any legal relationship between

Harry and Jimmie. Indeed, the lack of legal adoption made it necessary for Sullivan to make a special note in his will written in 1939: "Said James Inscoe Sullivan has resided with me since the age of about fifteen years, and has been, in all senses, a son to me, and has my love and affection as such."[74] But if their relationship was just like that of a father and a son, it seems peculiar that they did not become such legally, so as to avoid all the complexity. Along the same lines, it is notable that Jimmie never called Harry father when writing about Sullivan, but instead continued to use either "Harry" or "HSS." This raises a doubt that Jimmie was, indeed, "in all senses, a son" to Harry; it also makes one wonder if there was a disparity between how Sullivan felt about the relationship and how Inscoe perceived it. However, no one called attention to these contradictions to explore their lifelong partnership. Indeed, Sullivan himself was the first to make sure that no one did. He called Jimmie his son when he introduced this young man to his colleagues, not disclosing, even to his close friends, the fact that Jimmie was not legally adopted. Jimmie became "James Inscoe Sullivan," even though he was never a "Sullivan" officially.

Just as he tried to keep his relationship with Jimmie as lovers and partners secret, then, Sullivan kept private his unconventional approach to patients with homosexual conflicts. Meanwhile, he attempted to settle images of himself as Jimmie's doctor, employer, father, and guardian, all of which fitted nicely into the "existing social system." All this facilitated Sullivan's becoming known as an expert in the treatment of schizophrenia, but not as a critic of homophobia, because only the former had a place in his profession. Ironically, the "system" was precisely what Sullivan and some of his patients wished to overturn, by making a therapeutic community in which conventional sexual inhibition was to be abolished. And yet their critique of a society intolerant of homosexuality and their strong, intimate feeling for those trapped in such social prejudice remained insiders' talk, not something that they could bring out into the street. It is striking, to say the least, that Sullivan's "treatment" encouraging patients to accept homosexuality and his partnership with Inscoe began around the same time. Sullivan's (and perhaps Jimmie's) decision to create an image of Harry as Inscoe's father figure, no doubt one-dimensional but publicly presentable, illuminates the contested place of the connection between scientific work and subjective self. Such connection shaped, if obliquely, a crucial aspect of not only Sullivan's approach to homosexuality but also the science of homosexuality in general throughout the first half of the twentieth century. A number of researchers in human sexuality, including Jan Gay, Thomas Painter, Ruth Fulton Benedict, Margaret Mead, and Alfred C. Kinsey, grappled with this close connection between the subjective and scientific.[75] Sullivan certainly belonged to this cohort of scientists, and his response to this challenge traces one trajectory of human subjectivity devalued within modern, "objective" science.

Sullivan decided to leave Sheppard-Pratt rather than make a case for his private practice when the nature of his work became known to the hospital administration. Even though his approach to the issue of homosexuality was not acceptable in a hospital setting, he would continue to work out some elements of his method in his private practice in New York City. Here again, his partnership with Jimmie would remain in an uneasy, tense relationship to his private liberalism. At Sheppard-Pratt, we have seen that Sullivan began his career as a scientist, just as he began the same-sex personal relationship that was important to him. On the one hand, his partnership with Inscoe must have touched on issues raised every day in Sullivan's clinical practice, illuminating them and making them more real, more compelling, and more exciting. On the other hand, his private practices were potentially disruptive to his public self-image, and Sullivan concealed them using the same social proprieties he was working hard to dismantle in his clinic. As the next chapter shows, one public task on which he decided to focus, together with his colleagues at Sheppard-Pratt, was the making of a social and cultural critique that was related to their thinking about homosexuality, but was beginning to take up broader meanings than those immediately implied by "homosexual content." In this process of expansion, Sheppard-Pratt doctors' and patients' approach to 1920s social and cultural transformations and an emerging modernity was a driving force.

2

Illness Within a Hospital
and Without

One day in December 1926, a patient at Sheppard-Pratt described how he thought he had changed since coming to the hospital: "I studied . . . a lot of things I would like to know about myself as far as I'm concerned with other people—my relations to other people."[1] This would have pleased Sheppard-Pratt doctors, if the patient's understanding of his condition were indeed as thorough as his comment implied. As it turned out, his speech quickly became erratic and disturbed, suggesting that his appreciation of his newly found self-awareness had not taken such deep root. Nevertheless, it is important that the patient vocalized the lesson he thought he had learned, because it suggests the presence in the Sheppard-Pratt clinical culture of what doctors considered to be desirable signs of improvement. Patients' acquirement of a self-understanding, and their ability to explain just what this understanding meant to them in a reasonable, intelligent way, weighed much in doctors' assessment of patients' conditions. Patients were encouraged to pursue other goals as well in the course of becoming self-aware. Among these goals were to become "mature" sexually, as well as to become "independent" socially.

These therapeutic goals were deeply tied into the sociocultural changes of the 1920s, changes that doctors and patients together worked to grasp. At Sheppard-Pratt, an array of cultural issues in modern America—transformations in religion; the relaxation of sexual morals; profound changes in the meaning of personal and familial relationships; the influx of different racial, ethnic, and regional identities into urban life; and the changing face of youth—merged with physicians' and patients' aspiration to understand troubled minds and to grasp what seemed an inexplicable world in transition.[2] Sheppard-Pratt clinical records do not indicate that social and cultural changes were the sole cause of mental illness. But these records illuminate that the shifting social current was a crucial part of doctors' and patients' understanding of illness. This encounter between clinical and social concerns occurred in the subjective experiences of those who had serious conflicts with the era's cultural changes, as well as in doctors' attempts to respond to patients' struggles with personalized, and yet scientific, means. The people that the clinical records let us examine in depth were young men who tried to be "on their own"—who attempted to be independent of their families who insisted on traditional norms. Most of them single, these men had life experiences that reflected both familiar stories of growing up and the unique struggle of their generation bound to its time and place.

These men at Sheppard-Pratt illuminate key aspects of the emerging culture of the 1920s. These were people who told of being struck in unique ways by conflicting values that arose from modernity.[3] As youths, they pursued a new freedom in self-expression, while as males, they desired to meet traditional expectations of masculinity. These men, mostly aged between the late teens and the midthirties, aspired to be not only mature and independent, but also likable and lovable as friends, partners, and husbands. But in their own testimony, it was clear that the cultural flux around them made it hard to grasp a standard that satisfied both these aspirations. Because of—not despite—their status as mentally ill, many of these men spoke eloquently of the pain of failing in their hopes and responsibilities. They understood that their words might not be taken seriously—they were aware that they were seen as mentally unstable—and thus they tried even more urgently to make sense of their experiences. In their attempt to help these men, doctors, and strikingly, in many cases patients themselves, defined young men's overwrought concern about sexuality, and their attachment to their families, especially religiously devout ones, as a sign of "immaturity." And this lack of "maturity" was seen as the principal flaw that required medical treatment and social adjustment. Out of this effort emerged "life history" as a method of scientific inquiry and a means to encourage patients to make sense of their conflicting experiences and to become "independent." The doctor-patient exchanges, then, revealed not only ideas about maturity and independence as they relate to the era's changing sexual, gender, and familial relationships, but also innovations in the psychiatric means to capture and define these ideas through the examination of the subjectivity of men suffering from mental illness.

This exploration locates us at a different place from where we were at the end of Chapter 1. To be sure, as with Sullivan's approach to patients who had homosexual conflicts, the doctors in this chapter tried to help patients to come to terms with a "realistic" self-image, rather than attempting to make them fit better into the existing norms. But in a contrast with the relatively open-ended acceptance of homosexuality that was emblematic of Sullivan's "private" practice, the therapeutic objectives of the practice examined in this chapter came with more strings attached. Doctors here were more likely to qualify their practice with values they deemed scientifically and socially accountable. For instance, doctors encouraged patients to accept masturbation as common, normal sexual behavior, and yet "excessive," too frequent masturbation was considered to be a sign of illness. Doctors wanted to accomplish an appropriate degree of modern open-mindedness, but not an unlimited amount of it. Moreover, unlike Sullivan's one-on-one interviews, clinical dialogues between these doctors and their patients were not open to including or scrutinizing physicians' subjectivity. Doctors' effort to forge a useful link between the scientific and subjective was based on an assumed division between medical experts and lay persons. Patients were supposed to bring in raw material, and doctors had the task of turning it into a coherent medical record. Thus, in many cases, the link between patients' subjective experiences and doctors' interpretations was only in the eyes of beholder: doctors. Similarly, physicians' attempt to see a connection between individual and social problems was not always synchronized with patients' view of their struggle with illness.

This objectifying approach, compared with Sullivan's relatively open-ended practice, allowed clinical insights to go beyond the hospital's wall to create a bond between the medical and social sciences in "public." In this process of expansion, the liberal approach to homosexuality—the science of homosexuality taking shape at Sheppard-Pratt generally—was besieged by the developmental model of illness that set the sick, as "immature" individuals, apart from the healthy, "mature" persons. It was not surprising, then, that Sullivan would decide that Sheppard-Pratt was not an ideal place to continue his practice. Although the hospital promoted liberal approaches to a range of sexual experiences, it did not offer a space for a practice that pointed toward a full normalization of homosexuality; it did not accommodate the exploration of physician's subjectivity in medical practice, either. As a result, by the end of the 1920s, there emerged an increasing separation of public and private liberalism in the scientific approach to subjectivity in general, and in the science of homosexuality in particular.

Becoming Mature

The Sheppard-Pratt clinical records are filled with young men's worries. Doctors were concerned about worries that had "homosexual content," but this made it necessary to examine other aspects of patients' life histories as a backdrop of such content. Sullivan, for example, regarded a homosexual experience as crucial because it was related to a larger problem of a sense of lost manhood. Other incidents could generate a feeling of loss, the most notable of which were also matters related to sex: masturbation, premarital sexual relationships, and marriage. Young men at Sheppard-Pratt were concerned about these sexual matters because it seemed to them that one misstep could shatter their self-esteem, hurting their budding sense of being "mature."

How exactly was the lack of self-respect related to the loss of "maturity" in these men's thinking, and what does this suggest about the psychiatric approach to changing sexual and gender relationships in the 1920s? Throughout the decade, clinical records consistently included patients' remembering cautionary tales about masturbation they had heard from their parents and relatives.[4] A patient in his midtwenties recalled that when he was "a little boy [of] about 12, his mother pointed out an idiot who lived near them, and . . . told him [that] he got that way because he had done nasty things. . . . What she meant was masturbation." As the patient remembered it, the impression this remark had made on him was "tremendous."[5] No wonder, then, that another patient confessed, "When I came to 12, I had got the terrible habit of masturbation. Worrying about it caused my nerves to run down, and gave me lack of concentration. I had headaches." Such worry, in this patient's case, began when he read "a description in a scientific book in my father's library . . . about . . . masturbation leading to insanity."[6] In a more extreme case, another patient's mother, when she discovered that the patient had been masturbating, took him to a "genitourinary specialist." The doctor prescribed bromides and recommended a special diet and a special "sitting-up exercise" to be done twice a day. The patient took these recommendations seriously, because he was afraid that "his career for the future" would be at risk if he could not stop masturbating.[7] Yet another patient believed that his habit of masturbation had driven him to an "excessive sex life," and this had made him incapable of having "complete intercourse."[8] In these cases, guilt over masturbation led to a range of physical and psychological problems, which in turn prevented these individuals from becoming healthy, competent, and mature adults. Clearly, masturbation was something that doctors actively looked for, as it was part of their routine inquiry. Physicians believed that masturbation was likely to offer a clue to understanding mental illness, that is, men's fear that they were falling short of an image of mature men.

Some patients had keen insight into their own feelings, suggesting that young men, although wanting to adhere to "proper" sexual norms, were not adverse to change. A patient in his early twenties, for example, insisted that he would "stamp out all the sex" during his one-on-one interview with Sullivan: it was "better to leave the women alone," and he would not masturbate either. When asked by Sullivan what would happen if he could not eliminate his sexual desire, however, the patient did not have an answer. Their discussion continued as follows, showing that the patient was more aware of his unrealistic demand on himself than his apparent rigidity suggests:

SULLIVAN: So where are we? What's the answer in the realm of sex? . . . Can you juggle your conscience? Isn't it too tough to be juggled?

PATIENT: Maybe it is.

SULLIVAN: Isn't that pretty near what happened to you before? . . . Before you came here [to the hospital] the first time?

PATIENT: Well—it has always appeared wrong to me, and maybe that's the reason I have never handled the situation right.

SULLIVAN: And will you be able to get over that appearance of wrong in the future?

PATIENT: I think so. I am not so darned particular whether it is right any more or not.

SULLIVAN: I wonder if that's so?

PATIENT: Well—it is as prominent as it is in most people, I suppose, at my age.

SULLIVAN: No, I think your conscience is a little more rigid than most people's. And if it is—what are you going to do about it?

PATIENT: You have got me in a tight corner.

SULLIVAN: But it's a corner that life is going to present to you.[9]

Clearly, the patient understood that he would have to do something to modify his a-little-too-uptight conscience. The doctor, for his part, by referring to the "appearance of wrong" of sex matters, suggested that sex, including masturbation, should be an accepted part of a person's life. Given the fact that it was the patient's parents who had stressed the harm of masturbation, the doctor and patient can be seen as working together to alter or even eradicate traditional norms that spoiled modern adjustment.

Indeed, Sheppard-Pratt doctors, and Sullivan in particular, had no reservations about making a therapeutic effort along these lines. During a one-on-one interview with Sullivan, for instance, a patient in his late twenties said, "I would like to ask you . . . one question—and that is about—uh—masturbation. . . . I used to do it at home [and I] did a considerable bit of it. . . . I [am] still doing it and I'll continue to do it." The patient's worry was that "it" would annul his sex life altogether. In response, Sullivan said that he would not worry about it, adding that he was more concerned about the patient's wish to "get rid of the whole sexual business . . . out of [his] life . . . forever."[10] Apparently, Sullivan did not want the patient to attempt purging himself of sexuality, along with his habit of masturbation. To yet another patient, Sullivan said straightforwardly, "There comes to my mind a person who has masturbated all his life, as many as nine times a day, and he seems to be a fairly healthy individual," stressing the harmlessness of masturbation.[11]

In particularly interesting cases, doctors urged patients to see masturbation less rigidly by helping them to distance themselves from their religious upbringing. Given the relative decline of organized religion and the rise of scientific authorities as experts in mental problems during the 1920s, it is revealing, if not wholly surprising, that Sheppard-Pratt physicians made careful inquiries about patients' religious background.[12] Indeed, physicians' interest in patients' religious beliefs constituted more than a routine examination; it was a pointed scrutiny of a root cause of illness. Talking to a patient who had been worried that his sexual "sin" had made "the whole earth gone," Sullivan brushed off the religious assumption behind the patient's fear: "My dear chap, why should your sin have anything to do with the earth?"[13] Another patient was hesitant about discussing sex matters with doctors at first, because his father had "cautioned him not to divulge his sex life . . . on the ground that such a confession would . . . entail a permanent loss of his soul." But the patient decided to disregard this warning at one point during his stay at the hospital. After discussing his habit of masturbation with doctors, he told them that he discovered "it cheers him up when he is depressed," most likely reflecting a nonstigmatizing attitude that the doctors encouraged.[14] Yet another patient, who had been raised by "a very rigid Baptist grandfather," came to defend his habit of masturbation by claiming, "No one in my family died from doing it."[15]

These assertions are often fleeting ones in the records; thus it cannot be argued that the teamwork of doctors and patients necessarily produced a relaxation of sexual standards in these individuals. What these records indicate, though, is that Sheppard-Pratt doctors *aimed* to contribute to such a transformation from a religious to a secular approach to sexuality. In some cases, their aspiration seemed to make a difference beyond the clinical setting. One patient's family, for example, complained about his frequent masturbation, telling him that it would kill him if he did not stop. After he was released from the hospital as "unimproved" and still disturbed, the family faced the choice of either keeping him at home or sending him to a state institution. The family decided to keep him home for the time being with the hospital's assistance. Through talks with a social worker affiliated with Sheppard-Pratt, the family tried to learn how to accept the patient's erratic behavior. Their effort yielded some positive results. One report by the social worker indicated that the family began to understand that "it would be better to tolerate his interest in masturbation than to scold him about it or threaten him with bad results." Although not an open-armed acceptance (and only suggested in the social worker's words), this was a change that must have called for tremendous effort from all involved, especially given the family's long-standing affiliation with the evangelical Church of God in a rural area outside Baltimore.[16]

Even patients whose attitude toward sex seemed relatively relaxed and more experienced—those who engaged in both masturbation and premarital sexual relationships, for example—were often plagued by anxiety over religious teachings. Young men pursued sexual opportunities, but then felt that sexual freedom had done damage to their self-esteem. An unmarried man in his early thirties used to enjoy going to a dance club in Baltimore on Saturday nights. Occasionally, he and his friend would have a double date with "girls." When he had a fight with this friend, however, he stopped going out, and soon became "unduly interested in religion, talked of God and heaven." Clearly, he placed sexual freedom and the religious belief that prohibited it in contrast to each other. Both seemed to offer him comfort and confidence of a certain kind, but he could not decide which one of them would be a better place for him to be a man. The so-called loosening sexual standards in the 1920s could cause deep concern among young men, even as they lived by these standards. Even for those who had not been overtly religious, "God's prohibition" could have a considerable impact on their mental well-being.

Another patient's story illuminates both a young man's and woman's conflicted understanding of sexual relationships, within the institution of marriage and without. Both the patient and his wife had sexual experiences before marriage: he had been "in love with a half dozen girls," while she had been "so getting tired of running around on petting parties and the like." To her, "marriage . . . seemed something of an escape from a life that was growing monotonous," while to him, marriage was a ticket to a stable sexual outlet. On their honeymoon, the couple "had intercourse about three times a day." When they returned, "they rarely missed a day without sexual relations." To be sure, this could be seen as just an ordinary expression of passion. But the patient's troubled experience prior to the marriage suggests that for him it was not. When he was dating another woman before marriage, he related, he went to a dance with her and felt "ashamed of (or upset by) the effect the girls had had on his [genitals]." This was so disturbing that he "went to the cellar to the furnace, and tried to burn himself." He could not follow through because "his nerve failed him," but his guilt over any perceptible sexual desire did not go away. It was not entirely out of context, then, that the patient had a breakdown soon after the marriage, feeling that sex was not "anything but a concession to evil" and refraining from any sexual intimacy with his wife.[17]

Such cases suggest that at least some young men in the 1920s, though fully taking part in sexual opportunities that the era had to offer, nonetheless possessed deep anxiety immediately beneath a thin surface. In their actions, these young men seem typical of the sexually "freed" youth of the 1920s. But "freedom" is not the whole story if we look at young men's subjectivity as they engaged in what appeared to be liberating behavior. In some cases, what seemed to be a casual act of pleasure-seeking could ruin mental stability or sexual maturity that marriage was supposed to bring. Moreover, there was no clear social dividing line between those who were sexually open-minded and those who were not. Men who believed that everything sexual was wrong nonetheless went to dance parties and flirted with women. Women who went to a number of petting parties still thought of marriage as a place to settle down. Indeed, the aftermath of this couple's marriage reveals different paths that people could and did take in their exploration of sexuality. In contrast to the husband, who became incapable of sex with women, the wife went on to have a relationship with another man. What urged her to do this was her discovery that her husband's parents had not "lived together as a man and wife for fifteen years" and that this lack of a sex life had led to "a great deal of discord in the family." The wife decided that the patient was "exactly like his father [who was incapable of having sex] and nothing on earth would ever lead her to fall in the footsteps of his mother." She hoped to marry her new boyfriend after divorcing the patient. Clearly, she considered sex a natural and crucial part of marital life, which would have a singular impact on her future and happiness. Sheppard-Pratt doctors seemed to be fine with this, taking note of her statements without any hint of disapproval. The different paths that the couple took illuminate how categories based on behaviors, such as "partygoers" or the "sexually loose," are limited when we seek to understand the era. Those who shared a moment at a petting party might well have come from dissimilar backgrounds, with different expectations. What they took away from the party and what they did with it subsequently varied as well. At Sheppard-Pratt, the division between partygoers and others did not stand out; rather, clinical records highlighted people who moved uneasily on the border they imagined as existing between what was acceptable and what was not. This is the nature of modernity-in-the-making.

Not surprisingly, a person's experience of moving from premarital sexual relationship to sex in marriage was significantly gendered. For some men, the experience was a test of their sexual ability and maturity, while for some women, it illuminated their willingness (or unwillingness) to meet marital responsibilities. One male patient in his late twenties claimed that he had been engaged to a woman, primarily because he had been attracted to her "sex appeal." During their engagement, which lasted one and half years, they became sexually "intimate," embracing each other and "petting around." She masturbated the patient "to the point of . . . having an orgasm," out of which he "got enjoyment." But his pleasure was tentative and short-lived. Soon it began to cause "a very terrific strain" on him, and the "whole business upset [his] nervous system more than anything else." It was even more upsetting to the patient when the engagement was broken. This was not just because of the loss of sexual intimacy; he began to feel that his "sexual ability had been destroyed . . . [as] there seemed to be a rush of something from [his] balls to [his] body." This sensation lasted for a month, at the end of which he had a wet dream and was finally relieved from his worry.[18] Apparently, the failed prospect of marriage was an immediate threat to his sexual confidence, suggesting that even among those who engaged in premarital sexual relationships, marriage was still seen as a single acceptable setting to substantiate and complete men's sexual capability. This belief in the special meaning of marriage was so strong that a postponement of marriage, as well as premarital sexual experiences, could lead a man to feel that his sexual ability and maturity themselves were compromised.[19]

Sheppard-Pratt female patients were concerned about sex and marriage as well, but in different ways from their male counterparts. To be sure, women shared with men the idea that marriage was the only socially accepted setting for sexual relationships. But women at Sheppard-Pratt had particular problems with constraints that accompanied marriage. For instance, a married woman who was "reported as frigid with intercourse" felt that her "duty to her church and her duty to her husband" contradicted each other. This sense of discord was augmented by the fact that she was a "staunch" Catholic, while her husband was a Presbyterian. Because of this difference, she had been deprived of her right to go to confession and take communion. But this difficulty in sexual and religious matters did not lead her to think that she lost her sexual ability and maturity, as it did for a fair number of male patients. Instead, she began to feel that she was "unworthy": she was not good enough for her husband, because "he is so above me" intellectually. Moreover, she was "not domestic" enough and thus could not be a good mother to her child either.

What is striking in her case record is the sharp contrast between her idealized description of her husband's and doctors' response, indicating their disagreement with her self-blame. Taking note of her alleged frigidity, for instance, a doctor commented that she "made no complaint about her husband's excessive sex interest." Also, the same physician noticed that she "hinted at the fact that her husband makes only $25.00 per week . . . when she earned sometimes twice this." If these comments seem to encourage the patient to become more critical of her husband and his demands, others seem to push her to become more aware of herself as a sexual being. After discovering her "frigidity," the couple tried out cunnilingus and this, "with masturbation on the part of her husband," made her achieve an orgasm, a doctor noted approvingly. Also, during an interview with a group of doctors, she was asked if she thought that her "husband was really justified in bringing you here," as if to suggest that she think about her husband's having had a role in her breakdown. Just as they tried to make male patients become more accepting of their sexual desire in general and masturbation in particular, Sheppard-Pratt physicians encouraged female patients to explore more sexual possibilities—including those that might compromise men's demands. Despite the gender bias that excluded some women from in-depth analysis, one message that doctors tried to send to all patients, both men and women, seemed to be this: you should accept wider range of sexual expressions, because such an acceptance was the beginning of getting better.

More important, what "getting better" meant in a clinical setting was tied to what "becoming mature" required in life outside the hospital. Sheppard-Pratt patients' sexual concerns were inseparable from social concerns that accompanied the process of becoming an adult. Contrary to the image of the sexually liberated youth in the 1920s, young men's subjective experiences of masturbation, premarital sex, and marriage were filled with worries about their uncertain consequences. Can I be a successful adult even if I masturbate? Can I achieve a happy marriage even if I have premarital sexual experiences? Men who had homosexual experiences were no exception. Among the questions they asked was, Can I engage in homosexual relationships without being mentally ill? Doctors' responses seemed to be a definite "Yes, but only if you do not worry too much about sex." Because of their understanding that "compromised" sexuality was a threat to men's sense of maturity, doctors felt compelled to help patients relax the definition of "successful" or "full" sexual experience. Medical treatment could not stop there; the cultural flux of the 1920s demanded that doctors and patients discuss how, in real-life situations, young men could maintain their maturity sexually and socially. For example, some men's discussions suggested that their ability to get along with other men was intertwined with their ability when with women to be entertaining and a refined companion. Being a dependable employee (and a breadwinner) was one of their central concerns, because it meant, among other things, that a man had made a place for himself in men's world. If a place among men could not be established, a place for sexual relationships could not be either. Thus for some men at Sheppard-Pratt, when their career failed, their sexual gratification seemed to wane, too. But often, a man's effort to establish a respectable standing for himself was complicated by social changes beyond his control or comprehension—economic instability and job insecurity; a decline in agricultural business, especially in the South, along with the growth in corporate jobs in the North; and the increasing need to be college-educated to be successful. How could men handle these impersonal changes, if they felt them to be immediate challenges to their personal abilities as men, including sexual abilities? In their attempt to respond to the men's concerns, doctors were pushed to see close connections between sexual and social problems, both in their patient's subjective experiences and in the medical understanding of them.

Taking a patient in his midtwenties as an example, we can see the tightly knit connection between sex, marriage, and work as important components of becoming mature. What is striking in this patient's case, however, is more than this close connection between the sexual and social; it is also his unwillingness to live without what he considered to be a proof of his maturity, even when his life seemed to be full of the challenges that the culture of the 1920s entailed. Instead of seeing his life experiences—his encounter with a sweetheart at college, his worries about sex in marriage, his move from a southern town to an increasingly corporate and cosmopolitan northern city, and his struggle to succeed in his career when there was no familial connection to rely on—as something shared by many in his generation, he shouldered them as a purely personal challenge, a test of his maturity. The patient married young, at twenty-one, when he was a senior at a college in Atlanta, Georgia. His wife was nineteen, and the patient's parents opposed the marriage on the ground that he was not self-supporting. To this the patient responded by quitting school to take a job in a real estate firm in Washington, DC. He moved quickly, allowing only three months to pass between his first paycheck and the wedding. According to his wife, in the first few weeks of marriage the patient was "quite elated, and very much gratified to get away from his mother's domination." It is not clear what this "domination" entailed, but the consequence of being released from it surely included sexual freedom: during the first year of marriage he would "indulge in" frequent sexual intercourse.

Gradually, however, the patient's newfound sexual freedom began to erode. At the end of the first year of marriage, he started to lose his passion for intercourse. This, as the patient explained to his wife, was because "his manhood . . . and health might be undermined by sexual excess." Soon, the patient resorted to what doctors called "sublimation" of sex, something that gratified him without threatening his manhood. He became committed to his work more than ever, giving up his evenings and weekends to increase his sales. It seems as if the source of patient's maturity shifted from sexual gratification to career success. Strikingly, the wife made no explicit complaint about her husband's declining interest in sex (though her dissatisfaction might be implied by her telling the doctor), indicating that the couple was united in seeing that his career success was something that outweighed their sex life. But their attempt to reach this goal did not draw sympathy from others. For instance, the patient's business associate said dismissively that the patient had been trying to "keep up with the fast social group who far outstrip him in financial and political standing." Although only one person's observation, this comment shows the difficult situation in which this newcomer to urban life found himself. His independence from his parents, sexual satisfaction, and marriage itself were all at stake in this patient's success in a man's world. This immediate, almost suffocating link between a range of important events in life, without breathing room to put challenges that he was going through (in some cases quite successfully) into social and cultural contexts, seemed central to his struggle to become mature. In his making such an effort, freer sexual expressions, which Sheppard-Pratt doctors promoted as a foundation of mental health, could easily be sacrificed. Indeed, for many patients, it seems, it was the first to be jettisoned. To construct the foundation, then, doctors believed that they must dig into a range of social issues related to it. The examination of life histories was the means to accomplish this task, because these histories seemed to allow doctors to record medical and social interpretations, as well as individual experiences.[20]

Besides the difficulty of pursuing a career in an unfamiliar, often unkind environment, there are numerous other issues addressed by the efforts of Sheppard-Pratt doctors and patients to ensure men's health and maturity. Increasing demand for higher education, which was becoming prevalent in the 1920s, was one of the cultural shifts that complicated young men's struggles to establish a respectable standing in society.[21] One patient, a graduate of a polytechnic high school who wanted to pursue four more years of education at Johns Hopkins University, was a case in point. With his high school degree, he thought he was "sort of stopped and wasn't getting anywhere." He was more than anxious to "have something to show people," so as to "make a front" as a man. Doctors' responses to these expressions of ambition were mixed. On the one hand, the patient's feeling of being "inferior" to others and his desire to "correct it" were recognized by doctors as familiar. One doctor noted sympathetically how the patient thought that "[other] folks [are] all . . . ahead of me," how he wanted to "be alone and go my own way," and how he had been disappointed with being unsuccessful in doing so. On the other hand, doctors agreed that it is "unfortunate for people . . . [to] waste their time pursuing ever-increasing intellectual achievement rather than something . . . well within their . . . ability."[22] In their view, there was only one thing about the patient's desire for higher education that sounded reasonable: the patient asserted that a college education would not cost much more than staying at Sheppard-Pratt. Other than this, doctors seemed dubious about the increasing demand for higher education and the pressure that it imposed upon young men. The physicians' understanding seemed to be that such a social demand could propel some men in the wrong direction, which in turn could lead them to a mental breakdown. This shows how doctors were pushing patients to see themselves in social contexts, so that the latter would not have to take on unnecessary burdens.

In addition to the growing demand for education, economic instability in the 1920s affected young men's shifting grounds of self-respect. A single man in his early thirties, for example, developed an idea of persecution after working for a couple of factories as a strikebreaker. He did not feel particularly good about being a strikebreaker, but he feared unemployment when jobs were scarce. He had been without a job several times before, and he felt that "the neighbors and friends thought he was a failure." Here again, having a job and being successful were merged with a sense of maturity. Soon after the patient began to work for a second factory, however, he began to notice that "the picket workers were watching him at work, at lunch, and that they followed him home, [and] that . . . they said bad things about him." It is hard not to see a good reason for some of the patient's complaints. To be sure, part of his worries about the workers who were "watching him" could have been because of his illness. When he was in the most confused state of mind, he believed that one thousand members of the Ku Klux Klan had been following him. But most of his concerns seem legitimate, given the anxiousness he must have felt as a strikebreaker. Although Sheppard-Pratt doctors understood his complaints as a sign of illness, they also acknowledged the possibility that his worry about the strikers bad-mouthing him was just as ordinary as any worry. Thus doctors did not believe that illness came exclusively from within patients; it also came from without the hospital, where the economic fluctuations of the 1920s were a particular condition that shook young men's sense of being adults. Thus, specifically *when* the most recognizable concern about economy turned into a mental illness remained relatively unclear and certainly unmarked on the clinical records.[23]

Sheppard-Pratt patients' concern about job security was often complicated by the demographic shift that accompanied the growth of northern cities as educational and economical centers.[24] One patient from Richmond, Virginia, was from a well-respected, wealthy family. The patient took a job in an electric power company in Virginia after graduating from college, and his company soon consolidated with a larger one. This brought many new employees to the workplace, and it was then that the patient began to have a range of interpersonal conflicts. In particular, he noted that he did not get along with one man, "a fellow from up North," who came to the South but "did not understand the Southerners." The patient could not pin down just what he did not like about this man, saying vaguely that he "didn't like [this man's] attitude, and . . . his aspect [sic] toward the people he was working with." Although it seemed trivial at first, his frustration with colleagues of different backgrounds than his became intolerable. Soon he left the company, drank heavily, and eventually began to suffer from schizophrenia.

Although not in any way indicating that the regional conflict caused his illness, his record—more specifically, doctors' careful attention to a series of problems beginning with his frustration with his northern colleagues— shows how doctors considered such conflict an important reason for his illness.[25] For another patient, too, the regional differences were no small matter. A native of Mississippi, he objected to being placed in a ward at Sheppard-Pratt where the majority of patients were "Northerners." He felt that they were "not in sympathy with him," an unusually strong expression for someone whom doctors consistently described as "manneristic," "inaccessible," and "mute" throughout the preceding three months.[26] Indeed, this was the first and only complaint the patient made throughout his stay at the hospital, as far as his clinical record indicates. All in all, in both these patients, their general unhappiness was expressed as their dislike of northern style. Such regional friction was not uncommon in the 1920s as the southern agricultural economy declined and children of plantation owners moved to industrial and corporate positions. This transformation was, at least for some patients, disturbing enough to become a central part of their experience of mental illness. And doctors carefully took note of them, illustrating that a keen eye for the encounter between larger histories of social transformation and personal stories of illness was, indeed, essential to medicine in a border state.

In some cases, differences in patients' backgrounds informed conflicts that went beyond national boundaries. There were a considerable number of immigrants and their children in the Sheppard-Pratt patient population. One such patient, a twenty-year-old Russian man who had immigrated to the United States with his family at the age of eleven, illuminates what was a common experience for many who were new to the country in the 1920s.[27] As his personal history suggests, as a young child he did not have many friends: "The writer gets the impression that play activities were not deemed very essential to the welfare of a Russian child. . . . [As a result, the patient] did not adapt himself to extro-familio socialization," one doctor noted. When he came to the United States and settled down in Massachusetts, he could not speak English, causing him a "great difficulty getting on [at a school] for a short time." Although he quickly mastered the language and made impressive academic progress, he continued to fear that he might not be able to live up to "his pride and his ambition." Thus, when he took his first part-time summer job as a park keeper in Maine, he quickly became homesick, causing a "great jolt" to his self-esteem. To make things worse, he got a grade of C for his mathematics class at college during the semester he came back from the summer work. He felt deeply embarrassed about this, especially because he had copied some lines in a math examination from his classmate's paper. His reaction to his dishonesty was extreme. He felt that he was "immoral" and was afraid that "he would be deported from this country" because of the "sin" he had committed. For his doctors, it is unmistakable that his foreignness and the anxiety that arose from it were something that called for the most careful medical attention (although doctors did not seem to be aware of a cultural distance that might have contributed to his initial nervousness in speaking with American physicians).[28]

The increasing pressure from higher education, economic instability, and the growing presence of regional and cultural differences in cities, then, were problems that frequently came up in Sheppard-Pratt patients' life histories as important components of the process of obtaining and sustaining men's maturity. What is striking about these stories, however, is not simply their relevance to the cultural changes that have been associated with the 1920s. It is also what doctors understood to be patients' strong desire not to acknowledge these socioeconomic factors as their personal and interpersonal challenges, even as physicians encouraged patients to see these factors as relevant to their illness. For instance, the patient who wanted to go to Johns Hopkins, despite doctors' less than approving attitude, decided to hold on to his plan of getting a bachelor's degree. He did not believe that this desire itself might cause him stress. Likewise, the man who was a strikebreaker did not consider the possible link between his desperate need to stay on the job and his delusion of being persecuted. If anything, he was eager to deny such a connection, claiming that the job "was very satisfactory, and he was very much interested in it." When asked if he had been happy at Sheppard-Pratt, the patient's response was "If I could get back to work I would be." Also, the patient who had had a problem with his northern co-workers insisted, when asked by a doctor what he thought of his colleagues' unflattering remarks, that he did "not pay any attention to it." His colleagues "don't interest me at all," he asserted. Only when pushed by a doctor did he reveal his reasons for pretending not to worry about what people said about him: "What I do not know doesn't hurt me." These comments, which suggested patients' reluctance to acknowledge the connection between personal and social problems, frequently raised a flag in physicians' case analyses. In staff conferences, doctors discussed these statements as a sign of a lack of patients' self-awareness, something that stood out as a serious "problem" in their life histories.

Most likely, what doctors recognized in clinical records was different from what patients saw in their own life histories. Although it is not easy to see patients' subjectivity fully in clinical records, one can speculate that when a patient said that he wanted to go back to work, there was some self-awareness in his statement. It is a striking assertion, given the fact that he believed that he had been disliked and accused by factory workers. No matter how irritating the experience might have been, however, the job was still his in the midst of economic crisis. At least, it is possible that he was not simply being secretive or evasive, as doctors concluded. But it was not up to the patient to decide what he felt. In the view of doctors, the patient did not want to admit that a problem existed in his relationship with others, because to do so was damaging to his self-esteem. In this way, doctors believed, patients' desire to appear mature came in direct conflict with difficulties that the era's changing living and working conditions brought about. What all this suggests is that, in response to the sociocultural changes of the 1920s, medicine created a practice in which the most serious problem was young men's attempt to defend their budding identities as adults by an appearance of personal and interpersonal equilibrium. In this new practice, patients who refused to admit that their lives were affected by something much larger than themselves—something that went beyond their control—stood out as ill and in need of treatment. Thus, an awareness of a person in changing social contexts—a modern self-awareness—became a requirement for health at Sheppard-Pratt.

Becoming Independent

Just as much as Sheppard-Pratt patients held on to the belief that their world had not been shaken, their doctors worked hard to counter such a belief. For one, as we have seen, doctors were more than willing to tell their patients that the world in which masturbation and premarital sex constituted a sin against God was ending. It was a consensus at Sheppard-Pratt that almost any religious teaching prohibited sexual expression, imposing needless conflicts upon patients' mental well-being. Moreover, doctors were not shy about recommending that patients leave their religiously devoted parents behind. When they talked to young male patients, especially those whose parents were committed members of a church, doctors eagerly suggested plans to go away from home, find a job, and make a living on their own. Putting an old world behind and making a new life of one's choice were a virtue. But there was one condition that doctors demanded to see in patients before letting them pursue independence: they wanted to see that patients become insightful about changes that had been taking place in their lives. In addition, they wanted to confirm that patients become self-aware of their responses to these changes. Thus, to be independent, men were required to be open-minded and intelligent about themselves. There was one thing in particular that patients could do to prove that they had these qualities: tell a coherent life history that made sense to both a teller and listeners.

Given most doctors' interest in psychoanalysis, it is hardly surprising that verbal communication weighed heavily at Sheppard-Pratt. The hospital used other therapeutic approaches besides interviews, such as occupational therapies and recreational activities, and yet these did not count as much as patients' ability and willingness to communicate. Some patients showed notable progress in occupational classes and were reported to become more cooperative with other patients and attendants. But these improvements were not good enough to warrant further treatment at Sheppard-Pratt. Often the doctors' comments were explicit about this heavy reliance on interviews when they made crucial decisions such as approving a discharge from the hospital. For instance, one doctor said at the time of a patient's release from the hospital: "[The patient] will not, or cannot, delve deeply enough into his unconscious processes to make him a valuable case for research work."[29] This suggests that a poor prognosis, not an improvement, was a reason behind the release. Another doctor noted a patient's condition at his discharge disappointedly: "[Although] he was in excellent physical condition . . . [he] had very little, if any, insight into his mental disorders."[30] Again, although the patient was released from the hospital, his condition was not deemed optimal.

While these statements point to the fact that patients' self-understanding mattered in Sheppard-Pratt clinical judgment, others indicate that patients' willingness to explore their conditions jointly with doctors was as signifi-cant. Of a male patient who had "scant interest in anything psychoanalyti-cal" and was "scornful . . . of anything to be gained by personal analysis," doctors concluded, "The issue is not solved nor will it be solved without . . . intelligent co-operation on his part."[31] This assertion was notable, particu-larly because the patient was an academic (an anthropologist) and a writer who seemed to refuse to discuss his problems not because of his lack of abil-ity, but because of his dislike of self-analysis under doctors' guidance. This was also true of a college-educated female patient, who believed that she had been sent to the hospital by mistake and whose attitude seemed hostile. Even during an admission procedure, her responses to a doctor's questions were uncooperative, at least from the doctor's viewpoint:

DOCTOR: Do you know where you are?
PATIENT: Do you? (Pause)
> Patient suddenly smiled and in a relenting voice said, "I will answer for you Dr. Martin," and then in a loud tone of voice said, "I am at the Shep-pard and Enoch Pratt Hospital, Towson, Maryland."
DOCTOR: Why are you here?
PATIENT: (Again sullen) Ask Dr. Bird—a physician. (Sarcasm)

What is impressive here is not only the patient's anger with the doctor's questions, which she apparently considered demeaning; it is also notable that the typist took careful notes of the patient's attitude. Not only the words she spoke, but also the ways in which she uttered them, were watched and recorded. Her refusal to engage in a conversation with a doctor quickly made her an "undesirable" patient. Within three weeks after her admission, doctors held a staff conference concerning her, during which they decided that she had "no insight into the comparatively simple things that made [her] sick." Moreover, they concluded that they did not believe "she is at all sincere in her effort to get insight." In line with psychoanalysis's reliance on spoken words, then, Sheppard-Pratt clinical practice could not pursue treatment without patients' willingness to talk. The doctors wanted and needed patients who could respond well to what they considered to be an innovative method of psychoanalysis. Meanwhile, they were not hesitant to "get rid of" those who were unwilling to talk.[32] Sincerity—in this context, willingness to cooperate with doctors in a way doctors wanted—mattered.

Such a pointed attention to verbal communication suited some patients well, while it alienated others. For instance, most patients selected for one-on-one interviews with Sullivan were "suitable" patients in the sense that they had self-perceptions and were willing to communicate them. When talking to them during staff conferences—both before and after a selection was made for a special interview—Sullivan and the present team of doctors seemed generally sympathetic and understanding. Sullivan's attitude when he talked to his selected patients during one-on-one interviews was even more compassionate. Occasionally, he referred to patients by name, instead of official-sounding references such as "you" or "the patient."[33] A typical entry in these patients' files was "[The patient] has been quite uniformly co-operative. . . . [His] attention has been excellent, manner has been agreeable."[34] Or Sullivan found such a patient to be "intellectual," as if to suggest that spoken words fully represented a patient's intelligence.[35] One aspect of a record of a special interview in 1927, discussed in Chapter I, also reveals how Sullivan participated in clinical sessions with an unmistakably sympathetic attitude. When the patient told Sullivan that he would like to see all of the doctor's face to facilitate their talk, Sullivan turned to the patient as requested, asking if the patient wanted him to keep his eyes open. This was a voluntary offer, not something the patient asked for. This indicates Sullivan's openness to his selected patients, which he seldom revealed to others. In fact, the tone of his speech during conferences with nonselected patients differed much from that with the selected. The latter included accommodating expressions such as "would you mind telling me . . . ," "explain . . . if you will," and " . . . please," while the latter included little, if any, of them.[36]

Apparently, clinical experiences with cooperative patients were what Sullivan deemed the most desirable, as he incorporated them seamlessly into the published accounts of his practice. In a 1927 article, for example, he emphasized the importance of encouraging patients to talk without being intrusive:

The ideal interview is one in which the physician offers only the orienting questions . . . [about] topics on which he desires the patient to talk, and such provocative interjections as "And—," "And then," "Continue," "Which seems to mean what," and the like. With comparatively inaccessible schizophrenics it is often possible to obtain two or three thousand words in an hour without supplying the patient with anything of "explanation" or "interpretation."[37]

This description projects an image of a doctor as a willing listener, while it also highlights, when compared to his clinical records, what Sullivan did not choose to publish. Sullivan in many clinical records did not resemble the physician described in his own passages. Far from being accommodating to patients, he told a female patient that he "must interrupt you because you neglected to give me the answer to my question."[38] To another woman who complained about "the cold suavity of Dr. Sullivan"[39] and refused to explain her problems, he responded: "Then we will have to decide that you are so sick."[40] Typically, he described these patients as "evasive."[41] In the end, it was his belief that "if a person can't talk about what is going on in his mind, it is rather difficult for a physician to be very much good to him."[42] Thus, it was not only that patients who were not willing talkers tended to be discharged with poor prognoses. Even in the process of treatment itself, Sheppard-Pratt doctors could not effectively deal with those who did not take what doctors believed was the first step of therapy—to talk about their problems with candor.

Some patients found this requirement disturbing as well as limited. One male patient, for example, mentioned his drinking habit during an interview with Sullivan. Then an apparently futile discussion followed:

SULLIVAN: Why did you first take a drink?
PATIENT: . . . I was curious . . . I don't see why it is especially wrong.
SULLIVAN: Don't you? Then why bring that up?
PATIENT: Well, I have got to talk—I have got to say something.

Here, Sullivan suspected that patient was feeling bad about drinking but was not willing to discuss it. Meanwhile, the patient insisted that the topic came up only because he was pressed to say something. This discrepancy became wider as the interview progressed:

SULLIVAN: I haven't heard a thing yet that might give me light as to what ails you. I believe that you have spent about one hundred or five hundred words in mere talking, and you haven't told me anything yet.
PATIENT: I am not trying to conceal anything . . .
SULLIVAN: Well, then, talk, talk, talk about your illness . . .
PATIENTS: . . . you don't give a person a chance to answer a question—you always stop me just when I get started.[43]

Ironically, Sullivan's eagerness made him impatient, suffocating the patient's very words that he was looking for. Moreover, this exchange suggests that the quality, not just the quantity, of patients' self-examination was assessed carefully. Although this is not at all surprising or unreasonable in a therapeutic session, it is also true that doctors looked for a certain set of issues that interested them, not necessarily what patients were interested in discussing. What doctors demanded was a coherent story of illness and, better yet, a life history that illuminates a range of a person's experiences and brings them together in a narrative that makes both subjective (for patients) and scientific (for doctors) sense.

When patients lacked either ability or willingness to unite subjective experiences and scientific interpretations in their life histories, doctors were quick to decide that it was a sign of illness. The case of the Catholic woman considered earlier—the woman whose timid attitude to her husband Sheppard-Pratt doctors tried to eradicate—shows how the discordance between a patient's narrative and doctors' expectations was a serious obstacle in treatment. Assuming that the patient's illness originated in her marital frustration, doctors at the conference at first tried to make her realize that. But then a tension between medical interpretation and the patient's self-perception arose:

SULLIVAN: You have no reason for being here. . . . Are you getting even with anyone?

PATIENT: No—why should I want that?

SULLIVAN: Because you are human.

PATIENT: Why certainly not. . . .

SULLIVAN: This is a typical example of a person who has been taught to adjust to life by talking. Doesn't matter what she says—as long as she can make an impression.[44]

The doctor quickly shifted from a nonjudgmental to an overtly critical attitude. In the end, the patient's talk did not carry any importance, because she was not getting what doctors wanted her to understand: that she was punishing her husband by being mentally sick. The doctors who were present at the conference were, on the one hand, willing to assist her to become aware of what they considered to be unfairness in her marital relationship. On the other hand, they were also quick to dismiss her when she seemed incapable of seeing the unfairness so apparent to them. Sheppard-Pratt doctors' openness to fairer relationship between men and women could turn around and go against the very people they tried to help. This seemed to be the case especially when patients' discussions of their problems did not seem willing and insightful enough to physicians.

In a not dissimilar way, Sheppard-Pratt doctors' acceptance of masturbation was limited. While they tried to reduce patients' guilt about "self-abuse," clinical observations often included a critical note on a patient's habit of masturbation. To be sure, Sullivan asserted that a person could masturbate "nine times a day" but nonetheless be perfectly healthy. And yet at the same time, Sheppard-Pratt doctors, including Sullivan, took note of patients with an "excessive" masturbatory habit. It was usually listed with other behaviors that were apparently deemed pathological. In one clinical observation, a doctor noted, "[The patient] spent much of [the] time chewing his neckties, was seclusive [sic] in the day-time, indifferent to occupational therapy, and it is noted that he frequently masturbated."[45] In another case, a patient's masturbation was reported to worry his family "to such an extent that they were afraid that he might do harm to himself." The family took him to Sheppard-Pratt, and the hospital admitted the patient without a single comment about the stigma associated with masturbation manifest in the family's explanation.[46] The irony, of course, was that such a stigma was what doctors tried to eradicate in interviews with patients. While doctors' support for fairer gender relationships and freer sexual expressions made frequent appearances in clinical practice, their support for these ideals was not an open-ended acceptance in all settings. This sets the general clinical practice at Sheppard-Pratt apart from the private approach to homosexuality that Sullivan and his patients were shaping. Going against the prevailing homophobia, Sullivan's and his patients' discussions pointed toward a full normalization of homosexuality. Although their meetings did not generate public discussion of homosexuality, they contained explicit critique of, if not an overall reform of, the "existing social system." This feature was not shared by Sheppard-Pratt clinical practice in general.

Nonetheless, it is notable that certain aspects of Sheppard-Pratt clinical insights became closely connected to the sociocultural transition of the 1920s. In doctors' view, it was not healthy if a person pretended that nothing was wrong in the face of significant changes in social circumstances. A healthier attitude would be to accept the fact that the changes occurred and to do one's best to adjust. The adjustment would require a thorough reeducation thorough self-exploration, the kind that doctors hoped happened with schizophrenic patients, but that was also deemed to be desirable for all patients. If patients understood their personalities fully, it would not only help them recover from their current illness but also help warrant their mental health in the future when something unfamiliar and upsetting happened to them. In this way, self-awareness, self-examination, and patients' ability to vocalize them in a coherent life history would be a reliable means of prevention as well as treatment. Such reasoning was at the core of psychiatric practices in the 1920s, practices that doctors considered a clinical solution to social problems.

It is no wonder, then, that Sheppard-Pratt doctors were unwilling to send patients back to the outside world when the latter's self-awareness seemed either limited or nonexistent. This was a decision that helped some patients, but frustrated others who felt that doctors were not listening their side of their life history. But when patients seemed to make good progress in this regard, doctors would grant either a parole or a discharge, even when mild symptoms still existed. Significantly, Sheppard-Pratt doctors called this status "social recovery," suggesting that patients' ability to be aware and in control of their illness in day-to-day living mattered more than a complete disappearance of symptoms.[47] Once patients began to demonstrate signs of social recovery, doctors encouraged them to make specific plans for life outside the hospital walls. One thing that doctors tried to make sure in making these plans was that patients did not go home—the home from which they had come. Understandably, such a push for separation from a family was particularly strong when there appeared to be an unusual attachment between a patient and his parent(s). For instance, a male patient who was sexually assaulted by his father had the following conversation with Sullivan:

SULLIVAN: Supposing that you can't go home—in other words, you have got to
    stay somewhere besides home—that you have got to do something most
    of the time besides cutting up—what would you think of suggesting?
PATIENT: I don't know. Going home is all I want to do.
SULLIVAN: . . . What can you think of next?
PATIENT: No place I can think of besides home. . . . I don't see why I can't
    go home.
SULLIVAN: Well, it's a peculiar characteristic of the world that if one gets
    along badly enough in a place it's impossible for him to stay in that
    place. . . . Don't you ever suppose you could earn a living working for
    someone else?
PATIENT: I don't know. I would rather work for him [my father] than some-
    body else.
SULLIVAN: I am glad you are so fond of your working for your father, but you
    didn't get on too well at home.[48]

Rather than seeing the patient's habit of self-mutilation as a reason to keep him hospitalized, Sullivan urged the patient to find a place other than home where such a habit would not be necessary. The patient resisted, which is not surprising, given his age (he was in his midteens). The patient's hope was that "things have changed now." The doctor nonetheless refused to back off, insisting that the patient keep as much distance from his family as possible. Indeed, Sullivan did not want the patient's mother coming to see him frequently at the hospital either, calling it an "incest situation concerning the mother." No doubt Sullivan considered an immediate separation from the parents to be imperative. To achieve this goal, the doctor even took the patient to a public lecture on psychoanalysis (titled "The Genital Theory"), given by the analyst Sandor Ferenczi. Clearly, Sullivan's intension was to help the patient develop a better insight into his troubled relationship with the parents. Soon after this, Sullivan made a series of important comments about the patient's future plans during a staff conference:

> I recommend that he be paroled from the Hospital . . . as follows: that he is leaving the institution within the next few days to go to work on a farm which I am arranging until . . . he is called to take a position as a deck boy on a liner of the U.S. Shipping Board. . . . I want to see what goes on in a period when he is entirely on his own and wholly out of the influences . . . to which he has been subjected for years. His relations with me are colored by . . . transference and I would like to see his reaction to a third party. His work with me has been very gratifying.[49]

What stand out in this comment are the careful arrangements for a series of jobs that the doctor himself made for the patient. Literally, "social recovery" had to include the basic elements of a person's social well-being. Moreover, the comment on the "gratifying" nature of the doctor-patient relationship illuminates the doctor's more-than-usual involvement in the patient's case. It seems clear that the doctor decided to take this patient under his wing and that the former would see the latter's journey to the end. Such devotion ensured the doctor's decision-making authority, as he negotiated the discharge plan with the patient's parents. For instance, the patient's father insisted that he "didn't see why [the patient] couldn't go home" when he visited his son at the hospital. The patient and his mother wished to see each other every day. But the doctor pushed them back by highlighting an apparent contradiction in the father's behavior: he had an overt homosexual interest in his son, while he scrupulously monitored the son's church attendance and insisted that the youngster becomes a minister. What this suggests are different meanings that could be given to the patient's relationships: on the one hand, it exemplified a reasonable therapeutic approach to the seriously troubled family relationship. On the other hand, it was a story of medical professionals taking over a youth's education from the hands of a religious family, hoping to create a thoroughly renovated, modern lifestyle founded on self-awareness and autonomy. These meanings coexisted in tension, but without nullifying each other. Perhaps the patient and his parents themselves grappled with these meanings when they insisted on staying together as a family in the face of a history of abuse and mistreatment.

Some patients were not unaware of such a transition in power. In a strikingly perceptive memo he wrote to his doctors (some patients were asked to write their thoughts on their illness, which were kept in clinical files along with the standard eight portions), a man in his midtwenties revealed his view of the issue with much irony:

> "A Digging-up of My Mind-Soil for the Inspection of Drs. Corson and Sullivan." . . . In the old days, it was the Catholic priests that held the inquisition and applied the treatment and endeavored their utmost to save the soul; now "scientists" take the place of priests, theirs is the power and responsibility to make the mind of man normal, and harmless, and understandable and "usual." Being young, and helpless, and much impressed, I bow before this power and responsibility. My own ideas and morals are much too vague, indefinite, and ill-formed to stand before the weight of such accumulated authority. . . . You shall tell me which are "right" and which are "wrong." I might try to divide my morals in some such way as to religion, work, home, family, race, wife, etc., but they are so interrelated that a division would be impossible. I shall take them as they come to me.[50]

The patient was aware not only of the rise of the psychiatric profession as the authority on mental illness, but also of his own confusion about changing standards in a range of domains in his life. In particular, he was troubled by competing ideas about right and wrong in his religious belief and his marital relationship. Talking about the marriage oath, for instance, the patient claimed that he did not "believe in [it] . . . except that it says that a woman should obey a man—that is in the Bible too. It is an old fashioned idea—but I still hold to it." He did not know what to do with this conflict between his belief in Bible and his awareness that his belief was old-fashioned, except to resort to medical advice. But even that was not entirely satisfactory. Staying with his ironic tone, the patient questioned doctors' desire to "treat" him: "I didn't know how you wished me to be . . . normal. . . . I have no wish to be normal." He believed that he was not normal, but he resisted the idea of becoming normal. Sullivan's response was "I never offered to provide you with any standards of behavior—as a matter of fact I am very much more interested in unsocial behavior than social. But I would like you to have some coherence, to be able to get somewhere." This urged the patient to resort to normalcy, not to approve or even agree with it. A story that Sullivan was asking the patient to tell, then, was a kind of middle ground between the social and the individual, science's coherence and subjectivity's diversity. What Sheppard-Pratt doctors sought from patients was a life history that absorbed rich, fluid, and fragmentary experiences and translated them into a relatively simple, stable, and practical foundation for life outside the hospital.

Only after they confirmed such a facilitating life history in patients were Sheppard-Pratt doctors able to begin to make plans for patients' independent life after discharge. The doctor encouraged patients to consider leaving their families whenever possible, especially if their families were religiously devout. This was certainly the case with the patient who wrote "A Digging-up of My Mind-Soil." First, Sullivan suggested that the patient dissolve "the marriage and . . . live in such intimate relations with your wife," so that they could nurture sexual intimacy without constraints of the law. Although this plan did not materialize, the patient and his wife indeed decided to get a divorce. Second, a contact was made with a doctor in Washington, DC, Lucile Dooley, who agreed to take up the patient for extended psychoanalysis. Third, the patient would begin studying medicine, as the subject interested him and he might want to "use it some time in the future" as a means of supporting himself. During the last conference with the patient before discharge, doctors agreed that the patient was far from being well but "very intelligent and could probably get through medicine." Here again, what doctors deemed the patient's intellectual sophistication weighted much in their assessment of the patient's future. The patient's insights into his illness and medicine created optimism among doctors, despite his own claim that he was not "normal." Such optimism drove doctors to push a series of plans to help the patient to leave the dysfunctional family (through divorce), continue to develop self-awareness (thorough psychoanalysis), and acquire means of self-support (though medical education).

Sheppard-Pratt doctors tried to come up with plans for less intellectually inclined patients as well, as long as patients showed sufficient signs of self-awareness. Indeed, as was expressed in their doubt about the merit of higher education for all, doctors generally preferred plans after a discharge that did not include strenuous schooling. A clinical record of a male patient in his late twenties shows the hospital's approach to patients who were not interested in pursuing higher education but had skills and experiences that could be used for self-support. As such, his case suggests how doctors attempted to arrange occupational positions for as broad a range of patients as possible—not only people with serious problems with their families and those who were clearly educated and insightful, but also men who seemed to be more inclined to pick up manual jobs—so as to help them achieve independence. Since he was two years old, the patient had been living with his aunts, who had taken over his and his sister's care when their mother died young. As both the patient and his sister agreed, the aunts were religiously devout and highly successful in making him be afraid of his own sexual desires. Even his romantic relationship seemed to have been influenced by his aunts. His first engagement was broken because "he felt that his responsibilities at home would prevent him marrying. . . . He felt morally obliged to aid in the support of his aunts." Not surprisingly, Sheppard-Pratt doctors' therapeutic focus was on releasing the patient from these religious, sexual, and familial constraints.[51]

The patient's concern about his obligations proved difficult to overcome. Even as he tried to focus on occupational classes, he was preoccupied with how he would meet all his financial responsibilities:

PATIENT: [I am worried about] how I was going to get on my own feet after I got through here. I was going to pay the Hospital if I owned them anything over and above what I have been paying and how I was going to get straightened out afterwards.

DOCTOR: I have never known anybody being buried by Hospital bills. I doubt if you would be.

PATIENT: Those things always did worry me because I always did pay my bills promptly and always managed to get by some way or another. The fact is, before I came over here I was entirely out of debt.[52]

Similar to others at Sheppard-Pratt, this patient's sense of maturity and independence relied on his ability to stay on top of his bills. Although he gradually came to see this attitude as too demanding for himself, he was still so overwhelmed by the financial uncertainly that he was driven to self-mutilation. A month and half after his admission, he was reported to have "lacerated the right side of his neck with a piece of glass . . . [because] he had the idea that he was no good in this world; and only an added expense to his family." The longer he lived, the more hospital expenses he would have to pay.

Perhaps to lessen such a pressing burden, doctors allowed him to "assist with the work on the ward" once his mental status began to stabilize. It is likely that his work was meant to help him pay what he owed to the hospital. The similar arrangement was made for others with limited financial resources. This began to change the patient's condition. Soon, the patient "decided that it is impossible for him to resume life with his aunts—and that he is going to Philadelphia and to go to work there when he leaves [the hospital]." In his own account, the patient wanted to get away from Baltimore "because Baltimore has some rather sad memories for me and I would be better off—for me and my family if I were away from it." His father and his friends in Philadelphia promised to help him find a position, an arrangement that the patient appreciated. He was appreciative of Sheppard-Pratt doctors as well. His last word at the conference before discharge was "I wanted to say 'thank you very much.' You have been very nice to me since I have been here, especially Doctor Sullivan and Doctor Corson and others I talked to." Doctors were happy about the outcome, too. In the last one-on-one interview with the patient, Sullivan confirmed his hopeful thoughts about the outcome of the hospital's treatment: "You were in an emergency pitch—you felt as a man you were a total failure. I think you have done exceedingly well, Mr. ***." No doubt, the doctor's satisfaction here came not only from the patient's successful separation from his religiously and sexually prohibiting aunts but also from the plan that would most likely, in doctors' eyes, ensure his independence. Moreover, he seemed to develop an ability to be self-reflective. Thus this was a definite success story, one that fitted right into the hospital's therapeutic scheme.

A mutually happy end like this occurred only rarely at Sheppard-Pratt. Sometimes postdischarge arrangements were less specific, while other times patients' self-awareness was not deemed to be as thorough as it should be. Even when doctors categorized patients as "recovered," the former would still wonder about just how deeply that awareness might go. One doctor, for instance, noted his concern about a patient in psychoanalytic terms: the patient "had a considerable degree of insight regarding his illness, which is superficial however, and does not penetrate very deeply into his uncon-science [sic]."[53] Thus when a relatively clear-cut success that seemed to confirm both maturity and independence occurred, it was greatly appreciated as such by Sheppard-Pratt doctors. At the height of his professional satisfaction, Sullivan revealed that not only illness but also recovery was woven with patients' identity "as a man." Such reference stood out particularly because of the lack of the comparable gendered references in doctors' discussion of and with female patients. To be sure, sexual maturity, self-awareness, and willingness to share these qualities with doctors were important factors to measure patients' improvement, men and women alike. But with women, these qualities were not discussed as a means to restore "womanliness." This set women apart from their male counterparts, for whom the reconstruction of "manliness" was an outspoken priority.

In the Sheppard-Pratt clinical culture, then, manliness, not womanliness, became a distinctive ideal that must be therapeutically examined and repaired. The completion of the repair work was confirmed in coherent life histories that connected patients to normal life in society. Regardless of a range of skills and intellectual inclinations that male patients possessed, doctors were constantly searching for ways to relate men's qualities to social independence. In sharp contrast, womanliness—if there was such a thing at all in Sheppard-Pratt clinical practice—was something that doctors considered much more ambiguous and harder to conceptualize in patients' life histories. Compared with the numbers of men who were expected to pursue educational or occupational goals, for instance, a strikingly small number of women left the hospital with a specific arrangement for comparable opportunities outside the home. Sheppard-Pratt physicians encouraged female patients to be open to a range of sexual expressions, because it was part of the process of getting better. But unlike their male counterparts, female patients did not receive advice on how they might translate mental health into social independence. Women's life course did not offer a distinct arena in which their sexual maturity, self-reflection, and financial independence would carry socially desirable meanings.

The unique prescription of health, maturity, and independence, though distinctively gendered, places Sheppard-Pratt at an important place not only in the history of medicine but also in the larger cultural transformation of the 1920s. It captures a moment when the connection between medical and social problems became a central concern in clinical practice. At the same time as they offered medical treatment, doctors proposed different attitudes and a different life course that would allow young men, and to a limited degree young women as well, to negotiate old and new expectations. In an ideal scenario, men would achieve not only socioeconomic independence, but also a relaxed, open-minded, and even carefree attitude toward sex. Moreover, men would be reasonably insightful about and pleased by these achievements. In this emerging definition of modern masculinity, men who maintained close ties with their parents, were concerned about religious standards regarding sex, and were not aware of these social constraints were no longer well or mature citizens.

Sullivan's Departure from Sheppard-Pratt

The Sheppard-Pratt clinical records show how Sullivan was part of a team of doctors while at the same time forging intimate relationships with selected patients of his who had homosexual conflicts. Sullivan kept the latter apart from the former, trying to protect the critical approach to homosexuality from outside scrutiny. Certain aspects of his clinical approach—his critique of the religious stigmatization of sex and of the definition of homosexuality itself as an illness—were largely accepted among the medical staff, but other aspects of his practice could not be easily shared by his colleagues. Soon after he introduced a new method of therapy, perhaps as early as 1928, that involved physical contact between male attendants and male patients, it began to draw a critical attention from hospital staff. First, it was a rumor that the doctor was encouraging physical intimacy between patients and attendants who had been trained to be open to homosexuality. Then it became something more than that. Bernard Robbins, a psychiatrist at the hospital, recalled, "Actual homosexual activity between the attendants and the patients was not encouraged. On the contrary, when it did occur on accident, it was regarded as an exploitive situation . . . and the attendant was dealt with by rather forthright dismissal."[54] Despite Robbins's emphasis on the hospital's strict rule against homosexual relationships on its premises and Sullivan's attempt to be in compliance with the regulation, what also stands out in Robbins's comment is an indication that such contacts had actually happened. Perhaps on a limited number of occasions, the touching, holding, and kissing that Sullivan had encouraged developed into sexual relationships. Amid the mounting suspicion, Sullivan decided to leave Sheppard-Pratt. This highlighted the contrast between a certain kind of clinical insight that became part of public science and a set of ideas and practices that remained private.

Given the disapproving rumors about Sullivan and his patients, it seems reasonable to assume that same-sex sexual intimacy between medical professionals and patients was irregular. However, Sheppard-Pratt clinical records suggest a range of homosexual contacts that occurred at the hospital, helping us to understand these contacts in the hospital's clinical setting more generally. One of Sullivan's selected patients, with whom he had numerous one-on-one interviews in 1930, made a sexual gesture toward Sullivan, according to the doctor's note: "I went into the [patient's] room; he was lying quietly in bed covered up . . . suddenly flung back the covers completely exposing himself and showing me that he had nothing in the way of clothing on him, invited me to engage in sexual behavior with him. He then suddenly swung around, suddenly on his buttocks and flung his thighs around my neck."[55] The record of another patient, who was not in Sullivan's ward, also suggests that some patients made sexual gestures more openly at Sheppard-Pratt. According to a doctor's note, the patient had a disturbing habit of "grab[bing] for people's genitals around here [at Sheppard-Pratt] now and then."[56] These incidents were not confined to Sheppard-Pratt. One patient related that in another hospital where he had lately stayed, "he allowed . . . an attendant to do fellation [sic] upon him, and at this hospital there was a flurry of sex excitement on exerting force upon another patient, holding him on the bed, and again lying on a couch with a patient who stimulated him."[57] Yet another patient expressed his suspicion that, when he had been at Phipps Clinic before coming to Sheppard-Pratt, one of his fellow inpatients there "practically invited [me] to be homosexual."[58]

Although none of these cases indicates an actual homosexual relationship at Sheppard-Pratt, they show how homosexual tension, desire, and gestures were not an unusual part of life at the hospital. Sheppard-Pratt was a gender-segregated institution, where, not unlike the army, prisons, and reformatory facilities, men and women were kept in single-sex groups for a long period of time. Records of same-sex relationships in these institutions were not uncommon, particularly because of the heightened attention to these "problems" on the part of administrators. At Sheppard-Pratt, homosexual expressions were present not only among Sullivan's patients and attendants, but also among patients outside Sullivan's ward. It is not surprising, then, that the hospital's administration attempted to regulate homosexual contacts as much as possible, not because these contacts were an utter surprise to them, but because the incidents were known to happen. It was for this latter reason that Sullivan's use of "physical affection" became an object of the hospital's careful surveillance, generating condescending comments from the medical staff. "Miss Sullivan" as a reference to the doctor was one, while there were others that were more elaborate. William Elliot, a former attendant in Sullivan's ward, recalled derisively, "Sullivan was getting vicarious experience in working with these young homosexuals. . . . He was able to make the direct contacts he wanted. This is the only way he satisfied himself." Elliot added that people were aware that Sullivan "was in the ring but he wasn't playing." He was "just like a ringmaster. You jump but I am not going to jump."[59] In addition to Elliot's apparent lack of knowledge about (or disregard for) James Inscoe, these comments suggest how, even among Sullivan's own staff, there existed a doubt about his motivation. The line between personal satisfaction and scientific usefulness seemed too blurred. Thus, along with "Miss Sullivan," Elliot's comments suggest how Sullivan's method drew criticism not necessarily because it was seen to be a clear case of patient exploitation; it was considered dubious because his practice appeared to be shaped by the scientist's subjectivity as a homosexual man.

Of course, this does not mean that doctors at the hospital were not concerned about Sullivan's practice because it might invite patient abuse. Robbins's comment about the dismissed attendant clearly indicates that such a concern existed. The administration was doubtless aware that if sexual relationships between the hospital's staff and patients became known publicly, Sheppard-Pratt's standing and ethics would be questioned. The hospital's medical superintendent Ross McClure Chapman was particularly worried about Sullivan's method, because he was the person who had hired Sullivan and had given him unprecedented autonomy on his own ward. During a conference in 1928 for one of Sullivan's patients, Chapman expressed strong interest in the treatment the patient had received at Sullivan's direction:

CHAPMAN: Have you observed patients being treated in the hospital—is your observation pleasant or unpleasant?"
PATIENT: A pleasant one. . . .
CHAPMAN: Have you been treated with . . . courtesy or have there been exceptions. . . .
PATIENT: I was very much terrified and tormented by the Coronel [sic; refers to another patient], and wanted to be removed . . . from immediate contact with him; but, instead, I was put in more immediate contact with him. . . .

CHAPMAN: . . . Who worked that out?

PATIENT: Dr. Sullivan.

CHAPMAN: Dr. Sullivan put you there purposely for that?

PATIENT: That's what he said.

CHAPMAN: Have you been considerately treated or have you seen at any time any ill treatment of patients . . . ?

PATIENT: Nothing that could be called ill treatment.[60]

Chapman did not reveal the nature of "ill treatment" he was suspecting, perhaps because he did not want to alarm the patient unnecessarily. But Chapman later decided to let Sullivan leave the hospital, regardless of the nature of Sullivan's treatment that Chapman might have been alluding to in this exchange. In retrospect, Chapman justified his decision as being about Sullivan's temperament: "We must not forget that there was always a question . . . how long we could count on him? He had never been able to adapt himself to many of the people about him."[61] Thus, Chapman was worried about Sullivan's demand for more control and what many considered his uncooperative attitude. It is likely, of course, that Chapman was concerned about possible "ill treatment" of a sexual nature as well, even though there is no clear evidence of this. As for Sullivan, he was fully aware that he had been causing a problem for the hospital precisely because of his unorthodox therapy. When Clifton Read, one of the closest friends he would make in the 1930s, asked if Sullivan had written about "what went on in his ward," Sullivan "grinned and shook his head, [saying that] all he could do was suggest in a footnote."[62] Apparent in Sullivan's reaction is his awareness of the need to hide his clinical approach not only from the hospital administration but also from the broader psychiatric community. Thus, even to Sullivan himself, it was not clear that he could draw a clean line—a line he could uphold in public—between the unconventional but possibly effective therapy and an abuse of patients under the name of treatment.

In his clinical approach to schizophrenia and homosexuality, it was crucial for Sullivan to train attendants so that they applied what he believed to be the most effective treatment. By all existing accounts, it was attendants, not doctors, who engaged in physical contact with patients. The doctor's role was to talk about homosexual conflicts in depth during one-on-one interviews, not to be with patients when they acted out their concerns. Oftentimes, the doctor's subjective self became apparent in these conversations, partly because of their shared sexual experiences and identities. But regarding physical affection, Sullivan merely projected his beliefs through his attendants, rather than acting them out himself. But this scheme did not prevent his departure from Sheppard-Pratt. In March 1930, he sent a letter of resignation to Chapman, who accepted it immediately. Despite his successful treatment of schizophrenic patients and his willingness to further the hospital's application of the "new psychiatry," Sullivan stirred up the border between subjective and scientific aspects of clinical practice more than the hospital could tolerate or even bring to an open discussion. Once the hospital's staff became suspicious that his subjectivity might be shaping his scientific practice, it did not take a long time for the administration to become concerned about exploitive relationships between the medical staff and patients. In response, Sullivan tried to protect "what went on in his ward" through secrecy. This was in sharp contrast with the prescription of health, maturity, and independence that hospital doctors offered happily and eagerly under Sullivan's leadership as a clinical director.

Sullivan's work with his selected patients was based on a method of treating schizophrenia that challenged the social stigmatization of homosexuality and, implicitly, criticized the psychiatric profession, which had failed to address difficulties imposed upon homosexual men by a homophobic society. When this method seemed to his colleagues to be entangled with his subjectivity as a homosexual man, however, the social critique became hidden as well, even at a hospital where doctors generally promoted a better acceptance of a range of sexual expressions. The consequence of this suppression was twofold: not only did it make explicit, public critique of homophobia more difficult, it also made it hard to keep doctor-patient relationships transparent, so as to preclude patient exploitation. In this regard, it is important to note that, although sexual tensions and desires between persons of the same sex were not unusual at Sheppard-Pratt, Sullivan's practice was still considered to be unacceptable. For those outside Sullivan's ward, there was a huge distance between what seemed to be opportunistic actions of a homosexual nature and an attempt to use these actions as a therapeutic means. Understandable as this separation might have been, it left unexplored the question of what to do with the common acting out of same-sex desire. Indeed, the hospital's response to same-sex sexual expressions was almost nonexistent except for ignoring, repressing, and dismissing. While doctors freely discussed patients' anxiety over the changing mode of sexual expression as something that was connected to the social and cultural transformation of the era, this approach was limited to solitary or heterosexual sexual expressions told in life histories. When relationships included an acting out—especially that of same-sex sexual desire—it was not acceptable to deal with them in science. Thus Sullivan's story suggests how hard it was to publicly confront homophobia in the psychiatric world of the 1920s, even at a hospital where careful attention to the social and cultural origins of illness was the standard. Questions about the subjectivity of homosexual doctors and patients, unlike questions related to masturbation or heterosexual relationships, were not openly articulated in science, ultimately dividing the science of homosexuality into public and private practices.

Another important story embedded in the history of doctors and patients at Sheppard-Pratt was that they created new models of health and illness, even as they attempted to refute traditional models that they considered anachronistic. In their clinical work, homosexual experiences and feelings by themselves did not constitute an illness, while individuals who were overly worried about "homosexual content" were considered to be in need of therapeutic attention. The same emphasis on patients' worries about sexual acts, not the acts themselves, was apparent in Sheppard-Pratt doctors' approach to heterosexual relationships. Thus the message was, You can have almost as much sexual experience as you desire, but you should not be hesitant, uncertain, or secretive about it; to be healthy, you should be able to enjoy sex without care, and you must be willing and able to reflect upon it in insightful and comprehensible language in your talks with doctors. This capacity for self-reflection was expected to be used not only in sexual explorations, but also in interpersonal relationships in families, communities, and workplaces. These standards of health carried practical significance because they would help men to be successful in the emerging modern United States. Women were encouraged to acquire these "healthy" qualities as well, even though it was much less clear just what women were expected to do with their newfound open-mindedness and self-awareness when they were back to normal life outside the hospital. In this way, the hospital created a subtle, yet unmistakable, division between men's and women's mental health.

These new divisions of health and illness informed not only medical reasoning but also social scientific thinking of social problems in the 1920s and 1930s. Just as medical doctors were becoming newly aware of a connection between the social and individual, a number of social scientists were beginning to see this connection as a central focus of their research. To be sure, social scientists were coming to this observation along a different path from that of doctors. Some of the main fields of research for sociologists were urban neighborhoods, dance halls, and corrective institutions, locations that were much more open to the public than were clinical settings. Moreover, a number of anthropologists were interested in ethnic communities both inside and outside the United States as critical points of comparison to mainstream American culture. Increasingly, researchers in these social science disciplines regarded social problems as rooted in the troubled relationship between personality and culture. Thus, social scientists would collaborate with those whom they considered experts on personality—psychiatrists, psychoanalysts, and clinical psychologists. In turn, clinicians pursued interdisciplinary research programs with social scientists, so as to understand individual problems in a broad framework. In this process, clinical observations must go outside of a clinic and be discussed in models and language that made sense to scientists in different disciplines. Life history, which had potential for both coherency and complexity, became the most promising method in this regard.

3

Life History for Science
and Subjectivity

While Sheppard-Pratt doctors collected life histories as a promising medium for the scientific research of mental illness, some of the most influential social scientists of the time were beginning to use similar records in sociological, anthropological, and ethnographical research. Indeed, medical and social scientists' interests in this kind of source, unique in its intense attention to individual experiences and its resistance to categorical thinking, helped create one of the most prolific interdisciplinary collaborations in modern American history. This collaboration represented not just a series of interesting research programs based on multidimensional examinations of persons and cultures; it was a serious attempt to secure a place for human subjectivity in modern science, which had been, without doubt, moving toward favoring clear-cut, often dualistic modes of thinking. To be sure, scientists who were intrigued by life history sought to define it as a legitimate and dependable means of study, suggesting that they were in no way antiscientific. And yet many of them were fascinated by "others"—individuals who were mentally "sick" or sexually "immature," or peoples from cultural traditions that were not readily comprehensible to mainstream American observers—who compelled researchers to think hard about the fundamentally relative nature of human experience. Scientific research was not an exemption from relativism; thus it is not surprising that these scientists were particularly critical of biological, behavioral, and statistical methods that thrived in the early twentieth century. These methods seemed to promote a one-dimensional understanding of humans by removing them from their social and cultural contexts.

Although differing in their emphasis, what these scientists in the life history cohort had in common was an urgent sense of pervasive alienation, arising from a modernity that seemed to be obsessed with materialism, efficiency, and individual success. Indeed, one consensus among intellectuals in the 1920s was that the United States had lost touch with a crucial sense of self, as people became increasingly preoccupied with satisfying personal needs and desires that did not seem to have anything to do with the common good.[1] The increasingly influential Freudian theory of psychoanalysis only fueled this concern about a drifting self, as analysts "discovered" a domain in the self that was not accessible to the rational mind: the unconscious. The foremost features of the unconscious were its irrationality and uncontrollability, and thus it seemed to substantiate the fear that humans were becoming detached both from within and without. In this climate, individuals who seemed to be "maladjusted" to modernity (psychiatric patients, delinquents, criminals, homosexuals) and those who seemed to maintain a connection with uncontaminated human nature—the "primitive"—began to draw special attention from scientists. In some cases, scientists began to include racial minorities, African Americans in particular, among their research subjects, suggesting that scientific interest extended not only to psychological, sexual, and social "others," but also to those who were seen to be racially and culturally different. Barely hidden behind scientists' claim that their studies were meant to help these "others" to fit into society was their fascination with their research subjects, who offered, in different ways, a glimpse of what it is like to remain connected to the "true" self. Just as Harry Stack Sullivan was intrigued by schizophrenia and homosexuality as conditions close to "prenatal" status, many scientists in the 1920s and 1930s considered it crucial that their research helped preserve Americans' connection with the core of their selves, whatever that core might be. At the same time, they were concerned that their approach be fully scientific, so that their observations would have reasonable weight in academia. In this context, life history emerged as a promising vessel to carry out this dual task.

The interdisciplinary collaboration between medical and social scientists in the 1920s and 1930s, then, revolved around the development of life history. This story included intellectuals such as Robert E. Park, Edward Sapir, Charles Johnson, Harold Lasswell, Margaret Mead, and Ruth Fulton Benedict who, by bringing their inspirations and expectations to the formation of life history, defined the meanings and boundaries of the era's liberalism.[2] Because of their interest in understanding individuals and cultures in their own contexts, these scientists were pushed to be open to human differences. But just as Sheppard-Pratt doctors' approach to issues of sexuality was not an open-ended acceptance of variety, the scientists' interest in diversity was not limitless. Not unlike the way that Sullivan's critique of homophobia was expelled from Sheppard-Pratt clinical culture, the collaboration of medical and social scientists excluded certain groups of individuals from its arena of acceptance. Scientists, who were expected to be examiners (not subjects) of life histories, were excluded from scientific scrutiny, despite their aspiration to collect data through interactive, rather than unilateral, processes. Moreover, people whose fundamental character-istics as modern citizens seemed to be permanently injured—for instance, chronic psychiatric patients who did not seem to possess maturity, inde-pendence, self-awareness, and the ability to express all these qualities in a coherent narrative—slipped out of the scientists' vision of liberal reform. These are qualities that Sheppard-Pratt doctors attempted to reconstruct in patients in an early stage of treatment, indicating a strong connection between clinical and intellectual observations of individual experiences. Examination of the intellectual side of this connection, then, illuminates a larger picture of the division between health and illness. In particular, the development of the life history method shows how this clinical division expanded into a range of distinctions implicit in scientific analyses: "devel-oped" and "underdeveloped" personalities, "civilized" and "primitive" cul-tures, and "us" and "others."

The locations for research on life history were spread out from Wash-ington, DC/Baltimore to New Haven and Chicago, and researchers did not constitute a single group that remained intact throughout the decades and determined the direction of research. Instead, scientists from different loca-tions came together at conferences, colloquia, and seminars to form their ideas, collectively shaping a unique effort to remain close to human experi-ences in their scientific investigations. In helping to organize this effort, Sul-livan played the central role; his career in the 1920s and 1930s also suggests the fate of "private" liberalism after he left Sheppard-Pratt. His public profile became more prominent during these decades, as he promoted collabora-tions with leading social sciences as someone "who first made real . . . the possibility of a psychiatrist aware of culture," as the anthropologist John Dollard characterized him.[3] While Sullivan's public persona was burnished, his private liberalism did not find a place in the mainstream effort of the life history group. This was not because of a lack of effort on Sullivan's part: in an interdisciplinary conference, for instance, he tried to make a case for a more relaxed attitude toward same-sex intimacy in the United States; his first book manuscript, "Personal Psychopathology," suggested his support for a better acceptance of homoeroticism. Moreover, in his critique of rac-ism, he seemed to be criticizing prejudice in general, including homopho-bia. All these attempts to find a place for his private liberalism in public realms were shaped by the emerging interest in life history that aimed to be open to relativity, diversity, and a range of subjectivity. But ultimately, the science community at large did not recognize, let alone support, these attempts, making it necessary for Sullivan to pursue his work on the mar-gins. Thus, a full acceptance of homosexuality, as well as a careful scrutiny of the subjectivity of scientists and the chronically ill, failed to enter a more "public" liberalism.

The Beginning of Life History

In the interwar decades, an interest in life history on the part of medical and social scientists was driven by particular intellectual and institutional concerns within their disciplines. Life history in psychiatric practice, for example, flourished in part because of its connection with the "new psychiatry." Physicians in the new psychiatry considered the reeducation of a personality through the making of a coherent life history the most desirable therapeutic goal. Its usefulness for treatment, and its presumed link to social adjustment, made life history a signature method of the new psychiatry. The method emerged at a time of uncertainty in the profession, however. In fact, psychiatry in the 1920s was in its own identity crisis of sorts, which stemmed from its apparent lack of scientific credibility and professional respectability. The issue of scientific credibility had been a concern for a long time in psychiatry, dating back to the late nineteenth century. While other branches of medicine achieved theoretical and therapeutic innovations during the last three decades of the nineteenth century, psychiatry lagged behind in its pathology, diagnosis, and treatment. Psychiatry in medical communities was looked down upon as an immature science at best or, worse, a nonscience. The question of professional respectability was inseparable from this perceived backwardness. Because their field was considered to lack scientific sophistication, psychiatrists of the era had to work uphill even when claiming basic constituents of the professional standing. For instance, the American Medical Association did not count most psychiatric hospitals as educational institutions, discouraging medical students from getting psychiatric internships as part of their education. Moreover, with few exceptions, most medical schools did not house a department of psychiatry, limiting medical students' exposure to the field. It is not surprising, then, that while other medical fields established their boards of certificate for specialists in the 1910s and 1920s, psychiatry had to wait until 1934 to create its own.[4] In response to these challenges, some psychiatrists came up with biological explanations of mental disorders. Somatic theories that located causes of mental illness in the brain, nervous system, endocrine system, hormonal balance, blood circulation, or immunological system, to name a few, flourished in the first few decades of the twentieth century. None sufficiently proved to be theoretically coherent or therapeutically efficacious. Despite many surgical operations conducted on patients, including the removal of "infected" regions such as teeth, tonsils, uterus and ovaries, the statistics collected by the U.S. Bureau of the Census showed that the number of inmates at state mental hospitals, especially those who were chronically ill, continued to grow.[5] Not only did it alarm psychiatrists with the ineffectuality of their specialty, it also confined a great majority of them nationwide to what many considered backward state institutions. When other specialists in medicine engaged in potentially groundbreaking research and treatment in modern hospitals and laboratories, many psychiatrists found themselves spending most of their time in custodial care and administrative duties at hospitals where the doctor-patient ratio could be as high as one to two hundred.

Other psychiatrists sought out a solution to the problems of credibility and respectability in a new "science" of human mind, psychoanalysis, which was becoming popular in the United States, following Sigmund Freud's now famous lecture at Clark University in 1909. Although psychoanalysis did not use the established model of biological medicine, it offered a different set of theories, terms, and therapeutic techniques to help psychiatrists claim their distinct expertise. For its followers, Freudian psychoanalysis embodied the coming of enlightenment at last, letting them move beyond the age of ignorance and confusion.[6] But the majority of American psychiatrists remained suspicious of psychoanalysis precisely because of its idiosyncrasy. They continued to believe that it was crucial for psychiatric medicine to adopt biological and physiological models of explanation. Psychoanalysis might help them to better understand mental problems, but only with the risk of further alienating psychiatrists in the medical profession. In particular, psychoanalysts trained in Europe, many of whom were not medical doctors, posed a threat to the frail confidence of psychiatrists in their authenticity. To be sure, it was not until the late 1930s and early 1940s that American psychiatrists began to expel non-MD analysts from their professional organizations. But even before then, it was clear that psychoanalysis generated at best an ambivalent response from U.S. psychiatrists.[7]

For those who joined the new psychiatry, the questionable medical standing of psychoanalysis mattered somewhat less. The intellectual foundation of the new psychiatry was broad and eclectic, as seen in the thinking of Adolf Meyer, a leading figure in the field. Particularly after he cofounded the National Committee for Mental Hygiene (NCMH) in 1911 with an activist and former patient, Clifford W. Beers, Meyer became a driving force in the reform of the profession. Not only did he consider individualized treatment important, he also believed that mental illness should be understood multidimensionally from psychological, biological, and social aspects. Thus he disagreed with those who narrowly focused on biological factors, while by the same token, he was against the adherence that orthodox Freudians demanded of clinicians for a particular set of theories and techniques.[8] But the followers of the new psychiatry, as at Sheppard-Pratt, were not unwilling to adopt an analytic method as long as it was useful in exploring patients' life histories. Their priorities were to obtain data from a person's life with utmost specificity and to understand it in many different contexts. This guided the supporters of the new psychiatry to examine both patients' emotional reactions to experiences and connections between clinical concerns and social problems.[9]

Among these paradigms in psychiatry—biological theories, psychoanalysis, and the new psychiatry—the last was unique in its attempt to expand psychiatrists' professional authenticity by reaching out to other disciplines. Unlike biological and psychoanalytical theorists, these psychiatrists saw the possibility of a new science in interdisciplinary collaborations and integrations, not surprisingly so, given a holistic view such as Meyer's. Instead of isolating their field from others, psychiatrists in the new psychiatry chose to be inclusive of the natural sciences, social sciences, and humanities, in order to create a new discipline—a science of interpersonal relations, as Sullivan called it. While the most frequently noted change that the new psychiatry helped create was the deinstitutionalization of inpatients from state facilities and the expansion of psychiatric care in local communities, psychiatrists in the life history cohort were equally engaged in research-oriented, methodological explorations. Their concern was how they could achieve generality, applicability, and testability, all basic features of science, using highly personal, subjective records of life histories. The psychiatric researchers of life history, then, constituted a unique group that was most open to interdisciplinarity and individual subjectivity in the increasingly specializing field of medicine.

Social scientists' interest in life history came more or less from the opposite direction: from the general to the specific. Going against the predominant interest in statistical methods in sociology, for instance, John Dollard in *Criteria for the Life History* (1935) criticized scholars who, when wishing to "study the religious behavior of adolescents, for instance, . . . simply drop a statistical bucket into the well of adolescent experience and draw it out; they will view their bucketful of data as self-explanatory and not as a part of an individual unified life."[10] What was missing from such a study, he argued, was contexualization, a discussion of how a certain kind of experience made subjective sense to a person. Dollard went on to claim that any mass-oriented study must reject an approach that lacked contextual discussion:

> After we have "gone cultural" we experience the person as a fragment
> of a . . . cultural pattern. . . . A culture-personality problem can be
> identified . . . by observing whether a person is "there" in full emo-
> tional reality; if he is not there, then we are dealing with a straight

cultural or institutional history. If he is there and we can ask how he feels, then we have a culture-personality problem.[11]

In examining "culture-personality" problems, Dollard expected that life history makes individual, fragmentary, and emotional factors a more integral part of the cultural and institutional.

This interest in the integration of subjectivity into what was traditionally defined as objective data was not uncommon among social scientists. Indeed, the lack of qualitative analyses in qualitative studies was a vexing concern of American social scientists, especially among those whose careers centered around Chicago and Yale, and to a lesser degree, Columbia and Harvard.[12] Out of this concern emerged a fresh emphasis on the need for scientists to become more aware of the interaction between researchers, their subjects, and contexts in which they encountered one another. William I. Thomas in 1928, for instance, discussed what he called "a situational approach," claiming that the increasing interest among Chicago sociologists in the circumstantial factors of social problems had guided them to "life histories, personality documents and records with reference to the concrete trains of experiences." [13] Kimball Young, a Chicago-trained sociologist, had added to the discussion in 1927 by pointing out the value of examining research subjects' life experiences, especially those in childhood, in research of communities.[14] Trained at Columbia by Franz Boas and located then at the University of Chicago, the linguist and anthropologist Edward Sapir agreed, arguing that, in thinking of the link between individuals and collectives, he was "fond of Dr. Sullivan's pet phrase of 'interpersonal relations,'" as the exploration of such relationships helped him to "move forward to a realistic . . . definition of what is meant by culture and personality."[15] In 1935, Margaret Mead reiterated the significance of looking into "inexplicit unformulated . . . and uninstitutionalized" aspects of culture, such as child training and family relations, which had been excluded from the categories of issues that ethnographers examined regularly. Moreover, she said, it was crucial that researchers, when collecting information about these "inexplicit" aspects of culture, make "a much more extended entrée into the lives of the people, a much more complete participation in their lives."[16] Mead was not alone in stressing the importance of participant observation in collecting life histories. Harvard anthropologist Florence R. Kluckhohn, for instance, reported in 1940 on her experience of gathering data while she "lived" in a village in New Mexico. She did not reveal that she was an anthropologist, but attempted to obtain information of villagers' real "life-activities" as she assumed the personas of a wife and a storekeeper. Such participatory method would "provide a desirable balance between the . . . behavoristic [sic] type of investigation and the type which seeks some measure of insight into the 'meanings' current in the community."[17] All these approaches demanded researchers' attention to concrete, if often fleeting, details, and a fuller involvement in the situation where these details came alive.

Besides the heightened methodological debate over the place of individual experiences in study of collectives, Freudian psychoanalysis had augmented social scientists' interest in experimenting with life history interdisciplinarily.[18] Indeed, the American Sociological Society (ASS) and the American Psychiatric Association (APA) each created a special committee, in 1928 and 1927, respectively, to cultivate collaboration between the disciplines, influenced by an increase in the use of Freudian ideas in sociological research. The ASS committee appointed William I. Thomas as a chairman, and Kimball Young and Robert E. Park as its members, suggesting that there was an overlap between people who joined the debate over subjectivity and those who were curious about psychoanalysis.[19] Even before the committee was established, there existed a sociological interest in psychoanalysis. Park's *The Principles of Human Behavior* (1915), published six years after Freud's lecture at Clark University, discussed how people are often unconscious of their motives, suggesting the limits of sociological data based on what people could consciously recall in response to sociologists' inquiries. Trained at Columbia and teaching at Chicago, William Ogburn in 1918, too, used the Freudian concept of "unconsciousness" in his analysis of economy. Following up on this discussion, Thomas Eliot at Northwestern in 1920 discussed the development of a person from an individual to a collective mode of living, using psychoanalytic diagrams of personality proposed by a psychoanalyst Smith Ely Jelliffe. Building on Jelliffe's model illuminating that children's minds are "underdeveloped," Eliot argued that personalities of "savages," as well as those of children, are tied into "primitive, often unconscious, sources."[20] Clearly, Freud's ideas offered sociologists theoretical tools and metaphors with which to explore territories of human life that had been unfamiliar to them—factors that influenced human behavior, which, despite their importance, might not be easily observable.

What prompted social scientists to explore these unknown territories well before psychoanalysis became the mainstream in American psychiatry? Eliot's assumption about the close connection between youth, immaturity, and foreignness to Western civilization offers a clue. Such an assumption was hardly unique to Eliot. As is clear in the frequent use of the word *primitive* by the era's anthropologists and ethnographers when referring to non-Western societies, one of the shared assumptions in these disciplines was that such research subjects were throwbacks to prehistoric times. Indeed, anthropologists considered it to be an urgent mission to collect data before these non-Western cultures became extinct as a result of being exposed to modernization and civilization.[21] Although this did not mean that researchers did not appreciate the characteristics of non-Western societies per se, their value as research subjects lay in their assumed lack of modernity and civilization. Thus Elton Mayo at Harvard, in his 1937 article on the relationship between psychiatry and sociology, asserted that social maladjustments were rare in a "primitive tribe" because "the passage [from childhood to adulthood] offers no great difficulty." These communities had "established tribal beliefs and the routines, [which would] insure the effective collaboration of the group" in assisting their members' growing up. This was not the case in a more complex, "civilized society." As Freud had discovered, "defective social conditioning" had been causing a wide range of maladjustments including neurosis, promiscuity, and sexual "perversion."[22] The assumption here is that the more a society becomes "civilized," the more problems it begins to suffer. There was a clear parallel between "underdeveloped" and "developed" personalities on the one hand, and "primitive" and "civilized" societies on the other.[23] To better understand this difference between "primitive" and "civilized" societies, and more important, to find scientific solutions to modern problems through examining the difference, the psychoanalytic exploration of the "primitive" seemed indispensable.

The "primitive" was not confined to foreign countries; it could be found at home as well. Read Bain, a Chicago School–influenced sociologist who played a crucial role in the introduction of Freud to American social scientists, pointed to an increasing number of "psychopaths" in the United States. Refusing the idea that a person can be born to be sick, Bain asserted that "psychoses" such as "the homosexual syndrome" was a "masculine protest" against "women's clubs aping men and [men's] clubs." According to Bain, then, men who frequent "psychotic groups [such as] gangs [and] homosexual colonies" might be trying to escape pressures brought about by changes in modern society, such as increasing rights for women.[24] In addition to his rejection of feminism and his understanding of homosexuality as one of the ills of civilization, it is noteworthy that Bain, like Mayo, reiterated the contrast between the "primitive" and "civilized." Among social scientists influenced by Freud, a dualistic thinking that placed Western civilization, complexity, and maturity in contrast with savagery, simplicity, and immaturity of non-Westerners was potent. More important, the contrast existed within civilization as well. As modern society grew complex, there emerged a gap between those who were better adjusted to the complexity and those who were less adjusted, and it was social scientists' responsibility to understand the latter—the "simple," "primitive," and "immature" in a developed society.

This dualistic model brought social scientists near their "exotic" research subjects, at least as much as it created a distance between scientific examiners and examinees. Just as psychiatrists at Sheppard-Pratt were fascinated by schizophrenia and homosexuality as conditions close to the beginning of a person's self, social scientists were intrigued by cultures and personalities that seemed to offer a counterpoint to modernity.[25] While these points of reference were often romanticized (for example, "primitive" societies were deemed to be "preserving" human nature in its bare form), these cultural "others" could also be somewhat uncanny, especially when they were found within modernity. Criminals, delinquents, psychopaths, and perverts—all of whom were popular subjects of 1920s social sciences—seemed to represent just the kind of problems that modern, urban, and diverse America must confront. What was unique to the era's social scientists' response to these "others" was their embrace of—or their attempt to embrace—subjectivity, both for researchers and for subjects, which distinctively separated them from their predecessors who had not questioned the objectivity of their knowledge. Medical and social scientists, though from different paths, reached the same conclusion that life history was a method that opened up a place for both human uncertainly and scientific clarity. In turn, the work of scientists in the life history cohort illuminated concerns and prospects that permeated broader scientific communities cross-disciplinarily. We have understood how this took place within discrete disciplines. But the truly striking development in the life history method of this era was its diverse roots in a range of scholarship that cut across fields. These scientists expected that their diligent "spelling out" of all things possible would explain what seemed incomprehensible about a person and society. In a way not dissimilar from that of Sheppard-Pratt doctors who attempted to help their patients become more self-aware, the scientists in the life history cohort tried to get a grip on the changing reality by stepping into it with eyes wide open. Although these scientists were ultimately limited in accepting certain kinds of subjectivity—a scientist's subjectivity and the subjectivity of those who were deemed incapable of telling their life histories such as the chronically mentally ill—their effort created an opening for a kind of science that resisted systematized explanation in order to understand lived complexity.

The Tenet of Collaboration

The APA's and ASS's committees on interdisciplinary collaboration sponsored a brace of conferences called the Colloquium on Personality Investigation, in 1928 and 1929, creating perhaps the era's most important springboards for programs bringing people from different disciplines together. The ASS contingent included people from the Freud-influenced group, among them Ernest Burgess, Elton Mayo, Harold Lasswell, and Edward Sapir, in addition to the committee members who constituted the core of the life history cohort (and notably, Clifford Shaw as well). The APA representatives included William Alanson White as a chairman and Harry

Stack Sullivan as a secretary of the committee, along with psychiatrists such as David Levy, Lawson Lowrey, James S. Plant, and William Healy, all of whom were chief figures of the new psychiatry. In addition, there was Lawrence K. Frank from the Laura Spelman Rockefeller Memorial Foundation and the Social Science Research Council as a sponsor of the colloquium.[26] It was during these colloquia that some of the main concepts of life history were articulated, which in turn revealed how researchers of the era grappled with the meaning of subjectivity in science. Many scientists who attended these colloquia did not see subjectivity as simply individual; instead, it was an idea that scientists hoped would help Americans to make sense of who they were among "others." With this goal, scientists at the colloquia elaborated three main components of the life history method: "personality," "participant observation," and "social psychiatry."

One of these components, personality, appeared in Park's 1928 preliminary statement on the colloquium: "The task of the psychiatrist touches that of the sociologists," Park argued, because a "psychiatrist, on the basis of . . . medical knowledge, and with his opportunity to study personalities in hospitals, has access to aspects of human nature that are not accessible to the sociologists." Indeed, the concept of personality emerged in participants' discussion as an important bridge between sociological and medical thinking. Ernest Burgess called personality "a conception which a person has of his role and status in the group as influenced and modified in social interaction." Its characteristics, then, were best illuminated by personal interviews and life history documents. Mark A. May, a social psychologist from Yale University, soon to be the director of the Institute of Human Relations, agreed with Burgess, stating that personality was "the net result of your social interaction" and that personality types, "if there are such, are the result as well as the cause of different kinds of . . . social interaction."[27]

Intrigued by these dynamic definitions, Sullivan asked May to further explain what he meant by personality types. Their exchange illuminates a key intersection of medical and social scientific notions of personality:

MAY: By types [of personality], I mean types of responses. Therefore, personality is not something that is constant and carried around with you, but personality changes as you go from one type of social group to another. These changes depend entirely upon what goes on between you and the other members of the group. . . .

SULLIVAN: I am reaching for your idea which coincides with mine insofar as I stress the notion that interpersonal relations are invariably interpersonal; that the observer does not sit upon an ivory tower and gaze down at strange objects performing below him, but instead performs with them.[28]

Here, what May described as a person in a changing social setting was redefined as "interpersonal relations" by Sullivan, suggesting that in his definition, interpersonal relationships included not merely more than one person, but also social contexts in which an encounter between individuals occurred. Because of this inclusiveness, Edward Sapir would later see a "good meeting ground" for psychiatrists and social scientists in the concept of interpersonal relations.[29] Perhaps such recognition by social scientists pushed Sullivan to use it as a key term in his theory in coming years.

There are other ideas embedded in this exchange that became important both in Sullivan's interpersonal theory of mental illness and in the method of life history. For one, May's statement touched on what was to become one of Sullivan's unique theses: the idea that a person has a unique personality is "illusory" because a person cannot be scientifically isolated from interaction with others. Although May did not argue that individual personality is illusory, he came close when he said that a personality was not constant and could not be carried from one situation to another. Moreover, Sullivan's discussion of the role of the scientist in this exchange corresponded with "participant observation" that scientific interviewers were expected to make of interviewees when collecting life histories. Similar to the "interpersonal relation," the concept of participant observation was rooted in his clinical practice at Sheppard-Pratt; now it began to take new root in the interdisciplinary community. Surely Sullivan at Sheppard-Pratt understood that he could not perform his duties well as an interviewer if he remained in an "ivory tower." In this exchange with May, then, Sullivan can be seen as discovering a tie between the best of his clinical practice and social scientific inquiries. More important, "participant observation" became a reminder that scientists were not exempt from subjectivity. This worked against the dualistic distinction between interviewers and interviewees in the collection of life histories, producing a series of experimental, "participatory" studies such as Florence R. Kluckhohn's.

Yet another key concept shaped during the colloquia, that of the "social psychiatrist," illuminated the impact of the social sciences on psychiatry. Following the pattern of reform embraced by the new psychiatry, social psychiatrists were defined as new breed of psychiatrists who were specifically trained to understand mental illness in social contexts. Not surprisingly, psychiatrists at the colloquia proposed a plan to change the curriculum in medical education. Taking note of the lack of dependable treatment, for example, Sullivan argued that psychiatrists were "tangled up with the training of people whom we hope may solve" the problem in the future. Those who would find solutions to mental problems were "social psychiatrists," who, in his definition, were trained in "a good deal of what you [social scientists] have learned" in the course of education. Some participants suggested that, in light of this, there should be an exchange of professors between the fields: a sociologist lectures in a class on psychiatry at a medical school, a psychiatrist teaches in a course on economics, and so on. These opinions gained further momentum in the second colloquium, when educational reform became a focal point once again. Speaking for sociologists, for example, Ernest Burgess argued that students in the field should work with psychiatrists and psychoanalysts in a graduate course on life history. In response, Sullivan claimed: "The personnel that comes to us from any and all channels is not particularly good personnel [for social psychiatry] . . . [because] in the course of education the minds of this personnel are so systematized along certain lines that they become relatively incapable of appreciating the importance of data to which they are exposed thereafter." Here, Sullivan disagreed with Burgess's moderate plan: instead of making an exchange program in graduate school, Sullivan demanded interdisciplinary "departments in which general information rather than [the] highly specialized is the principle." These departments, because of their focus on undergraduate education, would encourage "people [to] get a good deal of knowledge without too rigid crystallization of ideas." This went beyond a plan for interdisciplinary collaboration. This was a plea for a new field integrating existing areas of expertise. Given the less than satisfactory status of psychiatry in medical education and the likelihood that most medical students did not take any courses in the social sciences and humanities in college, such a drastic change seemed necessary.[30]

Sullivan's proposal to create a new department in a university stimulated lively discussion among the colloquium's participants, suggesting the extent (and the limit) of their idea of multidisciplinary collaboration. Harold Lasswell, then a young political scientist and just back from a trip to Europe, during which he had met such psychoanalysts as Alfred Adler, Gregory Zilboorg, Sandor Ferenczi, and Wilhelm Stekel, was supportive of Sullivan; to create "a grand department of personality study" would be desirable.[31] On the other hand, Lasswell expressed his reservation as well, suggesting that this plan might belong to a distant future. The more immediate concern should be to create opportunities for researchers from different disciplines to learn about each other's interests. This moderate approach to cross-disciplinary collaboration, rather than something as dramatic as Sullivan's, was preferred by most participants, even those who clearly shared Sullivan's frustration with the lack of psychiatric education at medical schools. For example, James S. Plant, a psychiatrist from a juvenile clinic, criticized medical education in strong language: "Everything humanly possible is done to the [medical] student to keep him from thinking about things which he learns." By graduation, medical students would be soaked with specialized knowledge, and thus it would be simply impossible "to make them interested in various scientific approaches." But, like Lasswell, Plant was not taken by the idea of making a department of "social psychiatry." Instead, Plant's enthusiasm went into a plan to put students of Burgess, Sapir, and others in touch with Sullivan as a part of graduate requirement.

This discussion traced how Sullivan's long-standing interest in socio-cultural contexts of mental illness, nurtured at Sheppard-Pratt, began to be intellectualized and institutionalized. In this process, certain aspects of his practice were compromised. Compared with where his social critique had begun—one-on-one interviews with patients, during which he articulated the plan to take a "preliminary" step to change the homophobic "existing social system"—the colloquia for interdisciplinary collaboration was emotionally detached and more focused on professional, rather than personal, improvements. Although Sullivan's relative impersonality could be attributed to the academic setting, it certainly had consequences, including the moderation of ideas that did not fit into the colloquia's format. For instance, Sullivan's private liberalism was largely missing from his comments, with a notable exception of the following exchange with Edward Sapir. This exchange can be seen as verging on a critique of homophobia, although it was not explicitly expressed as such, and thus in fact highlights how Sullivan tried to negotiate a place for his private liberalism in public science. Prior to this exchange, Sapir had discussed a small group of men in an Indian tribe as an important social institution that helped men to excel as soldiers. Then, Sullivan asked:

> Dr. Sapir, you speak of this formation among these particular Indians, of groups of two and three who are sufficiently closely knit that a survivor would prefer death. That seems to me significant indeed for the understanding of many phenomena with which I deal. . . . I wonder if it would not be valuable to have your views as to just what constitutes these groups. . . .
>
> SAPIR: . . . The meaning of friendship among males . . . is . . . highly important in this society, just as it undoubtedly was in the society of the Spartans and among some of the feudal classes of Japanese. . . .
>
> SULLIVAN: Now you touch upon a problem which seems to be identical . . . with one . . . in the psychiatry of schizophrenia. The sort of rebuff which most of my patients seem to have suffered is in that very field of affection among males. They have not been able to establish the little group that they felt, for a reason that someone might tell us, they should establish. What is the anthropologist's approach to the understanding of that situation in American culture, let us say? How can we arrange any experiment for elucidating that matter?
>
> SAPIR: . . . One of the very distinctive things about modern American culture is the relative difficulty of establishing highly emotional friendships

between males, and between females for that matter. . . . But where society . . . favors that type of expression, certain individuals at least are provided with an outlet that perhaps saves them from the schizophrenic debauch. It is perfectly possible.

SULLIVAN: In turn the parallelism increases because that is precisely what we do in the mental hospital. We lead to complete distinction of the roles of the male and female and try to set up groupings between intelligent and sensitive employees and psychotic and sensitive patients of the same sex, and it seems to be remarkably successful in reducing the stress and strain of living, and thus in reducing the necessity for psychotic behavior.[32]

At first sight, this exchange seems to be a scholarly, comparative analysis of the sexes: some societies are easy about same-sex friendship, while others, including modern America, are not. Moreover, an extreme prohibition of intimate friendship between persons of the same sex could well be a cause of schizophrenia. Behind these lucid observations, however, was Sullivan's effort to integrate his private approach to homosexuality into a public critique of American homophobia. For one thing, while Sapir referred to the relationship between men in the group as "friendship," Sullivan called it "affection," a warmer, possibly sexual term. Although Sapir's example of the Japanese feudal classes (which were known for their approval of both sexual and nonsexual bonds between men) might have inadvertently invited Sullivan to mention same-sex "affection," it is nonetheless striking that Sapir continued to frame the same-sex emotional attachment as an expression of "friendship," as nothing explicitly sexual. The reason for this is not clear; perhaps homosexuality was not something Sapir felt he could connect to male friendship. But most likely, Sapir was aware that he was, indeed, talking about homosexual relationships. He had been a close friend of Sullivan since 1926, and he was one of a handful of people who socialized with Harry and Jimmie as a couple. Given this, Sapir had at least some sense of Sullivan's homosexuality and his clinical practice at Sheppard-Pratt. It is not surprising, then, that Sapir's response to Sullivan's question about the "experiment" included a discussion of "certain individuals" who, if "provided with an outlet" for same-sex intimacy, would avoid schizophrenia. For an anthropologist specializing in the language of Native Americans, one who was critical of the era's sexual "freedom" in general and "extreme cases" of homosexuality in particular (see Chapter 4), this was an extremely sympathetic observation. Without making it explicit that his discussion was about homosexuality, Sapir suggested that homosexual persons might benefit from better social acceptance.

For Sullivan, this whole exchange might have been a push-and-pull negotiation to secure a place in academia for his clinical approach to social

change. On the one hand, he pushed Sapir to make it clear that their discussion was about homosexuality. Sapir ended up referring to same-sex
"intimacy" toward the end of the discussion, which made his discussion
more suggestive of sexual relationships than of "friendship." On the other
hand, it was perhaps important for Sullivan that Sapir stayed out of an
explicit discussion of homosexuality by building his observations around a
more general concept of "friendship." In this way, Sullivan would be able to
use Sapir's comments to make the issue of homosexuality part of a broad
scientific concern about modern America. If homosexuality arose out of
social changes, it need not be seen as a peculiar pathological condition
anymore. It would be merely one of many problems that needed to be better understood. In this scheme, sociocultural changes, not homosexuality,
would be a focus of scientific inquiries. This would free homosexual persons from strains and stigmas that had long been imposed by homophobic
society. Although he was not explicit in his comments, it is hard not to
see these implications in Sullivan's discussion, given that his clinical practice at Sheppard-Pratt was based exactly on such a critique. The following
exchange between Sullivan and Sapir further illuminates Sullivan's tactic of
push and pull in his effort to incorporate his private liberalism into open
discussion of culture and personality:

SAPIR: It was necessary for those who entered on an expedition [of the Plains
    Indians] to confess all sexual irregularities. If one of the followers had
    committed adultery . . . he would have to admit that publicly, and no
    redress could be taken.
SULLIVAN: In the mental hospitals we again parallel these . . . primitive
    people in that . . . one of the most helpful things about treatment is
    the acceptance as having occurred of the sort of thing that your Indians
    might be confessing. In other words, in my particular group it becomes
    common property . . . that presumably these irregularities happen . . .
    and in psychiatric material it seems to relieve a vast amount of tension,
    with marked improvement of the patient's adaptability.[33]

Considering Sullivan's specialization in the treatment of patients with
homosexual conflicts by 1928, it is clear that "sexual irregularities" in his
"particular group" were homosexual experiences, not heterosexual adultery.
He made this shift from Sapir's example of adultery to his own of homosexuality without making the change of subject explicit. Here again, Sullivan
was pushing to make homosexuality and his private approach to it part of
public discussion of science and, at the same time, pulling himself out of
an explanation of what he was doing. But he certainly tried to make it clear
that sexual irregularities happen regularly, and thus it is important to accept

them. As he reiterated, confession would function both as a "device to bring social solidarity and as a device for discharging the feeling of guilt of the individual." Therefore, he implied, if in coded language, that homosexual men should be encouraged to talk about their homosexual experiences, so as to create a sense of comradeship. This suggests that he considered homosexual men to be members of a minority group, and that he hoped to see them become more aware of the presence of others like themselves. Confession— or telling of one's life history—would be crucial in this process of becoming self-aware. These views certainly shared similarities with the basic tenets of the gay rights movement in the 1960s and 1970s, although they were framed in the context of scientific examination of "psychiatric materials" at "mental hospitals." If the contents of Sullivan's argument seemed to point to bringing homosexuality out of the closet, the context of academic discussion in the 1920s required a careful enclosure of the subject within a broad concern about social institutions that dealt with "irregularities."

The fact that Sullivan was able to discuss the ideas of group "solidarity" and "participant observation" in the colloquium suggests a possibility he must have seen for expressing his private liberalism in a public setting. It is striking that he made these points without an apparent fear that his sexuality would be exposed as a result. Participant observation implied that the doctor listening to the patient's confession was part of a group, while he also made it clear that this group under his discussion was made up of people whose sexual behavior was "irregular." If he were to address an audience more discerning than the one in front of him, he would have to expect that his discussion would cause at least some people to wonder if he were referring to his own homosexuality. Indeed, this was the very question raised by one of his patients at Sheppard-Pratt when discussing why Sullivan had taken up his line of profession. But Sullivan probably did not expect his audience at the colloquium to ask such a question, one that would have been unwelcome and threatening to his reputation. He was likely confident that his coded language would be effective, causing no one in this particular audience to speculate about his sexuality. Thus, Sullivan was able to bring forward for discussion ideas and practices that, based on his experience at Sheppard-Pratt, he understood as too unconventional to be made public in most circumstances. Clearly, he had a sharp sense of different audiences— patients as insiders and intellectuals as outsiders—and offered a different explanation of his liberalism that he deemed most appropriate for each. His coded language helped him to make a seamless transition from one audience to another, while the huge gulf he perceived between insiders and outsiders made it possible to give a strikingly honest, if allusive, expression to his private practice. In this circumstance, a discussion of homosexuality between the lines, not a confrontational discourse such as the one that became predominant in the post-Stonewall era, was the most reasonable. Sullivan's discussion in the colloquium reflected what he considered to be the best tactic, not something that fell short of the activism that was to be materialized decades later.

The Sullivan-Sapir exchange also suggests a certain pleasure Sullivan might have taken in his pursuit of private liberalism. Sapir was a sympathetic outsider, a married man who respected Sullivan, regardless of the latter's "irregular" sexuality. Consequently, Sapir was a perfect choice with whom to discuss homosexuality. Sapir probably understood what Sullivan was up to, while Sullivan doubtless spoke as if Sapir understood that what was being discussed was, in fact, homosexuality. Sullivan allowed Sapir to stay with his safe choice of words while at the same time gently pushing him to see how far he would go. This process apparently remained undisclosed to the audience, a security ensured by its lack of knowledge, sensitivity, or both. In this way, subjectivity found a place in a scientific discussion. The "between you and me" situation that Sullivan shared with his patients at Sheppard-Pratt replicated itself in the Sullivan-Sapir exchange at the colloquium, if only to a limited degree. Certainly, Sapir was not an insider in terms of his sexual orientation, as far as we know, and Sullivan had to be careful not to make Sapir uncomfortable in front of his peers. However, in ways familiar to his clinical practice at Sheppard-Pratt, Sullivan's interaction with Sapir was based on a shared knowledge that something intensely personal was involved. Although it required careful protection, such an interaction could well offer its participants intellectual gratification unlike any others. Thus, Sullivan's private liberalism was not simply a collection of ideas and practices that could not be made public and as a result were repressed; it constituted an intellectual and cultural realm that paralleled and pushed public liberalism in science, a place to find a sense of belonging and satisfaction.

However implicitly, Sullivan's impulse to include human subjectivity in scientific discourse corresponded with the aspiration of other medical and social scientists to formulate life history as a legitimate method of investigation. The question that remained unanswered was what kind of subjectivity would be appropriate. Would scientists accept any subjectivity, or would they draw a line at a subjectivity that revolved around sexuality? What about homosexuality? The Sullivan-Sapir exchange suggests that Sullivan was testing the water to see if he could find answers to these questions. An urgent matter that also remained unarticulated was whose subjectivity needed be integrated into science. Would it be informants' subjectivity, or would it include, as the concept of "participant observation" suggested, researchers' as well? This was perhaps one of the most daunting questions for scientists, because of its immediate relevance to their data's validity. If they accepted their own subjectivity, how could they claim their data's authenticity? The most revealing of scientists' responses to this question can be found in one social scientist's support for life history in a psychiatric setting during the first colloquium. Surely unknown to most people in the room was the fact that he had been reluctant to offer his own life history when he was a patient at a mental hospital. He was hospitalized at Sheppard-Pratt between November 1928 and February 1929, with a diagnosis of schizophrenia. Apparently, he was able to maintain his intellectual life for most of the hospitalization (the first colloquium took place in December 1928, the second in December 1929). He was not the most cooperative patient, according to doctors' observations, however. About two months into his hospitalization, doctors still had to struggle to get him to talk. "During an interview of an hour or more, the patient talked fairly freely, but showed that in really intimate personal matters he was quite reserved," one doctor noted in the patient's record. When his condition was better, the patient's reservation became even stronger: "As he improves, he becomes impatient, and shows decided aversion to taking up his problems in any way which would imply close contact on the part of an outsider with his most personal problems. He holds that there are problems which are beyond psychiatry, which must be settled by one's self."[34] Contrary to his enthusiasm about life history as a social scientist, as a patient he was unwilling to have the method applied to himself. He protected his privacy, and he believed that subjective aspects of his experience should remain undisturbed by scientific intrusion. The disparity between his views as a scientist and as a subject of study revealed the difficulty of fully incorporating subjective matters into scientific materials.

Scientists supported life history's possibility to open up subjectivity, while their support strictly drew upon their established status as scientific observers. Scientists at the colloquia did not articulate what it meant to contribute a life history as an informant, as someone placed on the other side of a scientific inquiry. In theory, the inclusion of subjectivity in social scientific materials was unquestionably welcome. The problem was that, even when interviewers and interviewees became aware that they had things in common (homosexual experiences, as in Sullivan's case) in practice, such awareness remained on the periphery of scientific method. To be sure, as the Sullivan-Sapir exchange suggested, issues of homosexuality that received only an ambiguous recognition still occupied an important place in the history of the science of homosexuality; it suggests that although scientists mostly kept their sexuality and subjectivity private, they were sufficiently moved to see a public dimension. And yet, what emerged as a consensus was something less controversial; a recognition of a variety of human experiences and a need to integrate medical and social sciences to train researchers specializing in life history to examine these variations. Despite his explicit and implicit disagreement with this mainstream approach, Sullivan was not incapable of going along with this consensus. Indeed, many of his accomplishments in the 1930s—the making of the "science" of interpersonal relations, interdisciplinary research programs, and proposals for the reform of medical education—fit well with the public tenets of collaboration established by the colloquium. Even as some of his remarks in the colloquia pointed to the integration of his private liberalism into a public frame, then, he began to formulate an intellectual scheme that was mostly detached from his subjective experience as a gay psychiatrist.

Interdisciplinary Scientists at Work

Notwithstanding his failure in 1929 to obtain support for his plan to create a discipline of "social psychiatry," Sullivan was gratified that various endeavors were under way for interdisciplinary collaboration. For example, Harold Lasswell launched his research on personality at a mental hospital soon after the second colloquium, the result of which was published as *Psychopathology and Politics* in 1930.[35] Lasswell and Sullivan joined the seminar called "Culture and Personality" at Yale University in 1932 and 1933, funded through Lawrence Frank at the Social Science Research Council and organized by Edward Sapir. In Chicago, the impact of life history and psychoanalytic methods remained strong, producing some of the best-known sociological studies of urban slums, gangs, and immigrant communities under Robert E. Park and Ernest Burgess's initiative.[36] Chicago-trained sociologists Allison Davis and John Dollard in 1937 began a case study of "personality development from a combined psychological and cultural point of view," using African American children in New Orleans and Natchez, Mississippi, as their subjects.[37] Also, based on the discussion in the colloquia, Sullivan designed a new curriculum in psychiatric postgraduate education. When he established the Washington School of Psychiatry in 1936, he invited social scientists, including Harold Lasswell, Erich Fromm, and Ruth F. Benedict, as lecturers.[38] These social scientists also contributed to *Psychiatry*, an interdisciplinary journal that Sullivan started in 1938, drawing articles from psychiatrists, psychoanalysts, and social scientists.[39] Further, Alfred H. Stanton, a psychiatrist who would work with Sullivan at the Chestnut Lodge Hospital in the 1940s, and Morris S. Schwartz, a University of Chicago sociologist, collaborated in the 1930s on research on the impact of the institutional environment on psychiatric patients. Their work resulted in a landmark sociological study, *The Mental Hospital*, published in 1954.[40] Along with these developments, Sullivan's plan to transform the "existing social system" began to assume a new phase in the 1930s.

One of the earliest signs of this new phase of the interdisciplinary program was the establishment of his interpersonal theory of mental illness. While Sullivan's use of the word *interpersonal* remained somewhat fluid during the 1920s, it was clearly the most important concept in his theory by the mid-1930s. During the 1920s, he often used the adjective *interpersonal* interchangeably with *societal*.[41] Many of his unpublished manuscripts did not include the term, but instead employed descriptive explanations such as "[a person] govern[s] himself in accordance with the wishes of others"[42] and "cultural symbols . . . are derived entirely from events including other persons."[43] In other cases, he used a compound word, *inter-personal*, not the singular term *interpersonal*.[44] But in the mid-1930s, he came to use the adjective *interpersonal* more regularly in combination with *relation*, making it a key concept in his writing.[45] As he settled on this term, his theoretical scope was adjusted accordingly. In the early 1930s, his writing came to include a systematic discussion of stages of "normal" personality development, departing from his earlier focus on mental "abnormality." Similarly, in his published writing on interpersonal relations, the issue of homosexuality was not clearly demarcated as such for his readers.

This is nowhere better seen than in the pages of *Personal Psychopathology*, a book written between 1929 and 1933. Here, Sullivan offered his first comprehensive theory of personality development, in which he astutely embedded his critique of homophobia. In this, his first monograph, Sullivan made it clear that his subject was not a theory of mental disorders, but one involving "typical courses of events" consisting of "matters of common experience"—a life process in general. Thus he discussed developmental stages, beginning with "infancy." According to Sullivan, an infant is born into a "primary group" that consists of two people—an infant and a mother. In this primary group, an infant develops "facilities for communication," such as smiling, crying, and temper tantrums. These facilities are responses to a mother's emotional conditions: when she is happy, the infant feels secure; when she is nervous, her baby develops insecurity. This tight emotional synchronization he called "empathy" remains an important factor in any interpersonal relation throughout life. Infancy ends when "the young one begins to acquire the spoken language of his people" roughly at the age of eighteen months.[46] The next stage, that of "childhood," thus begins with the appearance of articulate speech, with which a child learns mores, habits, and fashions. In this way, a child's personality comes to be exposed to sociocultural factors, and a "certain . . . type of ideals and ambitions" emerges in a child's consciousness. A young one becomes a "creature of culture" in childhood, Sullivan concluded (40–41).

In the next stage, that of the "juvenile era," a child enters a "secondary group" which, unlike the primary group in infancy, includes people other than family members, such as teachers and classmates in grade school. With this transfer from the primary to the secondary group at about the age of six, "others" come to carry more importance. At this stage, however, the socialization with others is primarily egocentric. A child shows an appreciation of the needs of others only when they are favorable to his or her own interests (42). When the next stage, "preadolescence," begins at about the age of eight, the egocentric character of a child's sociality subsides. A preadolescent develops the need for an intimate playmate of similar age. In this need for an intimate interpersonal relation, it becomes more important to contribute to the pleasure of the other. Oftentimes, contributions to the self-esteem of a "chum" matter more than the satisfaction of one's self-interest. In this close association with a chum, "peculiarities of the home life . . . tend to lose their . . . effectiveness because they fall into unfavorable comparison with similar factors in the home life of the other." Thus the chum relationship is the beginning of a "social world," where conflicts brought from family relationships may be resolved as a "result of . . . new experience toward a rational integration." Consequently, the likelihood that members of a well-integrated social world grow healthily is high (164–167). In the next stage, "adolescence," a need for an intimate interpersonal relation is directed toward a person of the opposite sex. When one achieves a stable relation involving another person of the opposite sex, in which "sexual drives, desires, or needs" are resolved, this person enters into "adulthood" (44).

In *Personal Psychopathology*, it is unmistakable that all the stage markers in personality development are defined as changes in interpersonal relations. It is also obvious that the sociocultural factors that had an impact on personality development were more than those related to sexuality. Reflecting the expansion of his theoretical scope, which was pushed by his collaboration with social scientists, Sullivan's discussion in *Personal Psychopathology* included a range of interpersonally and socially constructed events. Embedded in this scheme, however, was his emphasis on the importance of broadening the realm of socially acceptable sexual relationships. Sullivan noted, for instance, the danger of the prolonged continuation of the primary group, because he believed that it created a warp in a person's personality that was "so great that [a person] cannot find anyone . . . with whom he can establish chumship" in preadolescence. Chumship in his definition was a close friendship between children of the same sex, insuring a sense of belonging that helped a child find a place in a larger group of same-sex friends. This larger group, sometimes called a "gang," often manifested sexual intimacies such as "mutual masturbation . . . and homosexual procedures." Contradicting mainstream psychiatric theories that defined this manifestation as a "deleterious" and "unfortunate . . . homosexual stage" (162, 165, 170), Sullivan

argued that these expressions of homoeroticism strengthened a bond within
the group and helped its members to adjust to heterosexual relationships
later in their lives:

> I have had opportunity to study one community in regard to the
> alleged evil consequences of these factors. . . . In this community—a
> large number of early adolescents participated in overt homosexual
> activities during the gang age. Most of them progressed . . . to the
> customary heteroerotic interest in later adolescence. Some of the few
> boys in this community who were excluded from the gangs as a result
> of their powerful inhibitions, who missed participation in community
> homosexual play, did not progress to satisfactory heterosexual devel-
> opment. (171)

Here, Sullivan's assertion was that homosexual experiences at a young age
were crucial for heterosexual maturity in later years. Such a developmental
conceptualization of homosexuality was challenged by many of his Sheppard-
Pratt patients who considered homosexuality a status in its own right, but it
nonetheless found a place in *Personal Psychopathology*. Even so, he pointedly
argued that, in a sexually rigid culture (such as modern American culture),
"there is generally sufficient personal frustration . . . [to necessitate] sexual
fantasy with almost any symbols" (163), including those of a homosexual
nature. On the one hand, his discussion of sexual problems would take the
form of a more general analysis of interpersonal relations. On the other,
his recognition of the importance of same-sex intimacy and his critique of
homophobia are palpable between the lines.

Only in moderate tone and language did Sullivan in *Personal Psychopathology* criticize the limited social acceptance of homosexuality. In the U.S.
general population, the proportion of people who "completed the evolution to the state of adulthood," an intimate relationship with a partner of
the opposite sex, was "not very great." Because of the popular belief that
"woman is declassed [when she has] sexual intercourse with a man, before
having married him, . . . a turning to the autoerotic or the homoerotic types
of interests" was common (43–44, 194). If these common interests were
socially accepted, the benefit could be immense. Indeed, as Sullivan argued,
"homoerotic interests in the female . . . encounter little social disapproval;
in fact, there is almost no attention given the erotic elements accompanying
such relationship." Compared with her male counterpart, a female homosexual achieved "an easier adaptation to her role" in her adult life (258).
Nevertheless, there remained the fact that his emphasis was framed by a
developmental theory that assumed that same-sex sexual relationships were
not part of a complete adulthood. The question of what should be done in a
society that did not allow a majority of its members to achieve full maturity

was left unarticulated. This was a departure from his recognition at Sheppard-Pratt that, because homosexual relationships are common, people with
homosexual conflicts should encourage society to better accept them rather
than wasting their time trying to grow out of homoeroticism.

Even this modified approach to homosexuality elicited his colleagues'
reservations about *Personal Psychopathology* as a scientific monograph.
Edward Sapir used it as a textbook in his seminar at Yale, and its members
thought that it was too centered on psychoanalysis, suffering from Freud's
apparently outbalanced emphasis on the importance of libido. If this suggested an uneasy status that both Freud and sexuality occupied in American
science, the title of the book fueled a rumor that the work was Sullivan's
autobiography. Eventually, Sullivan withdrew the book from publication,
noting that the monograph was only "privately circulated" (ix). In this way,
his attempt to include his subjectivity in science was circumscribed, even as
it was embedded in his professional concern for interpersonal relationships.
A scientist's subjectivity, especially that related to sexuality, was denied a
role in scientific theory. After the two colloquia on personality investigation
in 1928 and 1929, then, Sullivan embarked on more clear-cut, research programs that would not raise questions of subjectivity—at least not in the way
that *Personal Psychopathology* did. In 1932, he joined Sapir's seminar on culture and personality, making it a habit to travel to New Haven once a week.
By then, Sullivan was a close friend of Sapir, who had been at the University
of Chicago and had just relocated to the Institute of Human Relations at Yale
University. In addition to attending seminars, Sullivan often went to Sapir's
second house on a New Hampshire farm during summers, where Sapir spent
time with his second wife, Jean, and his children.[47] Through Sapir, Sullivan became acquainted with rising social scientists such as John Dollard,
Harold C. Taylor, and Hortense Powdermaker, as well as Mark A. May, with
whom Sullivan had had a discussion of the social context of interpersonal
relations at the colloquium.[48]

This group of social scientists offered Sullivan both intellectual inspiration and institutional grounds from which he could take leave of the sensitive subject of homosexuality and develop an apparently more mainstream
science of interpersonal relations. The group's research programs in 1932
and 1933 mirrored some of the recognizable trends in the era's scholarship,
while they also indicated a new direction of social scientific studies. Dollard, who was first appointed as a fellow and then as an assistant director
of the seminar, had been working on psychotic behavior from sociological
standpoints. His patron Ernest Burgess at the University of Chicago praised
Dollard's all-around training in "statistical, case-study, cultural and psychoanalytic techniques," suggesting Dollard's already strong interest in an
interdisciplinary approach to life history, which would soon materialize in

a series of works, *Criteria for the Life History* (1935), *Caste and Class in Southern Town* (1937), and *Children of Bondage* (1937).[49] Further, in his report on
the status of psychological studies of personality in Germany, Dollard took
note of Ernest Kretschmer's theory positing that "lower" and "primitive"
stages of cultural function appear in "higher" and "civilized" men, especially
among schizophrenics. Here again was the parallel between primitiveness and schizophrenia. Meanwhile, the work of Harold C. Taylor, who was
just completing his degree at Yale, suggested the prevalence of research
based on the gendered model of disease. Using "phonographic records of
the speech of twenty young men, picked from the most neurotic and least
neurotic freshmen of this year's class," Taylor tried to show that neurosis,
introversion, and effeminacy were correlated to unusually high pitch of voice
among men.[50] Along with these, Hortense Powdermaker's study of an African
American community in Mississippi seemed to have a considerable impact
on Sullivan's intellectual career. In her engagement with what she called
the first anthropological study of a contemporary community in the United
States, Powdermaker collaborated with black scholars Charles S. Johnson
and E. Franklin Frazier at Fisk University. Sullivan reviewed her proposal for
a Social Science Research Council fellowship to support her research, which
helped him to shape his own research agendas.[51]

By the late 1930s, Sullivan was working on several projects about a
great range of sociocultural contexts associated with mental problems. In
a 1937 article, he mentioned "reductions in employment, reductions in the
standard of living, and damage to the prestige of collective national, racial,
regional and class symbols" as possible causes of stress and conflict. Also, he
noted that psychiatrists needed to place these factors "in proper relation to
the total historical evolution of conflicting values."[52] To substantiate these
statements, Sullivan extended his examinations of social problems, some of
which were a direct outgrowth of the Yale seminar. In particular, his interest
in race problems in the United States became so prominent in his research
that it might be said that his focus shifted from homophobia to racism, at
least in his public discussion. In 1937 and 1938, for example, he collaborated
with Johnson and Frazier, who were by then investigating personality problems among young blacks under the sponsorship of the American Council of
Education (ACE). Sullivan's role in these studies was to talk to black youths
to determine the impact of their racial, class, and geographical environment
on their personalities.[53] Frazier had been focusing on the population in the
middle states, while Johnson's research had been about the Deep South.
Sullivan served as a consultant to both, interviewing no fewer than twenty
African American youths, mostly in Washington, DC, and Memphis, Tennessee, so as to offer psychiatric insight into the influence of racial tensions on
these individuals' personality development. He drew a couple of interesting

conclusions that suggested the new direction of his research. He noted, for example, that he did not find any "typical Negro characteristics" among his informants:

> The tragedy of the Negro in America seems to be chiefly a matter of culturally determined attitudes in the whites. . . . However, when . . . the techniques of intensive study of interpersonal relations have been substituted for those of a detached and generally preoccupied professional man, the presumptively "typically Negro" performances have been resolved into particular instances of the "typically human."[54]

Sullivan saw, for instance, that "fear" of whites, widespread among African Americans in the South, was related to the "great violence" done toward them, especially lynching. He did not attribute this fear to African Americans' race. He made a similar observation about young blacks in Washington, DC. He found that most of them were struggling with deep "rage" against whites, but was quick to point out that this rage resulted from inequality between blacks and whites in the city, not from a "racial" temperament. In life histories of his black informants, then, Sullivan found unambiguous evidence of social construction of so-called natural categories.

In this project for the ACE, Sullivan also discovered that this field of research—race relationships in the United States—was an ideal arena in which to apply the method of participant observation. Without doubt, he was aware of the limits of communication between himself, a white man, and African American individuals. One of his descriptions of an interview with an "outstanding" leader of the black community, for example, illuminates Sullivan's approach to the distance between the races:

> I think that this leader . . . progressed in our acquaintanceship only from a distrust of my motives, through a distrust of my judgment, to a vague wondering if I might actually be a detached observer without blinding preconceptions and group loyalties hostile to him and his people. He seemed to me one of the loneliest of men; a well-trained professional man of rather keen sensitivity, isolated in the nexus of several fields of hostility, so driven by some complex of motives (which proved mostly inaccessible to me).[55]

Here, Sullivan admitted that there were certain things about the interviewee that he could not grasp. Unlike his earlier, relentless insistence at Sheppard-Pratt that patients reveal all things possible to him, Sullivan let this informant remain "inaccessible." But he did not dismiss the value of information obtained. Instead, he drew the conclusion that the interviewee's lack of openness indicated the serious impact of racial antagonism.[56] Apparently, such a critique of race problems was far easier for Sullivan to publish than was his protest against homophobia. On the one hand, race problems allowed him to develop ideas that mattered to him: a critique of "culturally determined attitudes" that caused "tragedy" in those who were discriminated against; a better understanding of the "fear" of being open and honest, prevalent among minorities. On the other hand, he did not have to worry about being seen as too subjectively involved in his science, as he did at Sheppard-Pratt and in *Personal Psychopathology*. Indeed, his acceptance of "inaccessible" information suggests that he was, in fact, not subjectively involved in taking the life history of the black informant. With patients suffering from homosexual conflicts, he insisted that he know everything because he felt that he could and he must; with African Americans, he could leave things unknown. His subjects were racial minorities, not sexual ones, and his whiteness was obvious in a way his sexuality was not.

The study of race also taught him how to discuss sexuality in a more mainstream, less controversial way. In his observation of a sixteen-year-old black boy in Washington, DC, for instance, Sullivan revealed his sense of what he deemed a positive attitude toward sex among African Americans. This informant said that he had masturbated with his younger brother when they were small kids, seemingly without the feelings of guilt that Sullivan had seen too commonly among his white patients at Sheppard-Pratt. The informant also claimed that he had sexual intercourse with girls and talked to his father about it when he discovered that one of these girls gave him a sexually transmitted disease. His father did not punish him, but instead helped him to get the "necessary treatments" and showed him "how to relieve" himself. In response to these details of life history that he hardly encountered in his clinical practice, Sullivan argued, "Vividly outstanding factors in . . . many Negro family groups are superficially identical with those which in whites eventuate in arrest of heterosexual development and thus to obligate homosexual or bisexual patterns of behavior."[57] Here, "outstanding factors" in black families were a recognition of sex as an important part of human life. These factors were identical to white families' only "superficially," because whites turned the recognition of sex into strict sexual inhibitions. In this contrast between the races, then, Sullivan's critique of homophobia took a more general, recognizable form of an examination of white Americans' limited approach to sex.

This approach made sense in the intellectual climate of the 1930s. By the end of the decade, it was not unusual for physicians, psychologists, and sociologists to argue that seeing masturbation as a cause of mental problems was misguided.[58] In addition, as seen in studies of researchers such as Powdermaker, Sullivan, and Dollard, a cultural, rather than biological, understanding of race was becoming the norm among progressive medical and social scientists. In particular, African Americans in the South attracted these scientists' interest, as "others" who were nevertheless "within" American society—"American primitive(s)" who "promised both abnormality and authenticity" as research subjects.[59] In Sullivan's discussion, it is not difficult to see that he benefited from both the supposed abnormality and the authenticity of blacks. His characterization of African Americans as sexually "permissive" can be seen as being connected to the racist belief that all African Americans are "promiscuous." Indeed, he asserted, "there are many definitely promiscuous [black] people" and "this laxity arises from . . . a permissive culture." But he also disagreed with the misconception that all blacks are abnormal when he wrote: "I have to speak . . . against using them [African Americans] as scapegoats for our [whites'] unacceptable impulses; the fact that they are . . . poorly adapted to our historic puritanism is really too naïve a basis for projecting most of our privately condemned faults upon them."[60] This statement recognized that whites' fear of sex had indeed been projected on blacks, illuminating how African Americans were a "subject" close enough and, at the same time, different enough for white scientists to explore.[61] This mixture of fascination, respect, and prejudice lay beneath Sullivan's discussion of African Americans' attitude toward sex. It was precisely this mixture that made it easier for him to discuss sexuality within the context of race problems rather than as the problem of homophobia. Compared with white homosexual men, blacks were not close enough to Sullivan's subjectivity to force him to probe how it felt to be stigmatized. He could "participate" in African American life histories, highlighting injustice of both racial and sexual kinds, while keeping his own subjectivity at arms' length. In concluding his argument, he stressed that white Americans must "cultivate a humanistic rather than a paternalistic attitude" to blacks.[62] Reading this statement, no one would have wondered if he made a similar point about homosexual individuals (which he did at Sheppard-Pratt). This was because there was no hint of the scientist's homosexuality and subjectivity in this statement, even though the discussion was about sexuality.

It is ironic that, right around this time, he suggested that his white male friends sleep with black women to become free sexually (see Chapter 4). Moreover, less than two years after he drew this conclusion about the need for a humane attitude toward African Americans, he was involved in the psychiatric screening for the Selective Service, which accentuated racism (see Chapter 5). The lack of subjective involvement had its consequences, as much as the lack of public assertion of private liberalism. These consequences were most conspicuous in the ways in which Sullivan interacted with African American researchers in the 1930s. Working with Johnson, for example, Sullivan consistently arranged meetings in his office either in New York City or Washington, DC. When Johnson asked Sullivan to visit him in Nashville, Sullivan sent an apologetic letter noting that his "alleged financing

program has made no material progress [and he] see[s] no immediate possibility" of traveling. This prompted Johnson to reiterate that he would make
"available a fund for travel and expenses." Such an uneven relationship
persisted even after the completion of the research. In 1939, Johnson recommended an African American student at Fisk to meet with Sullivan, so that
the student could be trained in psychiatric techniques of personality study.
It took Sullivan three and half months to respond. When he eventually did,
he filled his letter with details of his busy schedule and his suggestion that
the student read his soon to be published lecture notes rather than attending his lectures at the Washington School of Psychiatry. It is not clear if Sullivan thought about the impact of inviting a black student to an all-white
institute. Regardless, Johnson's response was respectful, acknowledging "the
pressure on you" that must have caused "the long delay." But with two more
months without a word from Sullivan, Johnson wrote another letter to urge
him to set up an appointment with the student. Yet another month passed,
and Johnson's next letter suggested that the student follow Sullivan to Cin-
cinnati where he was scheduled to attend a conference. There was no indication that Sullivan ever responded to this rather urgent plea.[63] His critique
of racism, which he put out in public forcefully, did not seem to shape his
person-to-person interactions with his black colleagues.

Despite this standoffishness, which might or might not have been a
sign of Sullivan's awareness of race barrier but was most likely interpreted
as such by Johnson, their collaboration opened up an arena for a range of
skills and expertise to come together, putting psychiatry at the center of the
interdisciplinary scholarship.[64] Sullivan's theory of mental illness made a
notable contribution to the new psychiatry and the mental hygiene movement as well.[65] One important feature in *Personal Psychopathology* and his
articles in the 1930s was his assertion of a possibility for change in a personality throughout preadolescence and adolescence.[66] This was a positive
view, especially when it was applied to mental illness, because it suggested
a hope for recovery even at relatively advanced ages. In addition, Sullivan's
specialty since his Sheppard-Pratt days in the eyes of many had been schizophrenia. Schizophrenia was among the most serious of mental illnesses, and
it continued to be the single largest diagnosis given to inmates at state institutions throughout the 1920s and 1930s.[67] Sullivan's optimism, combined
with his ever expanding emphasis on sociocultural factors, pointed toward
the hope that even people with schizophrenia could be cured, if society
were different. Increasingly, it was his belief that society could dramatically
improve through intellectual and institutional innovations. And he had
many plans to change medical education; there were issues other than race
to be included in the interdisciplinary research programs. These tasks came
to occupy a considerable part of Sullivan's professional life.

Institutions for De-institutionalization

As seen in the discussion at the colloquia, the reform of medical education was a widely shared concern among psychiatrists, especially those who
supported the new psychiatry. In the early 1930s, Frankwood E. Williams,
William A. White—both representatives of the National Institute of Mental
Health—and Sullivan, fresh from his success at the colloquia, helped create a
Joint Committee on Psychiatric Education for the APA. Although the committee's work was much compromised as a result of negotiation with biological
theorists, the idea of educational reform began to gain the profession's support. Williams, for instance, pointed out medical educators' lack of attention
to "practical" issues that physicians were likely to encounter in their clinical
work. Using the prevalence of neurosis in forms of gastric and cardiac problems as an example, Williams claimed that all medical practitioners—not
just psychiatrists—needed to have some knowledge of psychiatry.[68] Sullivan's
proposal more clearly reflected his determination to secure psychiatry's tie
with the social sciences. Echoing the discussion at the colloquia, he criticized medical scientists that collected "objective" data in controlled environment. In contrast, he praised a student of psychiatry who observed his
subject while he "participates . . . in the data which he is assembling."[69] This
"participant observation" was one of the basic methods of examining current interpersonal relations,[70] while another method, "life history," recorded
a person's past interpersonal relations.[71] His plan for medical school curriculum, based on these methods, was demanding. In the freshman year, lectures
on cultural anthropology, sociology, economics, political science, literature,
art, and history would be offered. In the second year, students would be
required to examine their own life histories with their supervisors.[72] In
their third and fourth years, students would begin "supervised contact with
carefully selected clinical material," allowing them to practice participant
observation and life history method in a quasi-clinical setting.[73] It is apparent that Sullivan's curriculum was nothing if not radically different from the
standard. Most medical schools during the 1920s and 1930s offered courses
on biology, chemistry, physics, anatomy, physiology, pathology, and phar-
macology in the first years of medical education, but almost never the social
sciences and humanities.[74] But there were signs of change in medicine and
its allied fields. The Association of American Medical Colleges put together
a report on the lack of practice-oriented training in 1932. The American
Association of Social Workers published a series of reports on techniques
of communication with patients, pushing for medicine that would be more
open to human interaction.[75]

Sullivan's proposal found the first opportunity for institutional application at the Washington School of Psychiatry, established with Sullivan as a

head of the Division of Psychiatry, psychiatrist Ernest Hadley as a chair of the Division of Biological Sciences, and Edward Sapir as a director of the Division of Social Sciences. Soon after the school was established, an arrangement was made with the Washington-Baltimore Psychoanalytic Society for its members to take courses in psychoanalysis at the school.[76] Moreover, as Charles S. Johnson's recommendation of his student at Fisk University suggested, the school was open to social science students who desired to learn psychiatry.[77] The class titled "Non-Clinical Psychoanalysis" consisted of roundtable presentations: Sullivan's "Psychoanalysis and Social Sciences," Ruth Benedict's "Cultural Anthropology," Randolph Paul's "Taxation," Harold Lasswell's "Political Sciences," E. M. Jellinek's "Statistics," Howard Rowland's "Sociology," and Tom Gill's "Literature."[78] This was close to what Sullivan had in mind as a fully reformed medical education, while it looked somewhat out of place to those who were not familiar with the ongoing interdisciplinary collaboration. Indeed, one psychoanalyst, Douglas Noble, a graduate of the school, wrote in 1968, "Drs. Dooley [Lucile Dooley, a psychoanalyst who taught at the school] and Hadley . . . had tended to maintain a distinctly more orthodox psychoanalytic position. They were at the pains to clarify and preserve the distinctions between Sullivan's ideas and mainstream psychoanalytic principles."[79] Still, the 1930s was a time when psychoanalytically "oriented," if not "trained," psychiatrists such as White and Sullivan were influential in both psychiatry and psychoanalysis.[80] Leading analysts such as Karl Menninger, Clara Thompson, Karen Horney, Erich Fromm, and Frieda Fromm-Reichmann supported the consideration of social and cultural factors in psychoanalysis.[81] In this climate, Sullivan continued to promote his theory of interpersonal relations at the school, and also in the journal *Psychiatry*, established in 1938. In the editorial note in the journal's first issue, he explained the current development of psychiatry, illuminating his alliance with the mental hygiene movement:

> It [psychiatry] has extended from the asylum . . . through preventive programs in Child Guidance, School and College Mental Health Clinics, and Family Adjustment Centers, into practically every serious attempt at assessing group relationships, social organization and disorganization, personal success and failure. . . . It is becoming a science that is fundamental . . . to research into almost any aspect of people and interpersonal relations, broadly conceived.[82]

This conveyed one of the largest areas of Sullivan's thinking in the 1930s: scientific research into human relations at nontraditional institutions for mental health. These modern institutions needed intellectual and educational supports, which Sullivan hoped to offer through the school and the journal. In his so doing, his plans would contribute to the mental hygiene movement. The William Alanson White Psychiatric Foundation, created in 1933 by Dooley and Sullivan, offered a similar appeal to both the mental hygiene movement and the interdisciplinary scholarship on life history. Originally intended to gather resources to support Sapir's seminar at Yale, the foundation from the second half of the 1930s began to function as a fund-raiser for the Washington school, *Psychiatry*, and other interdisciplinary research programs. Soon after the foundation was established, for example, Sullivan, Sapir, and Lasswell contemplated the making of a research institute called the Institute of Ethnic Psychiatry. Its blueprint reveals much about the expansion of the life history method. In their plan, the institute was to further the "comparative analysis of personality development," especially with a focus on "difficulties [of youths] in adapting to the adult standards" in Western and non-Western societies. It would compare adaptive difficulties in different societies to understand "the depth of our entanglement in . . . a single culture." Such entanglements tend to make it difficult for youth in changing social circumstance to maintain mental health. Data from the "culture areas widely divergent from ours" would help individuals become aware of the relativity of their own culture and adjust to it in more flexible ways. The project's plan also noted that schizophrenia was "infrequent in some societies" and thus scientists needed to learn from such societies in order to design "therapeutic rearrangement of the cultural setting" in illness-prone societies. Clearly the project was based on the "civilized"–"primitive" dualism, and the assumption that studies of the latter helps the former. The fascination with "others" remained a strong force in the research agenda of the institute.

The blueprint of the institute also reflected the genuine urge on the part of scientists to make the utmost effort to better understand "others." For instance, the proposal noted political "unrest" as one good index of difficult cultural adaptation. Thus, the institute's research would focus on areas where political discontent was "active" or "inactive," in order to obtain the best comparison. The best contemporary example of the "active" was expanding communism in Soviet Union and its surrounding territories. By contrast, there were cultural situations in which political unrest was unusual, or "inactive," as in some Native American communities. Suitably, Lasswell was to take the initiative in "active" countries, while Sapir would be in charge of the study of "inactive" communities. Meanwhile, Sullivan would collect data from psychiatric patients from the United States for comparison. All these areas of study would be united by way of the method of life history, or "field survey" with a focus on personality conflicts and disorders. If this project reiterated their willingness to rethink American culture in light of "others," the fellowship program associated with this project suggested a result yielded by the decade-old discussion of "participant observation." In describing desirable candidates for the fellowships, the organizers noted, "Satisfactory candidates may appear from the more divergent groups in the United States, such as the Negroes and the American Indians. . . . The acceptance of some candidates who are foreign students of advanced educational standing [was] also desirable."[83] Compared to the mainstream scheme in which white researchers go to "primitive" societies to "examine" them, this was a more assertive statement of inclusion.

Although the institute did not materialize, perhaps because of a lack of financial resources, the work of medical and social scientists in the life history cohort in the late 1930s marked the height of a significant attempt to confront the limits of modern science. In many ways, this effort accomplished a revision of old institutions—state mental hospitals, medical schools, and disciplinary departments—that were impervious to aspects of 1920s and 1930s modernity. But the new institutions had blind spots of their own. The nature of participant observation raised questions about the assumed distance between researchers and research subjects, but its implications for the data's scientific validity remained largely unarticulated. Researchers who were open about their own subjectivity might risk their standing as scholars, as indicated by their response to Sullivan's *Personal Psychopathology*. It was not only Sullivan who experienced the harsh critique. Powdermaker's *After Freedom* (a result of her work in Indianola, Mississippi, that she began at Yale) in 1939 also drew comments such as "too personally involved," "too anecdotal," and "does not show grounding in the literature."[84] In this atmosphere, the life history method began to embody a certain disengagement with human subjectivity; it became exclusively geared to the subjectivity of the articulate. Already in the 1920s, Sheppard-Pratt doctors accepted life histories of certain patients—patients whom physicians deemed to be self-aware and willing to talk—only. In psychiatric practice in general, this could mean patients with mild or early illnesses, a perfect fit for emerging institutes for mental hygiene. Beneficial as it might have been to some, this focus drove the psychiatric profession's attention away from a great number of patients who were chronically ill and needed care and comfort rather than strenuous examinations of their life histories. As the profession became increasingly engaged in treatment of mild neurotic cases at counseling rooms and mental health clinics, in the 1930s, psychiatric medicine lost relevancy to patients at state institutions who were not willing or capable of talking. In these silent individuals, psychiatrists failed to discern subjectivity worth inclusion in science. Sullivan's increasing engagement in the institutionalization of research and education in the 1930s followed the same pattern. His belief in the curability of schizophrenia added a hopeful note to the reform impulse, but it was not practically applied to schizophrenic patients at state institutions.

Of course, like other psychiatric reformers, Sullivan believed that preventive mental hygiene was the best way to reduce the number of chronic patients in the future.[85] Theirs was a grand psychiatric project to create a healthier, better society, by eliminating problems before they became too debilitating. Certainly, psychiatrists' effort for prevention was not without its achievements: it disseminated psychiatric services and made them more accessible to people in need: in turn, it allowed psychiatrists to enjoy increased demand for their professional skills and knowledge. At the same time, however, the reform left out certain types of patients who did not fit their approach. Oftentimes, the lack of retrievable subjectivity coincided with patients in lower social classes. In many mental hygiene clinics, clients were financially comfortable, while the population at state institutions were largely from families with limited resources.[86] As if to mirror this, Sullivan's lifestyle after he began his private clinic in New York City became extravagant. His luxurious five-story townhouse on East Sixty-fourth Street, where Sullivan and Jimmie moved in 1936, was filled with sumptuous furniture and collectibles, vividly recalled by some of his friends long after his death.[87] Even though he was not without financial instability during his years in New York City, it was apparent that his move from Sheppard-Pratt to private practice introduced him to a life of affluence. In this way, the scientist's subjective experience of his own life history changed as well.

One telling sign illuminating the limits of liberal reform in psychiatry was a statistical one, a kind of data that researchers in the life history cohort deserted as old-fashioned, rigid, and even unscientific. As if to reiterate the fact that inpatients at state institutions were mostly forgotten, the U.S. Census Bureau's national survey continued to indicate a constant increase in their number, a problem that remained unresolved until the introduction of antipsychotic drugs and the demise of state institutions in the 1950s.[88] From these inpatients' perspective, life history might have seemed a method suited only to the privileged, suggesting the limits of liberal reform that sought out experiences of the socially marginalized. The unconscious, or "others" within "us," fascinated scientists, but their subjects had to have words to speak for themselves to remain in the realm of scientific research. Given this, it is striking that issues of homosexuality had a place at least between the lines in academic debate. The presence of these issues could be made public as long as it was not done too explicitly or subjectively. Ambiguous as this might have been, such an approach had the benefit of keeping the discussion of homosexuality alive, if under the surface. In Sullivan's vocabulary, for instance, "schizophrenic" could be code for "homosexual," making it feasible for him to move from one audience to another without changing his subject, just as he did in his exchange with Sapir. Likewise, his scholarship made a shift from sexual to racial tensions in the United States, allowing him to criticize the white mainstream culture that he considered to be the source of both homophobia and racism. As the next chapter examines, such fluid and fleeting presentation also shaped the scientific approach to sexual subjectivity and relativity in the 1930s.

4

Homosexuality

The Stepchild of Interwar Liberalism

Just as the life history method was a scientific response to the changing relationship between "us" and "others" in modern America, the science of homosexuality in the 1920s and 1930s reflected the era's shifting ideas about sexuality, gender, and culture. One striking characteristic of the scientific approach to homosexuality in these decades was a proliferation of different theories about its nature. To be sure, since the beginning of modern sexology at the turn of the century, constitutional and environmental views had coexisted, producing a wide range of theories about the cause of homosexuality, its dangerousness, and a debate over its malleability. But the interwar decades offered a particularly conflicted, challenging setting for medical and social scientists who together tried to make sense of homosexuality. For one, the scientists began to recognize same-sex attraction as a common phenomenon, especially among youth. Some went so far as to argue that homosexual experiences were useful components of a person's growth, not something that should alert doctors and teachers as a sign of deviation. Although still within the constraining developmental scheme of "maturity," this approach nevertheless was shaped by the possibility for the reconfiguration of sexual identities and gender relationships that the era embraced. The more visible this possibility became in American life, the more necessary it seemed for scientists to educate youth with realistic information. Moreover, there were scientists who began to define homosexuality in an entirely different cultural light. For them, homosexual men and women were artistic, cultured, and refined people who rose above the ordinary, because of their presumed openness to modernity. Unlike individuals who were sexually tense for whatever reasons, some homosexual persons seemed to represent some of the most exciting, if unsettling, elements of modernity—the pursuit of relationships outside marriage and reproduction,

membership in sophisticated urban cultures, and openness to sexual pleasure unconstrained by religious teachings. Although these scientists never
spoke for a majority of their colleagues, their voices became more audible
during these decades, a change no doubt influenced by growing urban communities of sexual minorities and scientists' aspiration to integrate diverse
experiences of "others" in knowledge.

This new model favoring homosexuality over heterosexuality in certain
ways contradicted the contemporary view of homosexuality as an illness or
a problem peculiar to modern society, suggesting how the science of homosexuality mirrored a transitional, conflicted moment in the history of American liberalism. How can a person be ill and at the same time extraordinary?
Drawing on a long-standing cultural imagination that connected creative
genius to mental illness, scientists in the 1920s and 1930s developed an
astute way of bringing these contradictory images together.[1] The defense of
homosexuality as possibly the most apt sexuality in modern civilization was
done through a discussion of homosexual persons as "others," exotic rather
than real-life individuals who belonged to the United States as full citizens.
In their public discussion of homosexuality, then, physicians argued that
homosexual individuals had desirable qualities even though the latter were
psychosexually immature and possibly pathological. Likewise, anthropologists suggested in their published writings that nonjudgmental attitudes
toward homosexuality in "primitive" societies offered a useful counterpoint
to sexually rigid America, which was, by consensus, "civilized."[2] While some
of these scientists worked to make Americans less homophobic, their argument was cast in terms of "us" speaking about "others," building on the
dualism between the "civilized" and "primitive" and the separation of scientists' subjectivity from that of their subjects. Ultimately, these conceptual
dualities contributed to an ideological distance that limited liberal science's
influence on achieving a better acceptance of homosexuality in the United
States. At the same time, the distance between researchers and their subjects shielded the former from the theoretical flaw that came from simulta-
neously approving and disapproving homosexuality.

This distance between "us" and "others" also protected scientists who
were sexual minorities from the danger of being seen as getting too subjectively involved in their research. While some of these scientists—Ruth Fulton
Benedict and Harry Stack Sullivan in particular—seemed aware of the meanings of their sexualities in their "private" lives, their "public" discussions of
homosexuality continued to keep a certain distance from issues surrounding
homosexuality in their contemporary United States. This was striking, particularly in light of the ease and confidence with which these scientists supported a fuller acceptance of sexual minorities when they talked with their
partners, friends, and (in Sullivan's case) patients. For instance, Sullivan's

clinical practice after he left Sheppard-Pratt in 1930 took on a more radical sexual phase, almost to a degree that it caused a serious concern and, in some cases, resentment among his patients and colleagues. Benedict, even when her exploration of homophobia was overshadowed by a critique of gender inequality in published writing, cherished her network of female friends and lovers, in which marriage and reproduction were less than central. This distance between private openness and public guardedness was observed by colleagues of these scientists, as they witnessed their friends' apparently contradictory attitudes firsthand. This was the case with Edward Sapir and Margaret Mead, who were close to both Benedict and Sullivan. These intellectuals' public and private approaches to homosexuality thus illuminate the science of homosexuality not only as it generated theories, but also as it shaped and was shaped by the subjective experiences of those who were involved in its making. The intense interaction between the scientific and subjective and, ultimately, an unbridgeable gap between public and private aspects of science further reveals the limits of liberalism between the wars, particularly in the context of Americans' self-conscious effort to conceptualize "others" both within and without the nation's boundaries. In a way not dissimilar to how scientists used life history to understand "others," scientific discussion of homosexuality opened up new ways to imagine possibilities in modern America amid increasing cultural diversity. And yet the emerging liberalism in the science of homosexuality was founded on ways of keeping a safe distance between researchers and their subject. Here again, scientists' own subjectivity, tied up with their private lives, became the most contested issue in their exploration of the era's transformation.

From the Immature to the Cultured

Among American followers of Freud, broadly speaking, homosexual men and women were considered to be immature people, those whose Oedipus complex remained unresolved and who could not establish a mature relationship with people of the opposite sex. Moreover, medical doctors often associated homosexuality with schizophrenia, drawing upon their symptomatic and etiological similarities. This pathological understanding remained influential throughout the 1920s and 1930s, although some scientists who supported it were not unwilling to note what appeared to be desirable qualities of homosexual persons.[3] Among the kinds of homosexual relationships that drew the era's scientific attention were those occurring in single-sex environment such as correctional facilities, urban "gangs," and single-sex educational institutions. Observers of sex segregation often claimed that it created "artificial" groups, making it difficult to for their members to achieve "normal" sexual development. Studying sexual problems at collages, for example, mental hygienist Ernest R. Groves noted the frequency with which sex caused "mental disturbance" among students. In particular, homosexual problems were difficult to resolve. But Groves did not blame individuals who engaged in homosexual relationships. Instead, he pointed to the presumed tendency that "if the college is . . . exclusively for men or for women the very artificiality of such a segregation . . . distorts sex."[4] Similar observations, clearly influenced by the era's feminism, which advocated the desegregation of the sexes, were made by sociologists as well. In their discussion, homosexual individuals were often divided into perpetrators and victims, suggesting the distinction between some who deserved to be protected from bad influence and others who were the source of such influence and beyond the reach of hygienic intervention. For instance, sociologist Winfred V. Richmond observed that from boys of the "gang" age, "the ranks of the homosexuals are every year recruited . . . who fall victim to their own half-understood desires and become the easy prey of the unscrupulous. Shutting our eyes to the problem, believing that only boys who are 'naturally' degenerate or abnormal can engage in homosexual activities, gets us nowhere."

Contrary to this alarmist concern about boys, Richmond's approach to girls was that a girl's "crush" on another girl represented a necessary transference of attachment from her mother, a useful "means of growth . . . in adolescent development."[5] Other researchers seemed to agree, although they certainly kept a careful eye on potential perpetrators. Writing about girls in correctional institutions, Lowell S. Selling, a Chicago sociologist, asserted that most inmates who experienced same-sex attraction were manifesting "pseudohomosexuality," something similar to affection between mothers and daughters and not necessarily sexual. Thus, like Richmond, Selling supported the possible usefulness of same-sex relationships for the psychosexual development of girls, while he also made a disapproving observation of "the Lesbianism," in which an "overt homosexual . . . relationship" occurred. In Selling's argument, those inmates who engaged in "the Lesbianism [were] considered pariahs and very much looked down upon by others . . . [and] not classed as [part of] the family [relationship]," suggesting his belief that a particular "kind" of female homosexuality was at the core of the problem.[6] It is clear that at times the perceived gender difference worked to domesticate (and thus to excuse) women with homosexuality, while at other times the difference seemed to vanish, highlighting what scientists regarded as the most problematic, "true" homosexuality.

Medical scientists were equally concerned to categorize a variety of homosexualities, reflecting the era's preoccupation with the question of who was responsible for this problem that was seemingly on the rise.[7] New York neurologist John F. W. Meagher, for instance, divided homosexual persons into two classes—"ethical homosexuals" who sublimated homosexual desire into socially acceptable outlets and "pervert homosexuals" who did not—to argue that the former, not the latter, was the group worthy of medical help. Mirroring the theory linking homosexuality and schizophrenia, Meagher claimed that when "ethical" homosexual persons became aware of their repressed same-sex desire, they experienced "panic," "paranoid reaction," and "dementia praecox." But "pervert" homosexual persons seldom sought clinical attention, because they—unethically—"justify their [homosexual] conduct." Thus, for Meagher, it was not the existence of "true" homosexuality, but a person's reaction to homosexual desire that mattered. To "ethical homosexuals," Meagher attributed a number of good qualities, although he was careful to note their immaturity: many homosexual individuals, men and women alike, "are intellectual and cultured, though sexually infantile."

Among those who acknowledged favorable homosexual characteristics, Meagher was moderate. John R. Ernst, a physician in Detroit, recommended that doctors always tell homosexual patients that "there is a large number of homosexuals . . . who are . . . artistic and creative, and that many of them are very clever and talented people." Los Angeles sexologist Aaron Rosanoff agreed, claiming that he had "the impression that intelligence above the average is more common among them [homosexuals]." Rosanoff also offered approving observations on the "culture" of sexual minorities, noting, for instance, that in their "dress there is much evidence of thoughtful and esthetic discrimination, careful choosing and harmonizing of colors, considerable individuality." George W. Henry, who led the famous study of "sex variants," observed that homosexual individuals "seem to be less prejudice[d] . . . against Negroes, Jews, and foreigners" than others, creating "something that bears a surface resemblance to democracy." As Henry speculated, this might be because of "the common bond of homosexuality [that] cuts across prejudices held elsewhere," indicating his awareness that there was a social bias that made homosexual persons an "underprivileged" population.[8] In addition to their apparent familiarity and comfort with these homosexual "characteristics," these researchers' comments suggest how medical scientists regarded homosexual men and women as deserving medical assistance. The consensus seemed to be that there were certain conflicted conditions unique to modern America—for example, the gap between the increased acceptance of sexual expressions on the one hand, and sex-segregated institutions on the other—and most homosexual persons were their victims. There might be some who were untreatable, but others could be helped. Indeed, focusing on this treatable group would bring a "solution" to a majority of homosexual individuals. The unique talents and tastes that many homosexual men and women seemed to possess were proof that they "deserved" to be treated. Once cured, they could well be useful citizens.

What, then, did doctors think needed to be done to treat "victims"? This was the question that brought physicians' attention not only to "others" in the United States such as troubled youth and the mentally ill, but also to "others" outside. Taking note of anthropologists' discovery of "the universality of homosexuality in primitive races," psychiatrist Donald M. Hamilton criticized how "the emotional attitude of abhorrence to homosexuality . . . so strong [in America]," caused embarrassment for even the most natural expression of friendship among people of the same sex. Such prohibition is damaging, especially because "in the highly civilized environment in which we live . . . psychological adolescence is prolonged." Because same-sex attraction is a dominant pattern of adjustment among adolescents, homosexuality naturally became frequent in this era of extended adolescence. Given this reasoning, the task of physicians was not to blame homosexuality, but to assist the patient in "sublimat[ing] his homosexuality to . . . [activities] in organizations in which he can be with his own sex." This idea of single-sex organizations was compatible with Sullivan's all-male ward at Sheppard-Pratt at least in its format, suggesting that his support for a more relaxed attitude to same-sex intimacy was not necessarily an isolated effort in science. Moreover, there were other observations that came close to Sullivan's resistance against the view of homosexuality as "sick." For example, Abraham L. Wolbarst, a New York psychiatrist, took the universality of homosexuality further, arguing that its presence in "the human race, savage or civilized, . . . [supports] that sexual variations . . . be regarded . . . as . . . normal." Although Wolbarst still commended treatment for homosexuality, and thus differed from Sullivan and some of his Sheppard-Pratt patients who desired a full acceptance of homosexuality, observations like his were notable because of their potential to materialize what he called "an enlightened social consciousness."[9] Such consciousness, as it expanded to the observations of the cultural institutions of "others," swing between the preoccupation with different "kinds" of homosexuality and the possibility for its normalization.

As seen in Hamilton's reference to "primitive races," anthropological studies were one of the sources of this emerging "social consciousness" among medical scientists. At the same time as they offered compelling information about homosexuality in foreign societies, anthropologists in the 1920s and 1930s provided medical scientists with a set of concepts that allowed the latter to see homosexuality as something larger than a person's condition: "primitive" sexuality, sexuality of "others," and proof of the human race's tendency to produce "abnormality." In particular, anthropologists who studied homosexuality among Native Americans offered a range of explanations that paralleled medical scientists' preoccupation with different "kinds" of homosexuality and, at the same time, their fascination with its favorable qualities. As seen in Chapter 3, many American anthropologists in the 1920s and 1930s began to question qualities of their own culture through the lens of others.[10] To be sure, similar to their medical counterparts, anthropologists who studied Native Americans' attitude toward homosexuality rarely pointed to the normalization of homosexuality in the United States (with the notable exception of Ruth Benedict). And yet some anthropologists broached a critique of gender inequality in the United States through their examination of homosexuality in "primitive" cultures, illuminating the extent—and ultimately the limit—of liberal "consciousness" regarding homosexuality.

Anthropological studies of Native Americans in the interwar decades took frequent note of "transvestites" and "homosexuals," and yet these figures remained ambiguous. This was in part because of the variation among different Indian tribes, and also because of the lack of clarity in Western understanding of sexual acts and identities. Sometimes these terms were used to refer to individuals who dressed, spoke, and acted like people of the opposite sex, while they were also used to denote same-sex sexual relationships. They could also be applied to people who possessed sexual organs of both sexes, as in the case of Navaho who were reported to use the term *nadle* to refer to both hermaphrodites and transvestites.[11] At any rate, anthropologists' attention was drawn to the permissiveness among Native Americans toward individuals whose gender, sexual identities, or both seemed different from the mainstream. For instance, anthropologist W. W. Hill observed that nadles played respectable roles such as mediators between men and women and guardians of wealth in their communities. No stigma was placed on nadles even when they engaged in usually prohibited acts such as promiscuity and homosexuality. George Devereux, the anthropologist who wrote perhaps most prolifically about homosexuality among Native Americans, offered a similar picture. He claimed that Mohave Indians had a ceremony for "transvestites" to officially declare their identity, after which they adapted the name of a person of the opposite sex; assume opposite gender roles; and be acknowledged as "homosexual" (*alyha* for men and *hwame* for women). They were allowed to marry, and their spouses were deemed "lucky in love" to be chosen. Often, "transvestites" (which Devereux used interchangeably with *homosexuals*) were from prominent families, while their spouses also had to possess special skills and abilities, including the spiritual power to cure diseases. To be sure, these customs were seen as being unique to "preliterate," "simpler," and "primitive" societies.[12] But the era's relativism and feminism made it a complicated issue, provoking a range of responses from anthropologists.

One response was to recognize the existence of institutionalized homosexuality, while defining it either as a phenomenon appearing only in "primitive" societies or as evidence of the universal tendency of humans to produce "abnormal" individuals. Emphasizing the "uncivilized" nature of societies that tolerated homosexuality, for instance, J. W. Layard argued that "the change of sex" (the term applied to men who assumed female roles and attires) was found in "tribes least affected by later infiltrations of culture." Moreover, regarding Pima attitude toward *berdaches* (a term used for cross-dressers), W. W. Hill asserted that these individuals were "disgraced" and "looked down upon," suggesting that even among Native Americans, homosexuality could be seen as a form of abnormality and could be a target of "ridicule and admonishment." George Devereux, in the same article in which he discussed the Mohaves' acceptance of alyha and hwame, also pointed out that their spouses, if not alyha and hwame themselves, "had to bear the brunt of the jokes that flew right and left in [their] presence." Thus, even as anthropologists observed the openness of Native Americans to cross-dressers and homosexual persons, they found ways to place it in the category of primitivity and abnormality.[13]

This could be seen as anthropologists' attempt to keep the critical impact of Native American acceptance of homosexuality on homophobic Americans at bay: rather than seeing Native American homophile attitude as a model to follow, scientists suggested that such acceptance was possible only because their societies were not exposed to civilization. The homophile attitude in "primitive" societies, then, did not indicate that homosexuality should be accepted in a "civilized" society. Nor did it suggest that homosexuality was normal. Such reasoning made it difficult for medical scientists who, inspired by anthropological studies of institutionalized homosexuality, began to take note of homosexual persons who might be more "intelligent," "artistic," and "democratic" than heterosexual individuals, to gain a coherent theoretical ground. Two conflicting images of homosexual persons—those who were abnormal and looked down upon and those who possessed extraordinary qualities and thus should be better accepted—did not seem to find a meaningful connection in the public discourse of both the medical and social sciences. Moreover, there seemed to be no clear connection between the sexualities of "us" and "others." Anthropological studies placed homosexuality in a broader scope of cultural comparison, but this did not change the primary distinction between those who constituted a standard and those who deviated from it.

There were reasons for this lack of connection, but it was not because of scientists' overall inability to compare American characteristics to their foreign counterparts on an equal ground. Indeed, feminist anthropologists delineated different "kinds" of Native American individuals who crossed gender or sexual boundaries or both, so as to criticize gender inequality in mainstream America. As early as the mid-1910s, Elsie Clews Parsons, who was soon to work with Ruth Benedict at Columbia, published a series of articles, claiming that Americans' aversion to both Indian "men-women" (men who acted like women) and American "tomboys" was "unjustifiable." The aversion was based on a belief in the rigid separation of male and female roles, no longer relevant or even "felt" by many in this era of increasing gender equality. Moreover, she pointed out how Zuni Indians were more concerned about gender roles than sexual roles. A change in gender attributes (which took place when a man cooked, for example) needed to be acknowledged socially, while "physical acts" of same-sex sexual relationships were simply accepted as a consequence of marriage involving men-women. Building on this observation questioning American conflation of gender and sexual categories, Oscar Lewis, another anthropologist trained at Columbia, argued in 1941 that "manly-hearted women" among the North Piegan—women who acted masculine—did not engage in homosexual relationships. With an unambiguous sense of fascination with the important social positions and strong personalities that these masculine women possessed, Lewis discussed how these individuals excelled both in men's and women's tasks, were wealthier and better dressed than others, were independent and assured in marital relationships, and were admired by other women as individuals who asserted "female protest in a man's culture."[14]

In explorations of different "kinds" of homosexuality like Parsons's and Lewis's, then, male dominance in the United States was scrutinized. In 1935 in her *Sex and Temperament in Three Primitive Societies*, Margaret Mead would follow suit, arguing that homosexuality in the United States originated in the extreme distinction between masculine and feminine traits. If society allowed individuals to pursue both masculine characteristics such as aggressiveness and feminine inclinations such as passivity, there would be no need for them to develop emotional or sexual attachment to a person of the same sex. Powerful as this argument might have been—especially to counter antifeminist arguments such as Read Bain's, which posited that feminism created more homosexual men (see Chapter 3)—the critique of homophobia in the United States became somewhat of secondary importance as the expansion of women's rights became the foremost issue. In their critique of Americans' preoccupation with gender divisions, the feminist argument allowed the issue of sexual desire to be absorbed by the problem of gender inequality. Homosexual persons in "primitive" societies entered American scientific thinking mostly as gender-atypical individuals; as the sexually atypical, they were not intellectually or politically exciting. They were "abnormal" persons who appeared "normal" because of their societies' primitiveness. In "civilized" societies such as the United States, they would be seen as "immature" individuals. Once scientists reached this consensus, there was nothing more to be compared and challenged. This reasoning disengaged the cross-cultural comparison of homosexuality from the question of why many homosexual persons, despite their supposed immaturity, seemed to possess desirable qualities. Ultimately, this disengagement made it difficult for anthropologists to fully confront social construction as the cause of the conflicting images of sexual minorities.

What stood out between the two main anthropological characterizations of homosexuality—that it was abnormal, if institutionalized, sexual expression of "others," on the one hand, and that it was a fascinating counterpoint of American sexism, on the other—was Benedict's focus on the bias against homosexuality as socially constructed bigotry. In unambiguous language, her 1934 article "Anthropology and the Abnormal" compared the less-than-desirable place homosexual individuals occupied in the United States to the respectable status that some Native American societies granted to homosexual persons:

> A tendency toward [homosexuality] in our culture exposes an individual to all the conflicts . . . and we tend to identify the consequences of this conflict with homosexuality. But these consequences are obviously local and cultural. . . . Whenever homosexuality has been given an honorable place in any society, those to whom it is congenial have filled adequately the honorable roles.

Compared to Hill's and Devereux's approach, which highlighted the mixed attitude of Native Americans, and to Parsons's and Lewis's focus on gender inequality, Benedict's focus was right at the center of the stigmatization of homosexuality. She did not say that homosexuality was primarily a problem of gender, nor did she refrain from discussing homosexuality in the United States, arguing that Americans' bias toward it must be changed.

Moreover, strikingly for an article written for a journal of psychology, Benedict was critical of the "treatment" of the sexually "immature," revealing her stance against anything that fell short of the full normalization of homosexuality: "Therapeutically . . . the inculcation of tolerance and appreciation toward its less usual types is fundamental. . . . The complement of this tolerance, on the patients' side, is an education in self-reliance and honesty with himself."[15] Nowhere here did she suggest that homosexuality needed to be treated; rather, acceptance by doctors, and self-awareness for homosexual "patients," was what mattered. Not in a dissimilar way as Sullivan at Sheppard-Pratt worked for self-acceptance and self-determination as members of a minority group, Benedict envisioned a society where mental hygiene involved full-brown individualism but no coercion or unsolicited intervention by others. Moreover, by claiming "honorable" roles that homosexual individuals would play in tolerant societies, Benedict came close to the image of homosexuality as extraordinary. Her suggestion of valuable qualities of homosexual persons, which she made without any reference to their supposed immaturity, set her apart from psychiatrists who, even as they discussed homosexuality positively, held on to an assumption that it was everyone's best interest to either treat or prevent the condition.

But ultimately, the positive image of homosexuality that circulated in public discussion of the medical and social sciences remained largely impersonal and unspecific, leaving Benedict's passage as perhaps the most explicit expression of antihomophobia in science. Her forceful discussion in 1934 appeared again in *Patterns of Culture*, but it did not develop into a coherent critique of homophobia, at least in her published writing.[16] Just as anthropologists did not confront two conflicting images of homosexuality, they did not make theoretical connections between gifted and well-respected homosexual men and women in "primitive" societies and intelligent, cultured homosexual individuals in "civilized" America. With the developmental scheme that was influential in the scientific understanding of both cultures and personalities, it was difficult to make sense of what seemed to be a striking similarity between such different societies. This dualistic scheme also limited medical scientists' application of liberal "social consciousness" to homosexuality in the United States. Homosexual individuals could be healthy, but only in "primitive" societies of "others." Their counterparts among "us," the "civilized," may appear healthy, but they could not be really healthy, because, in theory, they did not exist. Nonpathological homosexuality was the sexuality of "others." In this way, medical scientists insulated themselves from challenging the definition of sexual minorities as "patients" based on the observation that a number of these "sick" individuals appeared healthy, talented, and sophisticated. In medical thinking of the era, these individuals remained faceless, a population that existed elsewhere but never in front of physicians. Homosexual persons who were not "sick" were the ultimate "others," people who existed an abstract idea, not as real individuals.

One consequence of this distinction between "us" and "others" was that, instead of creating an explanation of the desirable characteristics of homosexuality in "public" discussion of science, the image of modern and refined homosexual persons flourished mostly in the "private" lives of scientists. Sullivan and Benedict offer the most revealing examples of this gap between the public and private. In Sullivan's case, one of the first signs of this public-private divide was his increasing categorization of different "kinds" of homosexuality in his published articles. Reiterating the connection between femininity and immaturity, for instance, Sullivan in 1925 asserted that there were certain individuals incapable of using language in a fully functional way. These were "females and biologically inverted males [whose command of language] . . . never develop[ed] much beyond the 'emotional' use of words." Thus, he went on to argue, it is safe to assume that, among women and men predisposed to be homosexual, "'primitive thinking' such as we see in schizophrenia" prevailed. While this assertion made a distinction between "inferior" and "superior" homosexual man, similar to Richmond and Selling's construction, another discussion by Sullivan made a unique distinction among homosexual men in 1929. In this argument, homosexual men who created "a stable relationship paralleling the enduring heterosexual couple" did not present social problems, while those who sought same-sex relationships only to secure "the attention . . . of as large a number of people as possible" were "dangerous" and often caused a "criminologic [sic] problem." Homosexual men who acted in a feminine, flamboyant way, so as to grab people's attention, were not interested in a commitment to a long-term relationship and thus were socially unacceptable.[17] Sullivan's interest in different "kinds" of homosexuality continued to develop in the 1930s, with the same emphasis on the connection between immaturity and effeminacy in homosexual men and their inability to form stable relationships.[18]

Interestingly, these distinctions were particularly conspicuous in Sullivan's circle of scientists. William V. Silverberg, Sullivan's friend and colleague in psychiatry, is a good example, as he argued:

> Non-reproduction by passive homosexuals [men who played the "female" role in sex] does not seriously menace the continuance of the race. They are not numerous and probably would not have offspring even if they did not practice their homosexuality. The real menace offered to society by these individuals is contained in their purpose to prevent from reproducing those who might otherwise reproduce; namely, just those who would be sexually most desirable to women.[19]

In this 1938 argument, it was "passive" and "feminine" homosexual men, not their "active" and "masculine" partners, who constituted a threat against society. Behind this argument seemed to be his desire to excuse "masculine" homosexual men from social accusation.

This desire might have carried a special significance for Silverberg, given the fact that he himself was gay. Silverberg took over Sullivan's ward after he left Sheppard-Pratt. Existing accounts suggest that Silverberg's work was largely successful, maintaining a high rate of recovery. Later when he moved to New York City, Silverberg had a male partner, a fact known to his family, friends, and colleagues.[20] Here again, "private" practices, both scientific and subjective, seem to complicate or contradict his "public" account of homosexuality. At the same time, it is striking, in both Sullivan's and Silverberg's discussion, that femininity constituted "inferior" homosexuality. This resonated the gender bias embedded in Sheppard-Pratt clinical practice; compared with men's, women's "maturity" remained underdefined and more easily connected to mental and social dependence. Moreover, Sullivan's and Silverberg's views showed different approaches to feminism in the science of homosexuality: among scientists who explored different "kinds "of homosexuality, some focused on "true" homosexual persons whose gender attributes were reversed: effeminate homosexual men and masculine homosexual women. Others, like Parsons and Lewis, criticized this conflation of gender and sexual attributes as a source of sexism, indicating how the science of homosexuality could either inspire or deflect gender equality.

Edward Sapir, another close friend of Sullivan, also expressed a discriminatory view of homosexuality in an article he contributed to the *American Journal of Psychiatry* at Sullivan's request as an editor. Criticizing the modern "cult" of sexual freedom as a reason for the lack of intimacy between the sexes, Sapir claimed that homosexuality was "unnatural," a striking view, given the fact that he socialized with Sullivan and Jimmie as a couple:[21]

> In extreme cases—one dreads to acknowledge how appallingly frequent these extreme cases are becoming—the constantly dampened . . . passion between the sexes leads to . . . homosexuality. . . . Love having been squeezed out of sex, it revenges itself by assuming unnatural forms. The cult of the "naturalness" of homosexuality fools no one but those who need a rationalization of their own problems.[22]

Clearly, it was utterly unproblematic for a scientist to dismiss homosexuality in the paper he wrote for his friend who was in a relationship with a man. What a scientist described as a "problem" of homosexuality academically was easily separable from scientists who were in same-sex relationships personally. Indeed, it seems as if making a critical observation about homosexuality was a way for gay scientists and their friends to accentuate the distance between their studies' subject and their own subjectivity: if they talked as if they stood outside the "problem" of homosexuality, then they were, indeed, not part of the "problem." The distance that scientists kept in their theories between "us" and "others," then, were indeed practiced in their relationships with colleagues. Added to this was the fact that scientists' personal relationships—the partnership between Harry and Jimmie, for example—were protected by socially acceptable images such as that of a father and a son, which in turn ensured that people did not raise uncomfortable questions about their relationship. Veiled in these images, it was not difficult for intellectuals to "accept" their colleagues who were sexual minorities at the same time as publishing unforgiving comments about homosexuality.

Sapir, for example, surely appreciated the carefully crafted distance between individuals who were personally close to him and the "problem" of homosexuality. His friendship with Benedict, with whom he shared a passion for anthropology and poetry, further illuminates how he negotiated image and reality. Throughout the 1920s and well into the 1930s, Sapir and Benedict exchanged their poems for mutual critique. In 1924, Benedict decided to share with him a series of poems reflecting her homosexual feelings. She was falling in love with Margaret Mead around that time, and poems were increasingly her vehicle for her thinking of how she might come to terms with her "unconventional" and yet powerful emotions. But Sapir's response was that, although these poems had "wonderful passages," Benedict's emotions seemed hidden. Thus Sapir did not—or did not want to—understand the homoerotic yearning that was apparent in her lines.[23] It is not clear if Benedict expected Sapir to understand her lesbianism, although, as we will see, it is likely that she did not. What is unmistakable, however, is that Sapir did not acknowledge homosexuality in his friend, either by choice or by lack of perceptiveness. Just as there was a large distance between homosexuality in a "primitive" society and "civilized" America, homosexual persons as a "problem" population did not have a link to actual, real-life individuals whom scientists befriended.[24]

This division ran deeply, among not only heterosexual scientists but also individuals who had same-sex partners. Mead, for instance, asserted in her letter to Benedict that the latter was not homosexual, if the term meant a person who could be sexually intimate only with people of the same sex.[25] Mead did not want the label of "homosexuality" placed upon herself either, because she felt that it contradicted her identity. Benedict, despite the network of women she nurtured, continued to call herself "Mrs. Ruth F. Benedict," holding on to her marital status long after it was dissolved. Similarly, Sullivan expanded his circle of friends who shared his high opinions of homosexuality, while he projected an image of a bachelor surrounded by rumors of heterosexual affairs. The concept of homosexuality articulated in science was not what scientists themselves wanted to embrace. The culture of the "inner circle" that Benedict created was strikingly different from Sullivan's, particularly because of her commitment to feminism. And yet Benedict and Sullivan shared something important; both engaged in "private" practices, with a clear sense of the needs, desires, and aspirations—things that were excluded from their "public" science—that these practices needed to respond to and articulate.

Benedict's Private Sphere

Ruth Fulton Benedict's same-sex relationships and their link to the intellectual and cultural transformations of the 1920s and 1930s have remained unexamined until recently. The sources that became accessible in 2000 on the centennial of her partner Mead's birth, as well as the scholarship that has explored their relationship, illuminate ways in which Benedict negotiated the public and private in her life. Benedict was a social scientist of Sullivan's generation (she was born in 1887, five years before Sullivan, and died in 1948, a year earlier) for whom homosexuality carried both scientific and subjective significance, and as such, she offers an important angle for comparison. In her relationship with Mead, junior to Benedict by fourteen years, Benedict relentlessly pursued equality, perhaps because their relationship started as that of a teacher and a student. Their relationship was in striking contrast to that of Harry and Jimmie, and to Sullivan's relationship to some of his patients and students, because in these relationships Sullivan assumed the power of the senior, better educated, and professional man. Despite this stark difference, the Benedict-Mead relationship, as much as Sullivan's relationships, was shaped by private practices shielded from public theories.

Benedict left sources of three kinds revealing how she grappled with her homosexuality: poems she wrote using the pseudonym Anne Singleton, letters she exchanged with Mead, and diaries and fragmentary notes. Among them, the poems are most expressive of her homosexual feelings. In one of her early poems, for example, she wrote, "I shall lie once with beauty / Breast to Breast," while in another, she wrote about a peaceful gratification she took from "sleep begotten of a woman's kiss." But these do not indicate that she spoke openly as a lesbian. She was aware of a literary convention of the time in which poems were written in a male voice, even when the author was a woman. In this light, homoerotic expressions in Benedict's lines could pass as something written by a man—or by a woman assuming a male persona—about an imaginary sexual intimacy between women. Benedict probably relied on this convention when she shared her pieces with Sapir, while she had another layer of protection, her pseudonym, when she published in literary journals. Thus Benedict was able to use her poems for relatively straightforward expressions of her same-sex longings without exposing her homosexuality.

When she wrote to Mead, however, such straightforwardness had to be modified—and not only because Benedict was aware that her letters embodied more pressing personal meanings to Mead. More than Benedict, Mead was uncertain about her sexuality, falling in love with men even as she pursued a relationship with Benedict. Indeed, when she became Benedict's lover in 1924, Mead was still married to her first husband, Luther Cressman. After divorcing Cressman in 1928, she married again—first to Reo Fortune, a Cambridge-trained anthropologist in 1928, and later to Gregory Bateson in 1936—all the while staying intimate with Benedict. Benedict was married when she was in a relationship with Mead as well, but her relationship with her husband, Stanley Benedict, including their sexual intimacy, appears to have been deteriorating. As her passion for Mead grew, Benedict became more certain of her homosexual inclinations. Benedict also was sure of her desire to shape a monogamous relationship with Mead, while Mead wanted to remain open to multiple relationships. As Mead explained it, she did not want to be "bread," a steady partner, to people she loved, but she wanted to be "wine"—someone who could bring inspirations, excitement, and freshness to relationships. Thus, in terms of both her sexuality and expectations she had of romantic relationships, Mead was not ready to fully commit herself to Benedict.

Mead's hesitancy and, ultimately, refusal to be a monogamous partner deeply disappointed Benedict, while it also marked the beginning of Benedict's effort to bring into alignment her sexuality, her personal relationships, and her professional life. What she tried to create—perhaps first uncertainly, but later with more confidence—was a lasting friendship with Mead as an intellectual and moral confidante. Hundreds of letters she exchanged with Mead while they were away from each other, which was not unusual, given Mead's frequent field trips in the 1930s, offer a clue to Benedict's journey. She would let go of her desire to be Mead's exclusive lover, while at the same time, she would not let Mead's ideas about femininity, maternity, and homosexuality—including those that were contradictory to Benedict's—undermine her decisions to live as she chose.[26] Indeed, what is striking in Benedict's letters is her resilience and confidence about her choice, which she described without an explicit defense of her decision to be a single, childless woman living with a same-sex partner. She was not shy about telling Mead about her love life, especially about her new partner, Natalie Raymond (a romantic relationship that began in 1931) and the happiness that it allowed her to discover. This was something that Mead reciprocated, with all details of her romance, marriages, and motherhood. And yet Benedict was largely silent about critical questions of how: How did she find happiness in the relationship that society abhorred? How did she bring her personal life and her thinking as an anthropologist together? And how did she process Mead's potentially imposing ideas about femininity and sexuality?

The fact that Benedict did not discuss these issues is, by itself, not surprising; what she wrote to Mead were personal letters, not something she felt compelled to rationalize in all details. Moreover, as the older person, she probably felt it awkward to be overtly assertive. And yet this lack of explicit self-defense is striking in light of Mead's incessant urge for self-justification. Explaining why she was falling in love with Gregory, for example, Mead in 1933 wrote to Benedict: "I've less a sense of his [Gregory's] youth than I've had before—and a more than ever vivid sense of his having authority of his temperament 'and of such is the kingdom of heaven.'"[27]

Taking note of the fact that Gregory was younger than she (he was three years her junior), Margaret emphasized how she nonetheless recognized "authority" in him, something that made it seem reasonable for her to pursue a relationship with him. To be sure, besides the age difference she had other reasons to want to justify her choice; she was still married to her second husband, Reo Fortune; in addition, she was working with him in New Guinea, which she worried might cause a dispute over intellectual property if their marriage were to fall apart. Nevertheless, in her explaining her decisions, it becomes clear that Mead was concerned about gendered conventions such as the belief that a husband must be older than his wife. A similar concern was evident in her contemporary published writing as well. In *Sex and Temperament*, Mead claimed that even in societies that did not impose a clear divide between masculine and feminine personality traits, one crucial distinction between the sexes remained intact: reproduction. She considered maternity a ticket to "full sex membership" in womanhood, suggesting her belief that certain fundamental differences existed between men and women. Thus in both public and private thinking, Mead accepted the difference between male and female even as she supported a cultural constructionist understanding of the sexes.

This, along with her analysis of homosexuality in a 1933 letter to Benedict, could have provoked Benedict's strong disagreement. In this letter, Mead argued that "the kind of feeling which you [Benedict] have classified as 'homosexual' and 'heterosexual' is really 'sex adopted to like or understood' versus 'sex adopted to a relationship of strangeness and distance.'" To think of it as a "man-woman relationship" or a relationship "within a sex," Mead went on to claim, "is a fundamental fallacy."[28] Here, Mead is suggesting that Benedict's homosexual feeling was, in fact, based on her attraction to someone similar to herself in temperament. It was of secondary importance which biological sex this person belonged to, and thus Benedict could not be homosexual. In so arguing, Mead was making a connection to her theory of masculine and feminine temperaments in *Sex and Temperament*.[29] Again, in Mead's letters it is difficult not to recognize the connection between her privately and publicly expressed ideas: she conceptualized sexual desire as something rooted in gender distinctions, just as she grappled with her attraction to both a man (Bateson) and a woman (Benedict) in her private life. Most likely this was related to her concern that if she were homosexual she might be incapable of obtaining "full membership" in womanhood. Indeed, in her published writings she began to note the importance of maternity as a foundation of femininity at the same time as she became certain of her desire for a child. In 1935, she was thirty-three, and she was worried that she might not be able to be a mother because of either her sexuality or her lack of reproductive ability. Such worry is unmistakable both in Mead-Benedict correspondence before 1939 when Mead had her first and only child, Mary Catherine, and in Mead's words of pleasure after she became pregnant. In

1937, concerned about the possibility that Mead could not get pregnant, Benedict asked if Mead was "still happy planning for a baby." Benedict hoped that it came true, but assured Mead that "all things will work together for good to you even if it doesn't happen." In a letter written in 1939, when she was finally pregnant, Mead wrote, "Yes, it feels as if the baby's moving were a bright spot in a dark world."[30] For Mead, the bond between motherhood and womanhood was unbreakable, offering no room for homosexuality. She regarded womanhood and homosexuality as mutually exclusive, a view that she upheld both in her public work and her private life, at the same time criticizing the extreme distinction between the sexes as a cause of social ills in "civilized" societies.

How did Benedict respond to these words, coming from her former lover? Her letters to Mead illuminate that she dealt with Mead's ideas by creating a sphere in which Benedict could express her views as a lesbian scientist richly, if privately. Although she was generous in sharing Mead's maternal pleasure, Benedict's observations on pregnancy and motherhood were not without a hint of irony. Similarly, although she was aware of the weight that motherhood carried for many women, she did not think that this should change her relationship to Natalie Raymond. Benedict's comment on the Sapirs in a 1932 letter to Mead, for example, suggests a critical stance Benedict took on motherhood:

> What do you think I got today? The announcements of a birth of a son to Edward and Jean Sapir. . . . I hope it will give Edward enough assurance of his virility to be worth the trouble of having a fifth child. Jean will be happier about it because she had made up her mind that there was nothing interesting . . . for her to do in New Haven.[31]

Ruth's friendship to Edward had been complicated for personal reasons by this time (Edward and Margaret fell in love in 1924, but the relationship ended in a bitter breakup in 1926—bitter not only for them but also for Ruth, who was close to both); thus her ironic tone here must be understood in light of her general impatience with Edward. Nevertheless, she clearly understood motherhood as a social construction, something that offered a man an assurance of his masculinity, and a woman a "fun" thing to do when there was nothing else to occupy herself with. For Ruth, motherhood was not fundamental to a "full" womanhood, as Margaret insisted.

Benedict could be playful, not just ironic, about people's preoccupation with reproduction, revealing that her observations were not based on jealousy or bitterness. Rather, her comments seemed to arise from her confidence and her desire for fairness among women. On Natalie, for example, Ruth wrote to Margaret in 1932:

It's a lot of pleasure to me to have Nat around, and I certainly get the heemyjeebies [sic] living alone. . . . Her boy-friend, the mild middle-aged psychology professor . . . has been here . . . and she has been dividing time. Poor man, he has good taste in going as far out of his proper line as daring to choose Nat, but the good taste is all wasted. . . . He's been married for twenty years, and is just out of it— childless—and ready to scrap anything and everything for children. But he's evidently not yet convinced that he can't persuade Nat. She's invented a "Mr. C" with whom she's in love, and he pictures his course as trying gradually to wear down her infatuation in favor of a real marriage with children.[32]

Here, Ruth admitted her fear of being alone, while at the same time, she made it clear that she did not see Natalie's boyfriend as a threat in that regard. On the contrary, Ruth regarded his desire for marriage and children as misplaced and amusing. His attempt at Natalie was something of a joke, not to be taken seriously by any of the women. Thus, she would not object to Natalie's spending time with him; Ruth could even complement his "good taste" to pursue Natalie, the person Ruth herself admired. What emerges is a person who was content and confident with the bond she had with women. With them, Benedict shared a world in which she expressed her irony and humor, which might not find a place elsewhere. She expected her partners to respond to her sensibility, while, unlike Mead, Benedict did not attempt to connect her private beliefs with her published ideas. This is striking, especially given the fact that issues of homosexuality were very much on her mind as she prepared *Patterns of Culture* around this time. In 1936, she was still interested in homosexuality: she told Mead that she had been reading George Devereux's manuscript "on sexual life of the Mohave, and it's a good piece of work."[33] This was when Devereux was still a junior scholar fresh from a postdoctoral position at the University of California.

The boundaries of Benedict's inner circle changed in the 1930s, sometimes including just Ruth, Mead, and Natalie, other times extending its welcome to others. In the summer of 1937, for example, Benedict spent two weeks at her "farm" (a farmhouse in Norwich, New York, where Ruth had spent her childhood and frequented as an adult on holidays) with Ruth Bunzel (Bunny), Ruth's friend and associate in anthropology at Columbia. Benedict described Bunzel as being "in love with me," although Ruth also noted that Bunny "accept[ed] the fact" that Ruth was not romantically interested in Bunny. What sustained this network of women seems to be an attempt to realize fairness—based on a full disclosure of one's feelings and a willingness to be open to others.' Between Benedict and Bunzel, for instance, there was a careful discussion of why Ruth was not attracted to Bunny.[34] Moreover, although Ruth could be terse about people's preoccupation with reproduction, she was not inattentive to her partners' desire for maternity. For one, Natalie wanted a child, and this was something she discussed frequently with Ruth. Writing to Margaret in 1932, Ruth explained:

> [Natalie] has been happy this year, as she never has been before. The only thing that troubles me is that she so obviously ought to have children; perhaps she could adopt a couple later. . . . She might fall in love with a man and have children of her own. Still, that's not likely while we are so happy together; she's naturally monogamous.[35]

Thus, even as she appreciated and felt mostly secure about the relationship with Natalie, Ruth did not look away from the possibility that it might change in the future because of the younger woman's desire for maternity. Benedict was never reserved in her recognition of Mead's belief in the importance of reproduction, either. Not only did Benedict offer an abundance of good words on Mary, but she also acknowledged the crucial place that reproduction occupied in Mead's thinking. In the same letter in which she mentioned George Devereux's work on homosexuality, for instance, Benedict drew Mead's attention to his findings about reproductive issues:

> You'll be interested in several points. Sex activities of all sorts are good. . . . But reproduction is serious. . . . Following out this idea, what the transvestites insist on is not recognition of their sexual perversion, but reproduction. . . . The male inverts fake pregnancy. . . . The female inverts insist on children too.[36]

This was not necessarily agreement, but it was a recognition that Mead's idea deserved serious consideration. Benedict was able to hear both Natalie's and Margaret's concern about their maternity, even as she separated herself from the world in which motherhood carried a special significance. For her as an older woman with a more established professional career, this was an unmistakable sign that Benedict desired fairness to those whom she thought were not as decided as she was about matters of gender and sexuality.

Benedict pursued fairness in relationships in other ways. It was important to her that Natalie, a graduate student at Cornell University in the early 1930s, succeed in her work. To have Natalie feel overshadowed by her famous partner was not what Ruth wanted. Ruth was not interested in being Natalie's guardian, either. In late 1932, Ruth claimed proudly that she was "no longer her [Natalie's] father to her. That doesn't mean that I am not quite as necessary—and as loved. . . . But it is different." This was an important change, because Ruth believed that Natalie first had sought out a fatherly figure in Benedict. But finally, Natalie was "convinced of my love for her" as a partner.[37] While this placed Ruth's relationship with

Natalie in sharp contrast with that of Harry and Jimmie, Ruth's intellectual collaboration with Margaret belonged to an entirely different realm from Harry and Jimmie's relationship, which implied inequality—doctor and patient, father and son. To be sure, because of Ruth's seniority, Margaret found it difficult to regard herself as Ruth's equal. But in their mutual critique of ideas, both seemed to uphold honesty and straightforwardness. For instance, Margaret was critical of Ruth's manuscript for *Patterns of Culture*, particularly its organization and texture (by which Margaret meant writing style. Margaret described it as sometimes "cryptic" and other times "uneven and choppy").[38] Ruth could be critical of Margaret's work as well, although Ruth was also generous in praising Margaret's accomplishments. The most revealing example of this is in a letter from Ruth to Margaret in 1936 when Margaret was away for her field research in the Malay Archipelago. In the letter, Ruth copied a letter from their common friend Jaime de Angulo, which had come to Margaret's New York address and was highly appreciative of *Sex and Temperament*:

> There was such a nice note from Jaime de Angulo. . . . "I have just finished reading Sex and Temperament. I have suspected that you [Mead] were the best functional anthropologist in America. Now I am sure of it. . . . Your other books were fine, but this is a masterpiece. . . . Now the whole question of sex and sex differences has been a passion with me all my life. I have thought and thought and worried over it. I have raged in turn at the virago and at the pin-headed female. Finally I solved the problem by turning myself into an androgyne. But that was no real solution. It did it for me, but I could see quite well that it was no formula for the public."[39]

In a way similar to the supportive way Ruth talked about Devereux's discussion of reproduction, Benedict in this letter mentioned "a nice letter" from the friend expressing full agreement with Mead's analysis of masculinity and femininity as a cause of homosexuality. Ruth's excitement was apparent in the fact that she copied the letter rather than forwarding it. And yet, again, this was recognition, not necessarily agreement. Indeed, given Mead's earlier comment urging Benedict to agree with the theory of temperament—that Benedict was not homosexual, but happened to be attracted to the kinds of temperament that American culture associated with women—it is striking that there were not clear words of agreement or disagreement from Benedict. Nowhere in Benedict's letters that followed Mead's 1933 assertion can we find a specific response. Similarly, nowhere in the 1936 letter did Benedict write that she, too, thought that Mead's theory of temperament made sense. This paralleled her published writing, which never grew into a full-scale analysis of homophobia in the United States.

Nor did it turn into a critical comment about the use of homosexuality in "primitive" societies to criticize a rigid distinction between femininity and masculinity in the United States—a position Mead supported publicly and privately. Most likely, this lack of critique meant that Benedict agreed with the gender equality that Mead, along with others such as Parsons and Lewis, was working for. And yet Benedict's silence in public also illuminates her way of protecting her choice to be a childless woman who had a same-sex partner and at the same time pursuing fairness in her relationships with younger women who might make a different choice—to be a mother, to be a wife. Benedict's critique of these choices was mostly enclosed in her humor and irony, expressed only as a private thought.

This approach and Benedict's lack of engagement with the questions of how—how she dealt with her feelings of being a lesbian—were frustrating to Mead. Ruth's letters in the 1930s were mostly about her friends and colleagues and Natalie's doings; Ruth's words about herself were scarce and fleeting. In 1938, Mead's frustration reached a point where it needed to be discussed; Margaret began to take the lack of personal details as a sign of a decline in their relationship. Ruth's following letter was perhaps the most straightforward expression of her feelings, although it probably did not take the form that Margaret wanted:

> I'm so sorry you got to feeling from my letters that I was so far away and maybe inhabiting a different sphere. Looking back, I can see how you felt so, for I've written about so many mere business details. . . . I've left out the things I'd have liked better to write. . . . But it's strange that in spite of all my busyness I have constantly freer and freer access to my obsessional self—and happier access—and you are the only person in the world who knows or cherishes that side of me. . . . I don't have devils any more; it's hard to put in words how completely they're gone. . . . I feel as if I lived in that country I despaired of for so long; none of the nagging things I have to do really touch me. I don't feel lonely either—not really, even with you away. It's like a little piece of eternal life.[40]

The "devils" that Ruth mentioned were most likely multifaceted. They could have been her childhood memory of her father who died when she was young (as Ruth indicated later in this letter), her fear of being alone, or her sense of being someone who chose unusual paths. Regardless, what comes across overwhelmingly is her sense that she reached a point where things did not have to be talked about. She felt that her self could resolve things by itself, without bringing them out to an open discussion. Even with her confidante Margaret, Ruth seemed to prefer to rely on unspoken understanding, because her status of being was "hard to put in words." By age fifty-one, then, Ruth had immersed herself in a private "sphere" in which there was no need to publicly assert her critical ideas about femininity, maternity, and sexuality. Both her struggle to come to terms with herself and her desire for fairness in her relationships pushed her to this equanimity. In this realm, she practiced her life, watching issues of importance carefully, but not feeling compelled to make her observations public. As the era's feminism and its critique of a division between male and female temperaments loomed large in many areas of American life, critical questions about homosexuality were in a unique, separate sphere in which intellectuals found unspoken answers. No doubt the making of this sphere contributed to the scarcity of open discussion of homosexuality in the United States. Benedict's story suggests that, at least for her, the making of this sphere, a sphere in which things remained silent, was accelerated by her diligent aspiration for equality for and among women. And she had good reasons for following such an aspiration. Even among the scientists in the life history cohort, femininity was frequently associated with primitive, inferior qualities, including homosexuality. She could avoid the label of homosexuality in public by being "Mrs. Ruth F. Benedict." She could not avoid being seen as a woman. Thus gender equality became a more pronounced, public cause, while a critique of homophobia was dealt with in private. This balancing between gender and sexuality was precisely what made her private practices both strikingly similar to and different from Harry Stack Sullivan's.

Sullivan: The Formation of an Inner Circle

One day in 1936, Sullivan invited his clinic's receptionist for lunch at his house at 158 East Sixty-fourth Street in New York City. The clinic was on one of the floors of his house, and he simply asked the receptionist to come up and sit at the table with him. The receptionist, Ralph Ellison, then a junior at the Tuskegee Institute in Alabama and taking a year off to earn money in New York (and of course, years away from his 1952 *Invisible Man*), was surprised when this prominent psychiatrist asked him to read his writing, and asked for comments. Ellison "could not believe that Sullivan really cared what he [Ellison] thought about it," but felt "very, very flattered." Ellison recalled that Sullivan was busy, getting a lot of long-distance calls from "well-known people." Ellison also remembered that the psychiatrist seemed lonely, living in a big house with Jimmie, a dog, and a housekeeper. There was no doubt, though, that Sullivan was living a luxurious life. Ellison thought of psychoanalysts as having lots of money, "lots of beautiful things around." He remembered a greenhouse on the top of the house, where Sullivan raised day lilies. There was an elevator shaft in this five-story house, although the elevator itself was never installed. Sullivan had a "hi-fi music [system]," one of the first at the time, which caught the eye of visitors to his house.[41]

Ellison's memory of Sullivan gives us a glimpse of Sullivan's life in the 1930s. He was an established psychiatrist, spending a significant amount of time taking care of administration. He was the president of a psychiatric foundation and postgraduate institute and an editor of two major psychiatric journals. He was often asked by the media for comments on social issues such as mental health, racial conflict, and the war in Europe, comments that appeared in newspaper articles or were broadcasted in radio programs.[42] He was known in intellectual and artistic circles. In some cases, he became acquainted with members of these circles through consultations he offered at his clinic. Some of his clients were well-known individuals. Dorothy Schiff, owner of the *New York Post*, was one. The dancer Katherine Dunham was another. Sullivan also consulted his friends' relatives, one example being Philip Sapir, Edward Sapir's son.[43] Their relationships also developed on social occasions. For instance, Sullivan was a regular at Clara Thompson's parties, which this sociable analyst held at her house on Sunday afternoons. Most partygoers were artists, writers, and intellectuals. Indeed, Ellison got his receptionist job through the sculptor Richard Bare, who frequented Thompson's parties. No longer was Sullivan a big name just in psychiatry; he was a public intellectual, a celebrity.

But when we look at what did not appear on his résumé, Sullivan in the 1930s seems more complicated. His sexual subjectivity continued to shape his scientific practices, leading him to go so far as to suggest that certain of his male patients and male students have sex with him. To what extent he thought that homosexual experiences were useful for treatment is unclear, but it is most likely that same-sex relationships were considered a necessary part of training within the small group of Sullivan's students. In any case, his private practices in the 1930s blurred the line between the scientific and subjective more problematically than they had in the 1920s, as Sullivan himself, not his attendants, began to practice his method, and his critical attention to his and his patients' subjectivity became less keen than it had been. But because his practices were not open to outside scrutiny, and because he cast a person's disapproval of homosexuality as a sign of sexual unsophistication, patients found it difficult to come forward with their complaints. We do not have Sullivan's clinical records from the 1930s, nor do we have personal letters between Harry and Jimmie. Nevertheless, records of interviews with his patients and students, collected by Helen Swick Perry and Michael Stuart Allen from the 1960s to the 1980s, reveal a separation of the public from the private comparable to that in Benedict's life.

Soon after Sullivan left Sheppard-Pratt in 1930, he decided to open his own clinic in New York City. He needed a setting—a more free-standing setting—in which he could offer what he believed to be the best to his patients. Fortunately for him, there was an increasing demand for psychiatric consultations in the metropolitan area in the early 1930s, allowing him to earn a sufficient income. His patients' main complaints were everyday issues such as anxiety, incapacity to work, and sexual inability and incompatibility, problems usually labeled neurosis.[44] Suitably, Sullivan's focus in New York was neuroses. He believed that patients with mild neuroses needed more attention because if they did not receive timely consultation they might collapse into serious psychoses such as schizophrenia. Sullivan's patients were middle class, people who could afford his then hefty fee of five dollars an hour for months and years.[45] This was the case with Sullivan's students, who paid ten dollars an hour.[46] Thus, Sullivan's patients in the 1930s were different from Sheppard-Pratt patients, who were mostly middle class but still included a significant number of working-class patients.[47]

As Sullivan shifted his focus from psychoses to neuroses in the middle class, his social and intellectual life became enmeshed in a growing community of psychoanalysts in New York. Sometime in 1931, he began a social group called the Zodiac with Clara Thompson and William V. Silverberg. Karen Horney and Erich Fromm joined the group later, holding sporadic meetings over drinks and dinner.[48] All trained in Europe, these were people who, as the first generation of U.S.-based psychoanalysts, substantiated the transplantation (and transformation) of Freudian psychoanalysis.[49] Among this circle of friends, Sullivan developed a reputation of being mysterious.[50] Lawrence K. Frank, who first met Sullivan at the colloquia on personality in the late 1920s and stayed in touch, thought that Sullivan "seemed to want to present the image of the psychiatrist, friendly and interested in people, but not intruding his own feelings too much. In fact, he [seems to have] maintained a mask."[51] Dexter Mean Bullard, Sullivan's longtime friend, who invited him to teach at Chestnut Lodge Hospital when he was leaving New York in 1939, believed that Sullivan "compartmentalized his friends, so that one friend knew one thing about him and somebody else knew something else."[52] What emerges from these comments is a mercurial, self-protective, and possibly insecure person. He disclosed a part of himself to his friends, but seldom was fully frank with any of them.

This complex pattern of friendship shows how Sullivan, like Benedict, kept his public and private lives apart . Both projected a heterosexual interest on their public personas, by the title "Mrs." in Benedict's case, and by the appearance of an attractive bachelor in Sullivan's. Harry Biele, a writer and a founder of the journal SAGE and a regular at Thompson's parties, recalled a telling episode with an erotic flair:

At a party, Clara [Thompson] was wearing a dress covered with dry sequins. She asked HSS [Harry Stack Sullivan] how he liked it. He walked over to her and shut his eyes, running his hands along the dress like a blind man. . . . [He said] "it's like moving your hand against millions of nipples at the speed of light."[53]

Here is the sense of humor and the sexual attraction between Sullivan and Thompson that Sullivan chose to reveal on a social occasion. In fact, Sullivan had quasi-romantic relations with some women in the 1930s, although none grew into a committed relation or, it seems, even an affair. The mutual attraction between Sullivan and Thompson did not seem to go anywhere.[54] Also, although some thought that Sullivan was attracted to Karen Horney, their relationship seemed to end abruptly. As Jean Sapir recalled, once Sullivan was accompanied by Horney when he came to the Sapirs' summer house. Harry's regular companion was Jimmie, and thus when Sullivan showed up with Horney instead of Inscoe, the Sapirs thought that it was unmistakable that they were romantically involved.[55] But soon after Horney moved from Chicago to New York, because Sullivan "summoned her," Sullivan "immediately terminated all relationship with her." The breakup caused Horney great confusion, because "she did not understand exactly what had happened."[56] These affairs and rumors created the image of a bachelor who was always in relationships with women—not an uncommon public profile for homosexual men of the time. Just as Benedict protected her reputation by suggesting her married status, Sullivan defended his by stories of heterosexual romance.

In sharp contrast to this public persona was what Sullivan disclosed to some friends in private. Clifton Read, a writer, was among those with whom Sullivan was open about his homosexuality. Read first met Sullivan in his clinic to consult about an individual close to Read, but later the men became personal friends as they began to meet for a drink and dinner.[57] Soon it became clear to Read that Sullivan had an exceptional eye for wine and food. Sullivan revealed more than his taste in food to this young friend. During one of their dinners together, for example, Sullivan "warned [Read] that if he went out to dinner with him [Sullivan], people would think he [Read] was homosexual." Read thought that it was "a small price to pay" for Sullivan's company. Also Sullivan told Read that he believed that "Maryland was the most civilized state in the union, [because it was] the only one with no law banning sex between consenting male adults." On another occasion, he referred to the Chinese as "the truly civilized" because he believed that they could enjoy "sex with both men and women." Thus, their relationship was formed in an air of refinement and avant-garde context, as if to suggest that, to selected friends, he personified the image of cultured and egalitarian homosexual men that floated in the public discourse of science.

Interestingly, Sullivan was also frank about his opinions of African Americans with Read, and with another friend, the painter John Vassos. Some of Sullivan's comments illuminate how, in the 1930s, his subjectivity merged with his science, in an even more complicated way than it did at Sheppard-Pratt. Once Sullivan said that Read might sleep with a black woman "if [he] had doubts [about his sexual performance]." Sullivan's reasoning was that "often whites could forget a mother's prohibitions [when they slept] with a black." This reveals how, in private, he believed that a black woman could be used as a therapeutic tool to reassure a sexually uncertain white man. This problematic approach was apparent in his comments about African American men as well. Speaking of the individual about whom Read consulted with Sullivan, the doctor suggested that the person "might improve enough under proper treatment to live outside a hospital, maybe on a small farm with a black man to look after him, someone he could scream at and even hit who wouldn't hurt him and would care for him whatever he did." Here again, Sullivan's personal bias—that it is appropriate to benefit white men at the expense of black people—influenced his professional opinions, as long as these opinions were offered in private. Clearly, the suggestions he made to Read differed from Sullivan's public approach to racism. Collaborating with E. Franklin Frazier, Sullivan wrote that white Americans must "cultivate a humanistic, rather than . . . an exploiting attitude" toward black Americans. Nevertheless his bias against African Americans, not the "humanistic attitude" commended in his published writing, found its way into Sullivan's therapeutic advice. Revealing the public-private divide both in his approach to homosexuality and in his race consciousness, Sullivan's comments also suggest the prevalence of the "us" and "others" dichotomy in scientific liberalism. The division between research subjects and those who examined them cut across cultures, sexualities, and races; and for Sullivan the distinction applied to race was more prevalent in private than in public.

To further complicate matters, John Vassos's following comment, made during an interview with Helen Swick Perry in 1964 (but never published by Perry), suggests that Sullivan might have hoped to apply this race-based therapeutic approach to himself—an indication that Sullivan's private practices encompassed his sexual subjectivity more directly than in the 1920s:

> V[assos] was committed to heterosexuality, so he never accepted Sullivan's advances. Also, Sullivan [was] interested in women too, but afraid. Always wanted to know about V's conquests. S[ullivan] advised him that Negro women had much to offer and V. used to go to Harlem for some, tried to get S. to go with him, but they "separated over Harlem," meaning S. wanted to go but couldn't. Afterward S. wanted to know about sexual position, etc.[58]

Beneath Vassos's boasts lies a picture of Sullivan trying to follow the same suggestion he offered to Read. No longer, it seems, was Sullivan a "ringmaster," as his colleagues at Sheppard-Pratt had seen him. As he "compartmentalized" his acquaintances into public and private spheres, his sexual subjectivity became more pronounced in the latter, expressed in both professional and personal relationships.

This shift occurred in his relationships to patients as well. Because of its sensitive nature, the information concerning Sullivan's sexual advances to his patients and students is scarce. But sexual tension existed inside and outside clinical settings, as some individuals who belonged to his inner circle recalled.[59] For example, one patient noted in a memoir written in the late 1980s a series of incidents at Sullivan's clinic in the late 1930s:

> One day he [Sullivan] got up from his desk and came and sat right beside me on the railing of the couch. He put his hand on my hand where it rested on my stomach. That was all that happened then. The next week when I went to Sullivan, he came over and got up in the couch with me and kissed me on the cheek. I was surprised. I don't think I was hurt nor disillusioned nor anything like that. I think I began to wonder whether he had ceased being the therapist and whether our fundamental roles were not changing. I felt no passion for him, although I felt very warm. I liked him very much and had grown to have great respect for him.[60]

Strikingly, during his interview with Perry in the 1970s, a decade earlier, this patient had described the same incident differently:

> One day, HSS came over and lay down beside [this patient] on couch, may have kissed [him] but definitely felt for his crotch. [This patient] was sexually sophisticated, would have known whether or not it was a sexual advance. When HSS lay down beside him, [this patient] thought that this wasn't part of therapy. He got up and said that he'd better be going. His memory was of being upset by this and of reporting it to [a referring psychiatrist] pretty promptly. . . . [This referring psychiatrist] suggested that he discontinue seeing Sullivan, but never said anything . . . against Sullivan, in fact she respected Sullivan as did [this patient]. . . . [This patient] had no feeling of aversion to Sullivan's advance. [This patient] had had no homosexual experience, but he knew that that was what it was. . . . [This patient] didn't like it because it was not appropriate to therapy.[61]

The patient seems more critical of Sullivan's behavior in the 1970s than he was in the 1980s. In the 1980s memoir, the patient emphasized the "warm" feeling he had toward his therapist, while in the 1970s interview, the patient made it clear that he felt "upset" and found Sullivan's advance "not appropriate." What is more striking is that the referring psychiatrist, to whom this patient reported this occurrence, as well as the patient himself, did not make a complaint or confront Sullivan concerning his behavior. It seems as if Sullivan's colleague and patient felt so much respect for Sullivan that no criticism could be made. Perhaps this image of the dignified doctor was reinforced in this patient's memory and helped make him stress the approving feeling he had toward Sullivan in the 1980s.

This seems to have been the case with another patient, who was in analysis with Sullivan in 1938, as found in Perry's record of her interview with the patient in 1971:

[The patient said] you know, he was homosexual, because you're just evasive if you don't. He said, I know this personally, because he made advances to me. . . . I [Perry] said, "Well, did he make a physical advance?" and he said, it doesn't matter. He said, "the same thing happened to a friend of mine, in a similar situation." This was before I [Perry] said anything about knowing Patrick Mullahy. In fact it was Patrick who told me a story like this. . . . Pat said that Sullivan made a physical advance.[62]

Perry noted that this patient seemed to remain "very, very angry" at Sullivan for more than thirty years after the incident. Also, both the patient and Perry knew that a similar incident that had been experienced by Patrick Mullahy, a philosopher who became a strong advocate of Sullivan's interpersonal theory.[63] Although the patient did not share with Mullahy such a pronounced respect for Sullivan, he noted that he recognized Sullivan's talent to "understand" and "stabilize" schizophrenic patients and that Sullivan developed "humane treatment for them," in his interview with Michael Stuart Allen in 1989.[64] As was the case with the first patient, Sullivan's sexual advances were smoothed out in this patient's memory, as these incidents were mixed with the image of the psychiatrist as a genius beyond criticism.

Also blended into memories of Sullivan was the image of a sophisticated man, making his sexual advances seem as if they were an invitation to a secret club of a select few. Even the patient who was explicitly angry recalled, with a sense of excitement, a time when Sullivan took him to an "esoteric" entertainment: "In NYC Harry Stack took us to a night club with transvestites and black female dancers. . . . He shocked me by saying that she was he!"[65] Soon after this visit to the club, Sullivan took another step to come closer to the patient:

He [Sullivan] came [to visit me] . . . we had dinner, at the end of the evening, he wanted me to come back to the hotel with him . . . just wanted me to lie in bed with him, it wouldn't be as bad as I thought.

He suggested that I would suck him, semen is just egg white, it's
O.K., he said. . . . I was not surprised that he was a homosexual, I had
assumed that because of his relationship with Jimmie. . . . He had
come hoping. . . . I refused and he left unhappy.[66]

Thus, although the patient "refused" Sullivan, he was not upset about
Sullivan's invitation. Indeed, what seems unmistakable in these passages is
that the patient enjoyed their time together and did not mind being introduced to gay culture, with which Sullivan was apparently familiar.

On this particular occasion, then, the possibility that the patient was
vulnerable to his doctor's demand—the possibility that existed both inside
and outside clinics—did not seem to concern either of them. Sullivan was
aware that the patient was going through significant changes in his life,
including his father's death, and that he was depressed when coming under
Sullivan's treatment.[67] Nevertheless, an ethical concern that might arise
from Sullivan's knowledge of these matters did not stop them from having
their night out together. If anything, the patient's description of Sullivan's
push for sex suggests that the patient remembered, or hoped to portray,
this incident as a man-to-man negotiation, nothing that should be seen as
abusive. Moreover, it is unmistakable that the patient in Allen's record did
not want to appear homophobic. The same sentiment was apparent in the
first patient's record: he was sexually "sophisticated" although he had had
no homosexual experience; he refused to sleep with Sullivan because of this
being inappropriate in a therapeutic setting, not because he was not sophisticated enough to be open to homosexuality.

In Sullivan's circle of analysts and analysands, too, an atmosphere prevailed that made it seem unsophisticated to refuse homosexual advances.
Otto Allen Will, Sullivan's student, recalled in 1973, as his interviewer Perry
recorded,

When he [Will] was in analysis with Sullivan, he told Sullivan of a
male friend remarking on a homosexual gesture of another male,
who touched a male's knee. And Will was very upset with his friend
for suggesting that there was not anything peculiar about this. And
Sullivan said quietly, "Maybe your friend was more sophisticated than
you were (or are)."[68]

Clearly, Sullivan was suggesting that Will would be more "sophisticated"
if he were open to homosexuality. This was in line with his belief in the
"civilized" Chinese he disclosed to Clifton Read. The image of homosexuality
as extraordinary was articulated both in personal and professional relationships in Sullivan's private practice.

The link between sophistication and homosexuality was further accentuated by Sullivan's belief that homosexual relationships facilitated a better understanding of schizophrenia. Benjamin Weininger, a student of Sullivan's who was under his supervision in 1937, claimed that same-sex sexual contacts happened because Sullivan and his students believed that "schizophrenics were homosexuals." In particular, Sullivan thought that Weininger "had a cured schizophrenia," and suggested that Weininger did "research" with Sullivan.[69] Allen related Weininger's recollection of this research:

[Weininger] had sex with Sullivan twice, in 1937. These two encounters occurred after a few drinks at Sullivan's New York City home. . . . Weininger, who identified himself as a heterosexual, recalled vividly that Sullivan was acutely sensitive to Weininger's anxiety about having sex with a man; so sensitive, in fact, that Sullivan . . . had premature ejaculations during both encounters.[70]

Notably, Weininger recognized Sullivan's "sensitivity" toward him, unlike the patients who were offended by the therapist's sexual advance. Most likely, this was because Weininger believed, like Sullivan, that their actions were related to scientific research. Indeed, he and "another heterosexual colleague 'tried it out' a few times with each other as a form of research into the cause of paranoid schizophrenia."[71] In this context, Weininger did not take sex with his supervisor as an imposition of a superior's subjectivity. Rather, it was seen as a form of training, something in which only dedicated, promising students were invited to participate.

That Sullivan's students shared a sense of being selected is further illuminated by a code that prohibited revealing such "training" to outsiders. When Will learned that Weininger had told Perry about Weininger's sex with Sullivan, Will became "upset" because he believed that the "sex life of a great man should be private."[72] Will felt protective of his teacher, and despite the fact that he considered Sullivan to be acting selflessly, he still thought that this method of training could not be made public. If it were, their scientific studies might be misunderstood as a pursuit of subjective satisfaction. In Sullivan's private practices, then, the borderline between the subjective and scientific existed only in the eyes of those who decided to see it. To those who did not, the distinction was nonexistent. But as with his students, his patients seem to have come to term with Sullivan's behavior, perhaps because they thought that a refusal and complaints might cause them to be labeled "sexually not sophisticated" and that a release of Sullivan's practice was code-breaking in itself. This was different from his clinical practice at Sheppard-Pratt: in comparison with his work in the 1920s, when he expressed a willingness to listen to his patients' opinions, his behavior in the 1930s seemed more self-serving and less concerned with how a patient might feel about the therapist's actions.

It might be tempting to consider that Sullivan's practice was a marginal, isolated incident. However, at least a few psychoanalysts associated with Sullivan seem to have used the same method. For instance, one patient of Sullivan's junior colleague at Sheppard-Pratt in the 1920s, during an interview with Allen in 1988, recalled how "frightened" he was when this analyst made an advance to him: "He [the psychoanalyst] lay down on the couch and offered to have sex with me. . . . I quit. . . . I felt disgraced. . . . It was a sexual maneuver, maybe inspired by an HSS theory."[73]

This patient, an openly gay man, remembered that he had responded with the most straightforward rejection. He considered the analyst a "very disturbed man himself," despite "his charisma and wonderful personality." The patient continued to socialize with this analyst, but never went back to him as a patient. It is ironic that, while Sullivan's approach seemed accepted among his students, patients often did not see its usefulness, including homosexual men for whom the approach was originally designed. It is more than ironic that the potentially offensive practice found its way out Sullivan's inner circle and was applied to an unknown number of sexual minorities.[74]

Sullivan's private practices in the 1930s illuminate their dangers as much as the possibilities he had seen in them. When he was at Sheppard-Pratt, he attempted to change the "existing social system," which was unfair to homosexual men. When he put his approach into practice, he decided not to care much about what outsiders might think; if he did, he would not be able to respond to his patients' real needs. Theirs, Sullivan articulated, were minorities' needs that could be met only in a protected environment.[75] In the 1930s, he developed an inner circle, in which homosexuality was given special significance. Particularly, homosexuality became highlighted as a key to understanding schizophrenia. Sullivan's associates "felt honored to be a member of his inner circle" and did not challenge his standards.[76] Thus, on the one hand, in the inner circle, the image of "civilized" homosexuals, which was unsubstantiated and faceless in public discourse, became more real. On the other hand, because Sullivan and his associates kept their practices closed to the public, such highlighting of sexual experience went unchecked. The blurred boundary between Sullivan's subjective life and scientific work, which had helped him to communicate with his patients in the 1920s, produced in the 1930s a series of practices in which doctors, patients, and students were expected to accept his beliefs, and in some cases desires, without asking questions. What all this means is that not only his patients' subjectivity, but also the scientist's subjectivity, became less examined in the 1930s. Unlike his practice at Sheppard-Pratt, which critically examined both the doctor's and patients' subjectivity in science, his practice in the

1930s allowed the scientific and subjective to merge without carefully scrutinizing whose subjectivities and what subjectivities were included—and in what balance. As a result, the subjectivity of the less powerful—African Americans, patients, and possibly some students—became trivial, while the scientist's subjectivity became untouchable as the most "civilized" and "sophisticated." Just as the dualism between "us" and "others" was prominent in Sullivan's racism expressed in private, sexualities were divided into the better kind (homosexuality) and the lesser kind (heterosexuality). This was in contrast with Benedict's private sphere, in which she questioned heteronormativity without privileging homosexuality. For her, this was fundamental to achieving fairness for women.

The limits of Sullivan's private practices were also apparent in his relationship with James Inscoe. Their partnership did not point toward fairness, but this was not because no one protested; indeed, Jimmie in the 1930s was not shy about expressing his unhappiness about people who thought of him as Harry's secretary or housekeeper. Throughout his New York years, it was known among Sullivan's friends that he lived with Inscoe. But when it came to the question of whether they were romantic partners, people had divided opinions. They agreed on one point about the nature of their relationship, however: Jimmie was a "discreet," "shy," "shadowy," and "fragile" person in need of someone's protection, and Sullivan's relationship with Jimmie replicated the therapist-client connection.[77] This image was enhanced by the support Harry offered to Jimmie, including financial subsidization and material comfort.

In return, Jimmie seems to have played the subservient role, as seen in a series of letters he wrote to Perry in 1971. For instance, as Jimmie recalled, he had been responsible for cooking for Harry's guests as well as Harry himself. He had to remember when to have guests, because "it would be I who would have to cook, make beds, etc."[78] In his letters Jimmie also revealed a sharp memory of the places he lived with Harry, giving great attention to details such as the exact sizes of rooms and windows, the number of tables and chairs, and ways in which they were arranged in a room.[79] This was because it was Jimmie who did the interiors of these places. Jimmie's responsibility included other intimate assistance of Harry: "[When HSS traveled he] always left packing to me. . . . In all of the years I was with him I had to lay out . . . his clothes he was to wear on a particular day. If I didn't pounce on his dirty underwear or socks . . . he would continue to wear them."[80] Regardless of what Jimmie might have felt about this chore, Harry doubtless appreciated Jimmie's devotion, once referring to Jimmie as the "protector of my peace and quiet." [81] But this did not change his status in Sullivan's public life. Indeed, Sullivan seemed embarrassed about Jimmie when he was with his professional associates. Jean Sapir remembered that Sullivan once "apologized for having Jimmie in tow," but said that it was necessary because "Jimmie was the worst case of demential [sic] praecox that he had ever seen."[82]

Despite his care for Harry, Jimmie also had some bitter feelings about his partner: "I have always greatly admired H.S.S. in his stand on patient treatment. But, I do wish he had left me better off—so much of my life was tied up with him in his work, and in his personal life."[83] It seems that they were both dependent on and bound to each other. They appreciated their partnership, but they also had moments of regret. Also, it seems that they both kept up an interest in women, even though it is not clear if the interest was genuine or a device to disguise their homosexuality. Although we do not know how Jimmie felt about Sullivan's affairs with women in the 1930s, we know that in the mid-1940s Jimmie himself made a proposal to one of Sullivan's female friends. It was a surprise to her, because they had not been in a romantic relationship at all. Revealingly, when Harry learned about Jimmie's proposal, Harry apologized to this woman, reiterating his role as Jimmie's guardian. Jimmie's "masculine" gesture, when it happened, was swiftly pulled back into the paternalistic dynamism in which he was expected to remain feminine and compliant.[84]

Harry's need to protect his self-image, even at the sacrifice of Jimmie's autonomy, then, arose out of a gender inequality that Sullivan assumed, as much as it did from his need to protect himself from homophobia. Not only in public, but also in private, Harry was concerned about his self-image as a paternal guardian, as Clifton Read's memoir suggests: "He [Sullivan] was scornful of fairies, effeminate men who pretend to be women—Sullivan projected a macho virility."[85] To be sure, this is one person's memory and might not prove that he was indeed contemptuous of homosexual men who projected effeminacy. Moreover, we do not know if Harry revealed a similar view to Jimmie. In any event, Read's memory seems ironic, because all who knew Jimmie agreed that he was "effeminate." Many remembered his youthful look, smooth skin with no hair, and his womanlike manner and gestures.[86] Also in Jimmie's pictures, he unmistakably projected a feminine image, wearing lipstick and assuming postures that seemed "playful, mysterious and homoerotic."[87]

Scientists' preoccupation with different "kinds" of homosexuality, which privileged masculinity over femininity, comported with an uneven relationship between Sullivan and Inscoe. Although this distinguished their relationship from that of Benedict and Mead, both Sullivan and Benedict failed to make critique of homophobia a public issue. Benedict's acceptance of homosexuality became a silent aspect of her life, while in Sullivan's private practices, the image of "superior" homosexual men prevailed. Because both practices were kept secret, a critical examination of sexual minorities' subjectivity did not occur in public. Moreover, as in Sullivan's case, private practices could absorb ideas and images that did not find a legitimate place in public—not only with issues related to sexuality, but also with issues of gender and race. Thus, while the era's scientific consensus moved toward racial and gender equality, Sullivan's private practices perpetuated racism and sexism. Consequently, desirable qualities of homosexuality, which was beginning to be seen as a reason to better accept it in the public discourse of science, became entangled with racism and sexism, which were increasingly losing their foothold in public. The consequence of this was revealed when Sullivan was asked to serve the government as the nation was entering World War II—particularly when he was compelled to make decisions about racial and sexual minorities.

5

The Military, Psychiatry, and "Unfit" Soldiers

Exploration of homosexuality by medical and social scientists in the 1920s and 1930s comprised "private" practices in which some revised or reversed what they claimed in "public." Whether it was an interaction with a patient in a clinical setting or a personal relationship with a friend, this private arena allowed scientists to imagine homosexuality in fluid, open-ended ways. The beginning of World War II dramatically transformed this pattern. The wartime national mobilization of science left no place for ambiguity and subjectivity, pushing a number of scientists to create clear-cut distinctions between those who were able to benefit the nation and those who were not. Not surprisingly, scientists in the life history cohort, whose fascination with seemingly endless varieties of human experiences had placed them in a unique position in U.S. science between the wars, were ambivalent about being implicated in the war effort. They were worried that involvement in national policy-making might change scientific inquiries in a fundamental way. In the end, however, many of them chose to join the unprecedented mobilization of science in the U.S. fight for the defense of democracy. Their choice was both pragmatic and naive, based on a belief that the free, autonomous pursuit of knowledge can be guaranteed only in a democratic society as they knew it. Many of the social scientists examined earlier, including Margaret Mead and Ruth Fulton Benedict, came to assert that ultimately a certain set of moral values—those informing mainstream American traditions—were not just one among many, but rather superior to others and requiring protection.[1]

The response of medical scientists to the war was similar, but the tempo in which theirs unfolded was faster, defining irreversibly the development of their expertise. The demand that medical and clinical theories be used to support the nation in wartime brought a number of scientists to the center of national and military policy-making as early as 1939, pushing those who had no preexisting professional connection with the government to work with policy makers, administrators, and army officers. One of the major products of the application of clinical medicine to public policy was the system to screen out "unfit" soldiers from the U.S. Army. Psychiatrists offered to use their diagnostic standards to determine who would (and would not) make a good soldier, a project that attracted the central administration's attention to their specialty's enormous, if unproven, potential as an agent of national defense. Harry Stack Sullivan designed, organized, and put into practice the national Selective Service psychiatric screening system, and he accomplished this within a narrow window of two years.

The making of the screening system constituted not only a crucial moment of change in American science in general, and psychiatry in particular, but also a significant turning point in the relationship between public and private practices in the science of homosexuality. Following the prevention model, Sullivan set his goals high to screen out all who exhibited signs of mental instability, which, if exposed to military life, could cause a breakdown. But obstacles quickly arose, illuminating ideological and practical problems involved in translating clinical insights into a public policy such as military screening. Moreover, Sullivan's ultimately unsuccessful attempt to shield certain of the men screened—namely, homosexual men—sheds light on how the making of a blanket policy circumscribed the liberal tradition in American science. This was a tradition that had been resisting simple categorizations and had rejected a belief in scientific knowledge as a collection of static facts. Also, this was the tradition that had been urging scientists to see sexual "perversion" as created by cultural experience, not as a sign of biological or psychological defect; some scientists had expressed their appreciation of "modern" qualities that seemed common among homosexual persons.

Sullivan tried but failed to use these positive observations in designing his screening system, and his work during the war exposes the result of a divide between public and private in U.S. liberalism, materializing in failure of scientists to create nonhomophobic, nonstigmatizing policies. Consequently, scientists enhanced the view that the mentally sick in general, and gay men in particular, hurt the national interest. In contrast to private science, which was nonstigmatizing of homosexuality but ultimately failed to influence public policy-making, the position on race that Sullivan supported in private—that white men's mental health should be protected at the expense of the well-being of African American men and women— openly influenced the selection of soldiers based on racism. This became apparent when many white Americans became concerned about the impact of war mobilization on American "stock": a number of physically strong, well-adjusted white men were sent to the war, while black men often failed to pass the screening because a large percentage of them were found to be "unfit," allowing them to avoid hazardous service. Scientists' response to this "problem" exposed the limits of liberal tradition in science in terms of its approach to both racial and sexual minorities. These limits foreshadowed U.S. international relationships after the war, in which the question of "us" and "others" became once again a central concern for American scientists.

Becoming a Military Psychiatrist

Sullivan's official relationship with the War Department began when he was appointed as a consultant on psychiatry to the director of the Selective Service in December 1940. He had already been determined to serve his country as early as October 1939, when he set up a committee of psychiatrists to promote the "utilization of psychiatry in the national defense."[2] In October 1940, he sent a memo to President Franklin Delano Roosevelt, outlining psychiatric considerations during induction into the army.

Working with the government in wartime was a new experience for most psychiatrists, and Sullivan was no exception. There had been a medical examination at induction during World War I, but a psychiatric component was often missing from the examination, in part because of the shortage of medical officers trained in psychiatry. Examinees who exhibited clear signs of mental problems were the only ones whose induction was considered questionable. Further, some evidence shows that the army rejected fewer than half of those who were found mentally deficient in the exam. Psychiatrists argued that this was because of officers' distrust of psychiatry. Because psychiatry at the time was believed to lack scientific explanations, it was not unusual for officers to assume that the mentally sick were fakers or that their problems, if any, could be corrected by army discipline.[3]

But at the end of World War I, it became apparent that the war had produced many men with psychiatric disabilities. The U.S. government spent more than a billion dollars to treat mental casualties, and it was widely recognized that the government had a responsibility to avoid a huge loss of men and money in the next war. When the Selective Training and Service Act was passed in 1940, it included the creation of the President's Civilian Advisory Committee on Selective Service (CACSS), which Sullivan soon joined as a psychiatric consultant. Besides Sullivan, the CACSS included representatives of the National Committee for Mental Hygiene (NCMH) and the American Psychiatric Association (APA), indicating the government's recognition of psychiatric expertise.[4] The committee's plan was ambitious: to eliminate before induction all who seemed mentally "unfit": all individuals who were likely to develop problems, as well as those who were sick. Such

a plan reflected psychiatrists' increasing focus on the prediction and prevention of mental illness in the 1920s and 1930s, and their peacetime optimism
that this focus helped create a better, healthier society.

Sullivan's interest in screening, too, arose from this belief in prevention
as a way to improve public mental health. Sullivan "extended the medical
model to an entire society" in his work for the Selective Service.[5] This was
because his attention to connections between individual and social problems guided him to "think hard about how America was to be mobilised [sic]
for war."[6] Thus, Sullivan believed that a medical model could and should be
applied to the general public and, by extension, to the screening of soldiers.[7]
In addition, there was an important ideological backdrop to Sullivan's interest, comprising his interventionism and his concern about his profession's
status, which helps explain the striking difference between the responses of
medical scientists and of social scientists to the war. Indeed, unlike most of
his cohorts in anthropology with whom he had worked in the 1930s, Sullivan
was a willing supporter of U.S. intervention of the war. In 1940, for example,
he criticized the national policy of isolation, making an analogy between
a mental patient and a country: "The people who really achieve isolation
come shortly to reside in penal institutions or in mental hospitals. Man is
profoundly and inescapably a social creature, and if he cuts himself off from
the communion with real people, then inevitably he . . . [loses] . . . healthy
touch with reality, and . . . sinks down."[8]

It was either intervention or the nation becoming mentally ill. This seamless application of the medical model—in Sullivan's case, his focus on interpersonal relationships as fundamental to mental health—to international
policies separated psychiatrists from anthropologists. Prewar anthropological studies had cultivated a critique of American culture. Moreover, unlike
psychiatrists, anthropologists had not had immediate, person-to-person
relationships with Americans whose lives would be significantly altered by
the war. These insulated social scientists from an immediate involvement
in national mobilization. To be sure, many social scientists in 1940 and 1941
supported the use of their expertise in predicting the Axis powers' course of
action and in helping to create antitotalitarian political sectors in Europe.
But revealingly, these social scientists called their method "the study of culture at a distance," upholding a certain degree of detachment. This detachment often revealed itself in their support for America's neutrality. As late
as September 1941, for instance, Ruth Benedict stood for keeping the nation
free to choose "pre-war 'peace,'" suggesting her preference of peace over war
even if, in the end, intervention might be necessary.[9]

Medical and social scientists diverged from each other in other ways.
For instance, as seen in Sullivan's 1940 statement about the organization of
screening, psychiatrists were pushed to war mobilization by a calculation

that the conflict would offer them a great opportunity to improve their status professionally:

> So far as . . . the Selective Service System is concerned . . . a great many candidates will be suspected of . . . handicap and referred for diagnosis to the advisory boards. There must be an adequate number of . . . psychiatrists on these boards. . . . To the extent that their work is thorough . . . human values will be conserved; a great burden of . . . compensation payments, hospitalization expenses, and pensions will be avoided—and the prestige and effectiveness of psychiatry, greatly expanded.[10]

No doubt Sullivan's desire to help his profession grow was a driving force behind his commitment to the screening. To be sure, the "new psychiatry" of the interwar years had broadened the profession through interdisciplinary collaborations. But compared with anthropology, a discipline that began to produce the second generation of homegrown scholars in the 1920s and 1930s, the APA at the dawn of the war still included a significant proportion of members who had been trained in Europe and U.S.-trained medical doctors without a certificate of psychiatry. Despite the increase in the number of psychiatric clinics, psychiatry's standing in universities across the nation was far from being established, making the mobilization of the expertise under the government's patronage seem an appealing opportunity for expansion.

As early as 1939, Sullivan was optimistic that the enhancement of American military through its not inducting the "unfit" would result in the protection of democracy. He regarded psychiatric screening as the crucial first phase in this scheme because mentally unsuitable personnel could be a serious threat to soldiers' morale. In his view, "men in the battle positions . . . are . . . conscious of their utter dependence on others"; "the solidarity that arises in the feeling of fraternity and collaboration [is] indispensable." When someone "break[s] down . . . and . . . [is] disabled by acute anxiety . . . , the so-called shell shock," this solidarity would be shaken, because these acute disturbances had "contagiousness." This would not only degrade the morale of the armed forces, but would also affect "the whole nation at arms, the worker and farmer, the parent and teacher, the civilian administrative personnel, the executive departments." Thus for Sullivan, the "protection of morale . . . [is] much more economical than are remedial efforts after disastrous failures at the front."[11] The impact of screening would be extensive, because the system was associated with the maintenance of national morale.

In Sullivan's reasoning, keeping morale high in the United States would aid an even larger cause; it would expand Western democracy and conserve what Sullivan called "human values." In a 1939 article, he defined "democracy as it exists today [as] a . . . process tending to the unfolding of greater opportunities for the achievement of human dignity, equality, and fraternity."[12] But he was concerned that democracy was declining. In 1938, he had written that the "sinking of Britain and France" marked the end of progress toward "a world democracy." He also argued that the United States, as a country that was "still relatively uncontaminated with the virus of the European and Asiatic disease," had the duty to "ward off the encroaching evils and insure humanity a continuing forward path."[13] Thus he assumed that Western democracy was a way to achieve universal values and that the United States needed to be its guardian. Military screening was not the least significant, as it contributed to worldwide protection of democratic, human values.

This heightened sense of responsibility, with a broad international aim, contributed to Sullivan's determination to continue the screening system even when it turned out to be ineffective. As he became aware that screening worked against the social acceptance of the mentally ill, it did not seem to occur to him that he might reconsider his involvement. Sullivan, along with a number of his colleagues, wanted to stay within the system so as to lessen its adverse consequences, even as he began to understand that the system was constructed on a shaky ground of scientific knowledge directly applied to public policies. Without doubt, this was a dilemma that many social scientists experienced in joining the war mobilization effort after Pearl Harbor. But the application of their expertise went largely into the concerted protection of democracy (and the demoralization of its enemies) rather than the division of American citizens into different categories such as "fit" and "unfit" soldiers. For example, Margaret Mead, drawing upon her understanding of an American "pattern of culture" as distinctively antiauthoritarian, helped create decentralized, grassroots nutrition programs to maintain high morale on the home front. Benedict took a position in the Office of War Information in 1943, beginning to look outside the United States to pursue national character studies (particularly of Denmark, Thailand, and Romania) in order to offer suggestions about psychological aspects of warfare.

These anthropological projects generally underscored and, in some cases, exaggerated unity among Americans. Mead's examination of American patterns of culture, for instance, included virtually no discussion of racial and ethnic minorities and the existing social schisms that had haunted the social scientists of the 1920s and 1930s. Instead, her characterization of the United States was often based on an assumption that the assimilation of everyone into mainstream culture is possible. Similarly, Benedict's *The Race of Mankind*, a pamphlet that she put together for the Committee for Democracy and Intellectual Freedom, posited that racial differences were superficial and culturally constructed.[14] This was a position largely different from the one that most psychiatrists took at the beginning of the war. Promoting the public's mental health, psychiatrists were trained to consider it their responsibility to identify a range of "problems" such as delinquency, immaturity, and maladjustments. Moreover, psychiatrists assumed that the identification of these problems helped the protection of the patient population and the public. Indeed, as one psychiatrist argued in 1942, war psychiatrists must counter "thousand of families . . . [and] physicians" who believed "that the discipline and the regularity of army experience will snap their sons out of their shyness and their day dreaming and put 'some real stuff' in them." What might seem minor problems must be "taken more seriously" in order to prevent the development of psychoses.[15] This particular way of defining public health made it reasonable for psychiatrists to work for the screening. Wartime psychiatrists shared with anthropologists a trust in democracy and a strong urge to protect it. But as psychiatrists stepped into the categorization of the U.S. general population, they confronted disparity and inequality within, from which anthropologists managed to look away momentarily.

The Panacea of Psychiatric Screening

The early phase of psychiatric screening reveals the plan's complexity as well as its ambitiousness. In the memo Sullivan sent to President Roosevelt in October 1940, he listed five major categories of mental handicap: mental defect or deficiency, psychopathic personality, major abnormalities of mood, psychoneurotic disorders, and pre- and postpsychotic personalities. Each category included a short description of suggestive signs. It is notable that his description of these signs was simpler and more inclusive than in the standard classification of mental illness issued by the NCMH and the APA. For instance, Sullivan wrote in the draft that mental defect or deficiency was "suggested by slowness or stupidity in complying with clear instructions,"[16] whereas the counterpart of this category in the NCMH-APA standard classification described its symptoms more particularly as "episodes of excitement or irritability, depressions, paranoid trends, hallucinatory attacks."[17] Pre- and postpsychotic personalities were not included in the NCMH-APA standard classification, but the screening draft posited that these personalities existed and should also be screened out.[18] As such, the screening criteria pointed to more extensive range of problems than the NCMH-APA standard. This was partly because of the need to suit the criteria to a snapshot diagnosis, in which little time was allowed to elicit symptoms, but it also reflected Sullivan's belief that candidates must be screened out as broadly as possible.

During the month after Sullivan submitted the draft, the CACSS met twice to go over it and subsequently issued Medical Circular No. 1 in November 1940. Although Sullivan was not officially appointed to the committee at this point, he participated in its meetings. When he joined the committee a month later, he proposed screenings at three points: at the local installation board, at the medical advisory board, and at the army induction center.[19] At a local board, an examiner was expected to detect "inadequate personalit[ies]" of all kinds. If the examiner were not sure that a candidate had a problem, he would refer the candidate to an advisory board psychiatrist. If a candidate were found to have no problem, he would be sent to an army induction center. Another psychiatric examination would take place there. Once the committee approved Sullivan's proposal, the medical circular was distributed to local board examiners. Sullivan agreed to organize a series of two-day seminars on psychiatric screening, beginning in January 1941. These seminars were designed to educate psychiatrists at advisory boards and induction centers about diagnostic standards.[20]

Sullivan knew of the need to educate examiners at all stages. He understood that most local board examiners were not trained in psychiatry. In 1941, there were more than six thousand local boards. But in his estimation, there were only thirty-five hundred physicians trained in psychiatry. Sullivan also decided that a third of these thirty-five hundred physicians must remain in civilian hospitals. In addition, there were about seven hundred advisory boards, each of which needed a psychiatrist.[21] The seventy-five induction centers needed psychiatrists, too. What all this meant was that there were not enough psychiatrists left for local boards. Yet as Sullivan explained, somewhat wistfully, his hope was that "many of the local board physicians will discover for the first time something of the place of psychiatry in medical practice."[22]

This screening plan was a complex project in ways that went beyond numbers. It was dubious how effective local board examiners, who were not trained in psychiatry, could be in sorting out the mentally "unfit." But Sullivan's plan relied on the elimination of such persons at the first and second stages of the screening. As he noted, "Psychiatric examination . . . require[s] an average of between 15 and 20 minutes per candidate. When the local and advisory boards have rejected most of the mentally handicapped, the average time per candidate . . . at this point of induction may easily fall to as little as 10 to 12 minutes."[23] He sounds optimistic, but it was unclear if local and advisory boards would function effectively to give psychiatrists at induction centers enough time to do their work.

Moreover, the effectiveness of psychiatric interviews at induction centers was doubtful. These interviews were supposed to sort out inductees who were likely to become problem soldiers. This was not a familiar assignment for psychiatrists, most of whom had positions as superintendents at state institutions. In many cases, inpatients at state institutions had advanced illnesses, and such cases did not offer psychiatrists opportunities to see mild problems. Sullivan was aware of this situation, but it did not seem to deter him. Even as he noted the difference between civilian and wartime psychiatry, he stressed the significance of the "detecti[on] of . . . early conditions" as something that would have a long-lasting impact on the well-being of the nation: "Either during the year of training . . . or in the demobilization and return to civilian status, or in the whole course of ten years following that . . . disability [will] expose all citizens to an increased burden."[24] Thus, mental health years after discharge was at stake. He did not believe that the preventive measure would be completely effective, but he felt that illnesses could be reduced by more than half.[25]

Despite these difficulties, Sullivan insisted that screening would be successful if examiners made good use of the available time. Ultimately, he argued, success depended on the examiners' ability to adopt the individualized approach that the new psychiatry had embraced. For example, observing how a candidate undressed could disclose if he was unusually tense. The first greeting, as well as the conversation that followed, also could be revealing. Slowness of speech at the beginning of the interview and a shift to an increasing somberness of expression could be a sign of mood disturbances. Extravagant statements, such as "I almost died from heart pain" or "I had frightful, splitting headaches," could be signs of psychoneuroses, especially the "hysterics." If a candidate demonstrated continuing insistence on a particular topic, even when an examiner interrupted, it suggested an obsession. Extreme sensitivity on the part of a candidate during an examination could be a reason to reject him. If he paid "much attention to [an examiner's] glance [and] bat [his] eyes immediately upon encountering [an examiner's] gaze,"[26] it could be a sign of a prepsychotic personality.

It is clear that Sullivan was envisioning interviews similar to those in small-scale clinics, instead of creating an entirely new set of procedures for the military. In his practice, as with most advocates of the new psychiatry, he had conducted careful examinations of patients' life experiences in intensive, one-on-one interviews. Even though interviews for military screening were shorter than those in civilian facilities, their goal was still to evaluate candidates' "personality . . . conditions," not to delineate symptoms.[27] In wartime screening, though, this approach met serious challenges. The number of psychiatrists who were familiar with the job, as well as amount of time available for each candidate, were limited. The application of clinical technique to public policy was on dubious ground from the beginning.

A related problem that concerned Sullivan and others who joined in the creation of the screening was the stigmatization of rejected candidates. This issue sharply crystallized in May 1941, when the medical circular was revised and reissued. It now pinpointed three additional categories of handicap that disqualified candidates from military service: chronic inebriety (drug or alcoholic addiction); syphilis of the central nervous system; and organic disease of the brain, spinal cord, or peripheral nerves. What is most striking, however, is the addition of "homosexual proclivities" in the list of deviations that should be referred to advisory boards.[28] In his 1940 memo, Sullivan had not made a direct reference to homosexuality, but instead mentioned the "impression of queerness" that certain psychotic personalities might make on examiners. He had recommended that examiners be alert, because some men "entertain . . . convictions as to bodily peculiarities or disorders which they attribute to excessive sexual acts."[29] "Queerness" could mean an unspecific strangeness in a person, but it could also imply homosexuality when it was used in specific contexts.[30] Sullivan's 1940 memo suggests that he was taking advantage of this ambiguity: given his claim that "queerness" was related to both psychosis and sexuality, it could well be a reference to homosexuality. But he did not say that it was, indeed, homosexuality. Sullivan, because he had worked with patients whose life histories included "homosexual contents," understood the stigmatizing effect of "homosexuality" both as a term and a concept. Perhaps this awareness made him choose the ambiguous and possibly less stigmatizing word *queerness*. In 1941, however, the advisory committee specifically spelled out that individuals with "homosexual proclivities" must be rejected by the military, shattering any effort Sullivan may have been making to shield homosexual men from the very label.[31]

The CACSS decided to try to screen out homosexual men before induction. The army's traditional procedure of excluding homosexuals was to charge men already in the armed services with sodomy and incarcerate them. But by 1941, that procedure did not seem plausible. With such a great number of conscripts, the army believed that it made more sense to reject the undesirable before induction.[32] The CACSS's decision to accommodate the army's demand created a dilemma for Sullivan. His precise role in this change of procedure is unclear, but evidence suggests that it was troubling to him. For one thing, he was well aware that rejection could stigmatize a person; he emphasized that the goal of the screening was to determine the "vocational appropriateness" of candidates, not to eliminate individuals as socially unworthy. In fact, he expected that examiners would reject more men overall than those they would accept.[33] The clear message here was that psychiatric selection was not for eliminating the unfit, but for selecting those who were particularly suited to military service. Along the same lines, Sullivan specifically called for educating the public to make people understand that the "unsuitability because of mental or personality factors . . . has no necessary relation to the worth of the registrant as a human being, or to his . . . ability to work."[34] But the reality was that rejection caused damage to those who were rejected.

To put the burden on the shoulders of the mentally ill in general and homosexual men in particular was not what Sullivan wanted. He had fought against this with his "schizophrenic" patients in the 1920s, most of whom he believed to be homosexual. Although his practice became highly problematic in the 1930s, his apparent intention—however misguided—had been to free patients from their conflict over their sexuality. In sharp contrast with his passion for protecting or privileging homosexuality was his argument in published articles and lectures. In his clinical records, there was no evidence suggesting that he made a distinction between different "kinds" of homosexuality; but in his published writings, his claims were different. Even as he struggled to minimize the stigma of rejection, then, by 1941 Sullivan had not publicly constructed theories from which he could argue against blanket homophobia. To complicate the matter, he recognized a certain medical need to screen out homosexual men from the military. Based on his earlier observations, Sullivan's belief in 1941 still was that homosexual men were at high risk of becoming schizophrenic.[35]

Sullivan was hardly alone in this belief. In 1941 during one of the seminars on psychiatric screening, for instance, Douglas A. Thom, then a professor of psychiatry at Tufts University in Boston, laid out his concerns about homosexuality in the army:

> Homosexuality is frequently associated with schizoid paranoid reactions. Persons with a strong homosexual component . . . find the Army a completely masculine environment. . . . Their own latent homosexual drives, for which they were able to find satisfactory sublimations in civil life, are often activated but denied outlet in Army life, which result in conflict, alcoholism and paranoid reactions.[36]

The single-sex environment, as well as the unforgiving regulation of individual behavior in the military, would push some people over the edge, even those who were well adjusted as civilians. This model of protection proved to be compelling, giving military psychiatrists a humane, legitimate reason for excluding homosexual men from the service. The model also allowed psychiatrists to maintain a sense of continuity: even as their expertise moved from the civilian to the military, their work still would be for the well-being of the vulnerable. Similarly, psychiatrists' persistent belief in the new psychiatry—that preventive measures were the best way to minimize psychiatric problems—served as an additional rationale for the exclusion of anyone who seemed suspect. Thus, on the one hand, Sullivan was pushed to accept "homosexual proclivities" as a risk to be avoided. On the other hand, he clearly understood that the inclusion of homosexuality in the list of deviations would fuel prejudice against it.

If we assume that Sullivan was aware of how the term *queerness* might provide a shield, then we can see him hoping to force the screening process to walk a narrow line between protection and rejection. Or he might have attempted to maintain the private sphere, in which he could take care of a range of problems without putting a singular, public stamp on them. Indeed, evidence suggests that he used screening to benefit individual homosexual men. In 1940, for example, he helped a patient of his friend psychoanalyst Clara Thompson to get out of the army. As this patient recalled, Thompson believed that "it would be disastrous [for the patient] to go in the army." She talked to Sullivan, and he used his "influence" to get the patient a rejection "without saying he was homosexual."[37] Sullivan's apparent intention was to protect the patient by avoiding a "diagnosis" of homosexuality. Sullivan thus tried to obscure the borderline between rejection and admission—or more specifically, the line between homosexuality and heterosexuality—in order to minimize the distress of those who were denied military service. Such vagueness had the potential to work against stigma, of course, but it was also likely to contradict his original plan of making screening as thorough and scientific as possible. More important, the protected environment he tried to craft for the rejected homosexual men did not have an impact on the screening policy, just as the full acceptance of homosexuality he articulated with his patients in his clinical practice never found its way to his published writings.

Whatever the particulars of Sullivan's views in this regard, the CACSS decided nonetheless to define homosexuality as a form of deviancy. Sullivan did not describe how he felt about the decision, but it is not difficult to speculate that the discriminative policy caused him a great strain. He was a homosexual man rejecting homosexuality, a status he probably had not imagined finding himself in. Because of his medical beliefs, he might have thought that certain "kinds" of homosexual men needed to be barred; still, the resulting overall stigmatization of homosexuality was inconsistent with his science of homosexuality, both public and private. But in the first half of 1941, he traveled around the nation to give seminars on the screening. Beginning in Washington, DC, he served as the main speaker and advisor in Boston, Atlanta, New York City, Chicago, Dallas, Los Angeles, San Francisco, and Buffalo. In these seminars and the selection of soldiers that followed, Sullivan's private practice of protecting homosexual men in particular, and American psychiatric profession's attempt to benefit the mentally vulnerable in general, entered a new phase of challenge.

Unfit Soldiers, Unfit System

Throughout 1941, both before and after the revision of the medical circular, Sullivan seldom made a clear reference to homosexuality. He believed that this term had "accumulated so great a freight of misunderstanding" that a better term should be invented.[38] He continued to use the terms *queer* and *schizoid*, instead of *homosexual*. For example, he described a candidate for induction whom he called a "schizoid" in his 1941 seminar on the screening:

> An unduly mature-looking, serious, quietly alert, carefully-spoken registrant but recently discharged from [a mental] hospital as a social recovery from a severe schizophrenic psychosis, catatonic type—a fact unknown to the referee—gave so good an account of himself . . . that the officer was loath to lose this excellent "first sergeant material" in class 4-F. In general, a schizoid with a college education is apt to make a better than average college-graduate impression, if he is not obviously a "queer duck."[39]

Given Sullivan's belief in the link between homosexuality and schizophrenia, it was likely that Sullivan believed that the "schizoid" candidate in this quote had homosexual tendencies.[40] But Sullivan said that the candidate was a "schizoid," not a "homosexual." He chose not to single out homosexuality as an independent reason for rejection.

Such carefulness stood in sharp contrast with a direct reference to homosexuality such as Douglas Thom's, although Sullivan was not necessarily alone in offering nuanced descriptions of candidates. Dexter Mean Bullard, who was at the analytically oriented mental hospital Chestnut Lodge in Rockland, Maryland, gave lectures in the Selective Service seminar series. His discussion of "schizoid" individuals who should be screened out was strikingly similar to Sullivan's, although Bullard was far more explicit about what he considered to be underlying sexual conflicts of these individuals:

> More difficult to gauge are the modestly unobtrusive, quiet and gentle mannered chaps . . . of rather youthful appearance with sensitive features and an air of refinement, sometimes with slightly effeminate mannerisms or gestures. How will they like the idea of a common shower, of having no privacy? . . . Are they disgusted by dirty stories whose point is strongly oral or anal? . . . Have they failed to break away from the early attachment to the mother and to find a substitute?[41]

Framing the candidates in the psychoanalytical theory of personality development, Bullard was no doubt talking about people whom he believed to be homosexual. But, like Sullivan, Bullard avoided a direct reference to homosexuality.

Thom, Sullivan, and Bullard were all giving seminars in the first half of 1941, suggesting a range of approaches to homosexuality among psychiatrists before the revision of the circular. Some had no reservation about singling out homosexuality, while others were cautious about the use of language. Among the latter, *schizoid* was used as a label that included *homosexuality*. Compared to *queer*, an ambiguous, nonmedical term, *schizoid* was a more pointed and certainly medical term that could signify homosexuality. And yet *schizoid* was not equivalent to *homosexual*. Unlike *homosexual*, *schizoid* could include a range of problems that had no direct connection to homosexuality. Although it is unclear to what extent psychiatrists used *schizoid* with an intention to protect homosexual persons from stigmatization, there is no doubt that *homosexuality* was a term about which psychiatrists had no clear consensus before the revision of the circular. Moreover, it was also unclear if it was a medical condition that could be translated into a single diagnostic term. Of course, the term had been used in clinical practice, and it had been regarded as a form of mental illness by mainstream psychiatric theorists. But in early 1941, *homosexuality* was not part of the official diagnostic terminology, certainly not in the same way as it became one when the *Diagnostic and Statistical Manual* was issued seven years after the war ended. The manual defined homosexuality as sociopathic personality disorder, a definition based on wartime use in the military. War mobilization put an effective limit on the relatively flexible interpretation of what constituted mental illness in clinical settings.

In this regard, it is noteworthy that both Sullivan and Bullard in early 1941 described "schizoid" individuals as people with many favorable qualities, some of which echoed the image of "sophisticated" homosexual men that floated on the periphery of scientific discourse in the 1920s and 1930s. Most likely, it was this image that helped psychiatrists in the war seminars to stress the desirable qualities of candidates who were "unfit" for military service. Indeed, mirroring the prewar characterization of homosexual men as intelligent, Leo H. Bartemeier, a psychiatrist who lectured at one of the seminars, suggested that a "schizoid" man was often a "valuable citizen" who had grown up as a "model child." He might never have "gone out with girls" and might still be single at the age of, say, thirty-four, but this was "because he was more interested in study." He might even spend "his spare time reading Spinoza and fantasying about the solution of world problems." These comments were made without a hint of condescension. Rather, the point that Bartemeier tried to make was that even though this thirty-four years old "would probably acquire a psychosis . . . if compelled to live closely with other men in the Army . . . it seemed reasonable to suppose that left where he was he might continue to function adequately on his job."[42] This model of the protecting the vulnerable, combined with the assumption that homosexual men had numerous desirable qualities, occupied a notable place in the rationale of screening in its early stage.

On the other hand, just as Sheppard-Pratt patients who suffered from "homosexual content" were diagnosed with "schizophrenia," people with admirable qualities discussed in the screening seminars were "schizoid," not "homosexuals." This lack of a clear definition in public cut in both ways. While the ambiguity could help prevent the stigmatizing isolation of the "problem" population, it also made it difficult to create a coalition among scientists to speak against hardnosed hostility against sexual minorities. In 1929 during the Personality Colloquium, Sullivan used a similar tactic of protection for patients who could not be intimate with persons of the same sex. Then, he compelled Edward Sapir to argue that American culture was punitive of same-sex intimacy. Again in 1937, Sullivan confided to his friend that openness to a range of sexual expressions was a sign of civilization. But in 1941, particularly after the revision of the circular, the same approach hit a different kind of wall.

During a Chicago seminar that took place immediately after the revision of the circular, for instance, Colonel William C. Porter from the U.S. Army made a callous comment about homosexuality, quite unlike remarks by Sullivan and other psychiatrists:

> We feel that the homosexuals, if they are overt in their manifestations, can do inestimable harm in the Army of the United States by seduction of youths who are not homosexually inclined. That has been our experience. We find that the American culture will not admit social intercourse with known homosexuals: that the homosexual becomes a pariah and an outcast in his organization. His life is made miserable, and the morale of the organization of which he is a member, if known, is lowered. Therefore, we feel that . . . a known homosexual . . . should be excluded from the military service.[43]

Not only is this harshly dismissive of homosexuality, Porter appears to have given not the least thought to the consequences of being excluded from the army. His comment also demonstrates a set of widely held preconceptions concerning homosexual men: they were seductive, promiscuous, and antisocial and as a result did not fit into any organization.

Notably, Sullivan responded with a defense of not denoting homosexuality, asking for the "liberty of being heard a little more" on homosexuality:

> There may be a hesitancy on the part of local board and advisory board examiners to label a selectee as having . . . a homosexuality, on the basis of what at best is an inadequate examination because of the liability of malpractice suit to which the physician exposes himself. Not only for that reason, but also because of this business of refined

diagnosis, the great deal of time it takes, and perhaps irrelevancy of the results, we have been urging that causes for rejection shall be answered . . . in terms of group so and so.[44]

Sullivan went on to say that by "group so and so" he referred to any of the eight categories of mental handicap defined in "Medical Circular No. 1, Revised." None of the categories in this document included "homosexuality"; instead, "homosexual proclivities" was mentioned in the supplemental list of "deviations" that examiners should look for. By recommending the use of the "terms of group so and so," Sullivan was pushing for a rejection of homosexuality without making a direct reference to it.[45] He was saying that examiners must screen out homosexual persons because it was required, but that a psychiatric examination is not at all reliable in detecting an examinee's sexual preference. This contradicted his 1940 statement on the possibility that the screening increases psychiatry's prestige. When it came to the issue of homosexuality, he had to say that the screening itself was not dependable. He was deeply conflicted.

During a seminar in San Francisco later the same year, he emphasized that the rejection of homosexuality was not a biological, but a cultural, demand, indicating his continued reliance on the relativism that shaped the scientific thinking of the 1920s and 1930s. He reiterated that American culture "require[d a man to have] a strong interest in a member of the other sex." He then began to tell a fictional story of a homosexual man, in order to encourage better understanding of homosexuality among his audience.

> He realizes that he hasn't the skill to maintain the show of being a man. . . . [He] discovers he can't make the grade and be a real he-man as he-men should be. At that unhappy state—driven by all the drives that man acquires by development and aculturation [sic] . . . ; that means combing your hair straight back . . . marrying at the appropriate age . . . anything you know that is the right thing for you and your family to do—[he] also observes that all the other things that he had been doing aren't quite right, they just aren't quite right.[46]

Here Sullivan seemed to express his sympathy for homosexual men, although his comment notably lacked the word *homosexuality*. He felt he had to say this at the seminar because he realized that the screening defined homosexual men as unquestionably misfits. He wanted to stress that homosexuality was socially and culturally constructed and that being unfit for military service was not inherent in homosexuality itself. But all these points had to be made without using the word *homosexuality*.

What is equally striking is that Sullivan tried to lessen the screening's undesirable consequences rather than resisting discrimination itself.

Certainly, the prevailing homophobia, particularly in the military, played a part, as did Sullivan's fear that if his own sexual preference came to light he would lose his standing. Another important reason for the lack of explicit critique was the overall limits of liberalism in the science of homosexuality in prewar years. In the 1920s and 1930s, Sullivan excluded the insights that he had gained from private practice from his public writing, while he continued to stress that certain kinds of homosexuality were less mature than heterosexuality. With such a circumscribed view, he could not counter the growth of homophobic policy after mid-1941. Sullivan's use of unspecific diagnoses and unspecific reasons for rejection during wartime was of a piece with his and his profession's propensity to deal with the issue of homosexuality mostly in private. This containment shaped a system that deprived many healthy sexual minorities of the right to serve the nation. When the budding egalitarian view of homosexuality conflicted with the official view of it as an illness, as it did in wartime, liberal scientists were ineffective in creating a nonhomophobic policy.

As 1941 progressed, it became more difficult for Sullivan to protect homosexual men in subtle ways. His strategy might have been effective in the small circle of psychiatrists he associated with during the 1930s. They would have understood that his story of a man who could not "maintain the show of being a he-man" was, in fact, a criticism of social pressure on homosexuals. But such a story did not appeal to the larger audience he now addressed, who did not belong to Sullivan's circle or even profession. It did not function as a counterargument against the view that homosexual men would do unquestionable damage to the U.S. armed forces. As Colonel Porter's comment shows, the army concluded that it would not suffer the "harm" caused by homosexual men who "seduced" heterosexual soldiers.[47] For those who believed in the application of psychiatric insights to patient welfare, this was a definite turning point.

How did this change in policy affect homosexual registrants? For one, there was not much consideration about the impact such rejection might have on individuals who had not "come out" before registering. Some homosexual men and women came to induction without a faintest idea about what "homosexuality" meant. It was not a term in universal use, and when denied an induction because of their homosexuality, the rejectees had to first grapple with its meanings, and then figure out if and how they were going to tell their families, friends, and employers. For others who had known the term, the policy of elimination caused a dilemma: should they admit their homosexuality, to be honest about themselves, or should they deny it, in order to be patriotic and faithful to their sense of duty? To some, the scantiness of the screening offered a reasonable, if incomplete, solution: an examiner would ask if a homosexual registrant liked girls, and he would answer yes without even having a chance to reveal that he liked boys as well. Indeed, countless homosexual men, and beginning in 1942, homosexual women—eager to serve the nation just as much as any others of the generation—got into the army and served their full term.

For others who were "found out" to be homosexual, either in the screening process or after induction, the experience was just as memorable and often lastingly painful. Those who got in and were found out to be homosexual were sent to the army's prisons or rehabilitation centers, depending on the nature of the charges and when they were made (the army shifted its policy from internment to reclassification based on psychiatric evaluation in 1943). Eventually, most were discharged without honor (the so-called blue discharge), stripped of recognition and compensation. In some cases, a soldier reported that his problem originated in his homosexuality to an army psychiatrist, only to find out that the doctor reported that to their unit's commander. This damaged the relationship between medical officers and soldiers.[48] The experience of registrants who were screened out before induction could have been equally difficult. Sullivan's plan to have examiners use ambiguous group designations did not produce the expected effect. Many psychiatrists took the liberty of putting down the word *homosexuality* as a reason for rejection. Moreover, in practice, it soon became known which code referred to which problem. Some group designations accompanying a rejection—"psychotic personality" for example—came to be used as a contemptuous code-name for homosexuality, when a person showed no apparent mental abnormality.[49] In addition, those rejected for psychiatric reasons included many individuals about whom examiners at different stages of the screening disagreed. This led to recall and reclassification, confusing and frustrating candidates and their families. The suspension of their status often created a problem in the workplace as well. Some employers complained that they could not interpret their suspended employees' status, hurting stable business operations.[50] This applied not only to those who were found to have homosexual tendencies, but to virtually everyone rejected due to a psychiatric reason. Psychiatric screening accentuated bias against rejectees in many different ways.

One social bias that was illuminated as a result of psychiatric screening—prejudice against African Americans—calls for special attention here, not only because of the sheer weight it carried in changing race relationships during the war, but also because the screening of African Americans offered a sharp contrast to the elimination of those exhibiting "homosexual proclivities." Soon after the screening began, it became clear that African Americans were rejected at a disproportionately higher rate than that of white candidates. The predominantly white board of examining psychiatrists failed to distinguish differences based on culture, class, and the level of education from mental deficiency, leading to a rejection rate of 23.8 percent for whites and 45.5 percent for blacks, according to a 1943 study of eighteen- and nineteen-year-old draftees.[51] This imbalanced rejection concerned white physicians and black leaders, but for entirely different reasons. For many African American observers, the high rate of rejection was yet another piece of evidence that racism replicated itself in military service, while for some white critics, it meant the risk of disproportionate sacrifice for whites. Some of Sullivan's comments on screening were made with a clear intention to respond to the latter. For instance, in a press release in October 1941, Sullivan indicated that the number of candidates who fell within the categories of "psychoneuroses" and "peculiarities of personality" were greater among whites than among blacks. Sullivan did not explain the reason but suggested that, using these categories, psychiatrists were helping "young Whites [to] be retained in the home front" and more blacks to be sent off to battle.[52]

In a way this was a strange claim, given the fact that, in total, black candidates were rejected much more often than their white counterparts.[53] Nevertheless, Sullivan highlighted those categories that helped to keep more whites than blacks at home so as to assure people who were concerned about "the 'cream' of American youth [which apparently meant whites, as well as individuals who had well-developed physical and mental abilities,] . . . being skimmed off for the combat forces, to the serious detriment of the 'stock.'" Clearly, Sullivan was trying to make sure that people understood that psychiatric screening was not a threat to "the biological soundness of the [white] American people."[54] Although such an attempt contradicted his egalitarian approach to racism in the 1930s, Sullivan did not seem to notice the contradiction, just as he did not see a problem in the prejudice against African Americans he disclosed to his friend Clifton Read. This lack of recognition, on the one hand, illuminates the distance between the public and private in the culture of science: scientists could claim one thing in the former and assert another in the latter, even if the two came into conflict. On the other hand, the fact that Sullivan's private beliefs about both sexual and racial minorities were articulated in public, if mostly in coded language, illuminates how there was constant interaction between these different spheres. Sullivan's positive description of homosexual candidates, as well as his characterization of African Americans as those who must be recruited more to protect America's "biological soundness," were what he tried to bring to the public arena from his private practice.

On another occasion, Sullivan's assertion that "cream" population must be protected was tied into the increasingly problematic realm of eugenics. In late 1941, stressing the need to create an army with mentally fit soldiers, he wrote:

I pray that we may avoid any further worry about the evil effects on
the future American stock of the first little intelligence that has gone
into sorting out people for military service. Let us be clear on the fact
that we are under infinitely greater, more real and immediate threats
to our future than eugenic considerations will ever bring us, so that
anything that we can do to make the army a success becomes a simply
imperative necessity.[55]

Here, he did not question "eugenic considerations" themselves, but
rather argued that psychiatric screening was too "little" to produce a negative effect on the U.S. biological "stock." Just because screening helped to
keep a large number of "unfit" individuals, including African Americans,
at home, it did not follow that the future of the United States was at risk.
This logic, in effect, endorsed the existing bias against minorities. Echoing
a sentiment common to military leaders and policy makers during the war
years—that "war was no time for social experiment"—statements like this
reveal how, in the face of national crisis, certain scientific assumptions
about "us" and "others" were left unchallenged.[56]

At this point, psychiatrists in general and Sullivan in particular were far
away from where they had been in the 1920s and 1930s when they had collaborated with social scientists. In a 1941 letter to the social psychologist J. L.
Moreno, Margaret Mead expressed, in sharp contrast to Sullivan's lukewarm
attitude toward eugenics, an unmistakable concern about the uncritical
acceptance of racial differences:

I feel that to emphasize hereditary factors more than is absolutely
necessary for scientific accuracy may be doing incalculable harm.
The first response of the average person to any accepted scheme of
temperamental classification is to construct "we-groups" and "you-
groups." . . . It is most important to avoid at present, especially within
the social sciences, any sort of schism. I believe that if this theory
were advanced now . . . it might do great harm.[57]

To be sure, this deemphasis of biological differences tended to generate an idealized image of America as a united nation. It is notable, however,
that Mead took it as her responsibility to counter biological theories that
assumed essential differences between humans. She did not want her theories of cultural and temperamental diversity to be interpreted as suggesting
irresolvable distinctions between races and peoples. As psychiatrists such
as Sullivan grappled with the selection of best-fit soldiers, it became difficult for medical scientists to remain on the same ideological and rhetorical
ground as social scientists. Although scientists from different disciplines

had created collaborative programs before the war, and again worked together after 1945 in the creation of international organizations, the routes taken by medical and social scientists in the middle of the international crisis were distinct from each other. The national mobilization of science, by assigning different tasks to different fields (and by setting the stage for scientists to take on responsibilities that carried national significance) put the multidisciplinary science community on hold.

The isolation from social scientists made it easier for psychiatrists, at least for the time being, to be insulated from an adamant critique of race problems such as Mead's. To further complicate the matter for Sullivan, the less than egalitarian attitude toward race might have seemed a way to protect homosexual men. Indeed, one of the categories of problems into which more whites than blacks fell, "peculiarities of personality," included many men who were found to have "homosexual proclivities." Given this, Sullivan's recommendation that "peculiarities of personality" be used as a means to retain whites at home can be seen as his unpronounced desire to protect white *and* homosexual men, possibly at the sacrifice of black soldiers. To be sure, he probably did not believe that he could persuade the general public that the retention of people with "peculiar personalities" helped the preservation of the "cream." But he might have thought that those who appeared "mature" and "serious" and often made a good impression on examiners, but were rejected because of their "peculiar personalities," were in fact better than average. Indeed, since the beginning of his career in the 1920s, he often expressed his high regard for the intelligence and sensitivity of schizophrenic patients. In his description, those "sensitive individuals" frequently manifested some of the best personality traits.[58] When these individuals recovered from mental illness, it seemed to him that they "grew wise enough to be tolerant of the imbecility surrounding them, having finally discovered that it was stupidity and not malice."[59] In the 1930s, as we have seen, the depiction of homosexuality as "sophisticated" continued to prevail in his private practices. Instead of making it explicit that he was protecting schizophrenic and homosexual men, he might have chosen to protect the larger racial group, "young Whites."[60]

He did not explore why more whites fell in this category than blacks. Nor is there evidence that the statistical difference between blacks and whites made him wonder if it was because of racism—a kind of question that his public thinking on racism in the 1930s would have raised. Almost all the patients Sullivan was acquainted with were white, as far as we can tell from the records, and perhaps this made it easier for him to speak on their behalf. Moreover, as seen in Chapter 4, his critique of the bias against African Americans was an extension of his critique against heterosexism.

The latter preceded the former in his thinking, because for Sullivan, race issues offered a more mainstream, more effective means to address what he saw as the root cause of heterosexism. In his collaboration with Johnson and Frazier in the 1930s, these critiques coexisted without conflicts; his critique of heterosexism remained mostly confined to the private sphere, while his liberal approach to race problems was published as part of the project sponsored by a public organization. By the end of 1941, however, with the war on, the relationship between sex and race became more complicated. At this point, it was clear that his effort to translate his private critique of homophobia into a public one to reduce the adverse effect of screening was futile. Meanwhile, the prejudice against African Americans he had expressed in private during the 1930s became more prominent in his public speeches in 1941, so much so that it seemed to overwhelm the critique of racism he had presented in public before the war. Private practices of science played a considerably shrunken role in the protection of homosexuals in wartime; with regard to racial minorities, in contrast, a certain kind of racism that had been kept in private—that blacks could be "used" to benefit whites—seemed to flow effortlessly into the public.

As a result, African Americans as a particular kind of "others"—whom white scientists understood to be a mistreated population, but whom they did not approach with a sense of subjective involvement—became an easy scapegoat during the first few years of the war. It was easy not in the sense that blackness was more stigmatized than homosexuality; both suffered from injustice, if in different ways. Rather, it was easy because, among psychiatrists who contributed to the creation of the screening, there was no private effort to counter the assumption that African Americans constituted an inferior race. When blacks were rejected more than whites, most psychiatrists considered it to be because of their poor quality. When certain categories were found to reject more whites than blacks, it was seen as a convenient means to preserve "sound" materials in the "stock." Such racial reasoning became predominant in part because the relation between what should be discussed in public and what should remain private was stirred up in a new way. As the United States moved deeper into the war in 1943 and 1944, this changing relationship between public and private brought about strikingly different consequences for homosexual and black citizens. For African Americans, there was a relatively quick rise of resistance against such an obvious contradiction of liberalism as it had been shaped in public. For homosexual individuals, there was a longer process of creating a public forum to counter homophobia. But before African Americans and homosexual men and women began to witness these consequences, the screening system had to go through another phase of challenges.

The Demise of Screening

In addition to the stigmatization of homosexual individuals and African Americans, the screening system in 1941 began to face a host of other pressing problems. As soon as the system was put into practice, psychiatric interviews at induction centers revealed their limitations. In addition to psychiatrists' unfamiliarity with the task of singling out latent problems, they confronted the pressure of time. A succession of short interviews and quick decisions resembled, as one psychiatrist had warned during one of the two-day seminars, the work of an immigration inspector. Examiners were expected to discern problems speedily, and they came to realize that this was not possible in practice. Lawrence Kolb, a representative of the U.S. Public Health Service and a psychiatrist with long experience at a state hospital, pointed out:

> I have often thought in my state hospital experience . . . how many of those people, if they should come by our immigration line, we would actually detect, and I had to . . . say that perhaps most of those, if they were not obviously doubled up with catatonia or something like that, would get by. The line of inspection is a good thing, but it will not get more than a very small proportion of potential psychotics, neurotics, and psychopaths.[61]

If the illnesses of inmates of state institutions, who often demonstrated advanced symptoms, were difficult to pick up, what could be done with candidates with minimal signs? More important, if superintendents at state hospitals, who were familiar with cursory examinations, found the wartime screening too short and too demanding, who would be able to achieve satisfactory results? The answer was, virtually no one. Thus when the induction began, examiners quickly became skeptical of any attempt to understand the candidates' personalities, resulting in countless interviews that consisted of a few formulaic questions such as "Do you have any worries?" "Have you visited a doctor often—and for what?" and "Have you ever had a nervous breakdown?"[62] In most cases, the length of the interview fell within the range of between twenty seconds and five minutes.

Objections to the screening, from both within the military and without, multiplied. Some complained that there were too many rejections and that the army was denied a chance to induct sufficient personnel. This objection became more frequent after Pearl Harbor, when the army could not afford to be too selective about draftees anymore. Others argued that the dual screening system harmed local physicians' reputations because their decisions were often overridden by psychiatrists at induction centers. The rate of rejection at induction centers tended to be higher than at local boards and caused embarrassment for physicians who had passed those who eventually were denied induction.[63] Many families became upset when their loved ones were rejected because they were "feeble-minded" and "imbeciles."[64] Meanwhile, the War Department became suspicious of examiners who generated high rates of rejection. Some psychiatrists, like Sullivan, helped their clients obtain a rejection. Clara Thompson and Janet Rioch, prominent psychoanalysts, were among them. Another psychiatrist found himself followed by the Federal Bureau of Investigation because he helped many to get out of military service.[65] Tensions between the military and civilians, the medical profession and the public, and general physicians and psychiatric doctors were revealed.

Sullivan responded that these critiques were "none-too-material" and often based on "erroneous" arguments.[66] At the same time, he continued to stress the current geopolitical importance of psychiatric screening. He claimed that the Axis powers were an "immediate threat to the capitalistic-democratic social order," attempting to provoke "social upheaval" to destroy "everything that has been built up in the past 3,500 years," such as "human achievement and realization of the true and the beautiful."[67] More specifically, he insisted that Hitler was expanding a sinister "interpersonal operation," as the dictator encouraged alienation and suspicion among people. Hitler did this by attacking "people's faith in any essential meaning of life." He destroyed organized religion and governmental organizations, and "widen[ed] all the cleavages that exist in the group" with his religion of race.[68] Psychiatrists, who specialized in the "science of interpersonal relations" as Sullivan defined it, had a unique responsibility to protect the allies from demoralization.

But Sullivan had reservations about his own arguments. Even as he upheld the larger purposes of the war, he began to acknowledge that his views embraced contradictions. For example, in the same 1941 article in which he discussed Hitler's interpersonal operation and psychiatrists' responsibility to confront it, he addressed the following problems he saw on the home front:

> [First, t]he army of a democracy cannot be democratic. . . . There is no . . . place for an equal voice in the government; and often no freedom of decision but rigid discipline and unquestioning execution of orders. Second, the civilian population of a democracy on the verge of war cannot remain free to question the necessity for . . . universal effort for the national defense. . . . Painfully banal as these two thoughts may be, I fear they need very much wider acceptance.[69]

Perhaps it was Sullivan himself who needed to confront these "banal" thoughts for the first time. While psychiatric screening was supposed to protect democracy, he began to fear that the operation of democracy could actually work against it. Often he projected his frustration on the public: "The public . . . must be educated if we are not to let our schizoid people be destroyed, whom we want to preserve, because they are destroyed by accident by the community."[70] Sullivan's deep commitment to the protection of "our schizoid people" suggests once again his strong desire to shield schizophrenic and, by extension, homosexual persons.[71] What is also apparent is Sullivan's belief that these individuals were victims of American intolerance toward those who deviated from the "normal"—something that American culture created almost "accidentally"—and thus needed protection from ostracism resulting from rejection by the army. His thought was going to the problem that the system he had created began to generate.

By late 1941, then, Sullivan's earlier, positive views on democracy and its ability to protect "human values" had become sharply compromised. What impressed him now was the paradox of democracy. In a war to protect democratic traditions, the nation had to restrict some of its most important procedures. This recognition clearly signaled an important setback for the liberal tradition in science. Sullivan, along with others, had believed that the application of clinical insights in the screening system helped not only to further democracy, but also to keep morale high in both the army and the public. But the difficulties of mass screening required psychiatrists to downplay its undesirable effects so as to at least maintain the system. To make matters worse, psychiatrists began to disagree about the best way to contribute to national mobilization. Seeing the numerous obstacles of the screening, and responding to public sentiment, which was turning against an "excessive" elimination of registrants, an increasing number of psychiatrists grew suspicious of the idea of prevention of mental illness itself and began to look for something that worked therapeutically, rather than preventively.

Sullivan's goal of prevention seemed ever more implausible after the United States entered the war in December 1941. The army quickly relaxed its screening criteria in 1942, so as to induct candidates with minor defects such as mild stuttering, even though homosexual persons continued to be screened out at least officially.[72] Disappointed as Sullivan might have been with this development, many psychiatrists of the time remained enthusiastic about the national recognition they had obtained through the screening. At the APA's annual meeting in 1941, the president, George H. Stevenson, gave an address that included a long quote from a letter from the president of the United States, expressing the "grateful acknowledgement of the splendid cooperation your organization has extended in our program of national defense."[73] Papers in sessions addressed challenges in the Selective Service psychiatry, but what dominated the meeting was excitement about being endorsed as an agent of national defense.[74]

Sullivan quit the CACSS in early 1942, but the screening process survived, albeit in a modified and limited form. Apparently, he resigned because he did not get along with the new director of the Selective Service, Major General Lewis B. Hershey. Hershey believed that a standardized psychological examination (the Army General Classification Test) administered at an induction center was more efficient and dependable than the psychiatric screening at local and medical boards.[75] Psychiatrists continued their campaign to support the value of the screening, but opinions began to diverge. According to William Clair Menninger, a chief consultant in neuropsychiatry to the surgeon general of the army from 1943 to 1946,[76] "Zeal[ous] psychiatrists promised more than they could deliver" between 1940 and 1942. In particular, "induction-center elimination of men with minor symptoms of instability [was] overcautious and wasteful of man power."[77] Here Menninger is criticizing the members of the CACSS, perhaps Sullivan in particular. While Menninger valued preventive psychiatry, he would not boast of its effectiveness when there was less than sufficient knowledge, equipment, and personnel.

As if to mirror the change in leadership from Sullivan to Menninger, the focus of war psychiatry gradually shifted from prevention to treatment. At the end of 1942, admissions to hospitals for neuropsychiatric disorders reached more than 25 percent. The clear implication was that the stress of being in combat, rather than having inappropriate personalities, was at the core of the problem. In an important report issued in 1944, John W. Appel and Gilbert W. Beebe concluded that neuropsychiatric casualties were inevitable. Various factors, such as long time spent in the military, continuous exposure to combat, loss of friends, insufficient information on operations, and lack of confidence in commanding officers, could cause anyone to have a mental breakdown. Thus the authors stressed the need to improve evacuation screening, intended to determine if a casualty was to be treated and returned to full duty or to limited service or rather be discharged from the army. Appel and Beebe did not disregard the preventive induction screening, but they also called for more prompt, symptom-based diagnoses and prognoses at the war front for the efficient use of manpower.[78]

By 1942, Sullivan himself had to admit that "the elimination of all or of even two-thirds of those who [would] break down in the service" was "what [could] not be done." There was "in several places in the War Department a conviction that psychiatry was given a chance to show what it could do in selecting men for the service, and that it failed."[79] Sullivan's disappointment was clear in his report to the board of trustees of the William Alanson White Psychiatric Foundation after his resignation from CACSS as a psychiatric consultant: "There remains but the passing of the torch to hands that are ready to seize and carry it. Your president [Sullivan] has in large measure failed in his efforts to illuminate the field of the national emergency. The course of events was unpropitious and the opportunity has passed."[80]

This was perhaps the first major failure in Sullivan's career. Earlier, as seen in his talks and writings, he was confident that he was making a constructive critique of psychiatric practices. Such confidence is utterly lacking from this statement. Not only had the screening he advocated failed, but it also accentuated the preconception that homosexual persons were unfit to serve. These failures occurred because the war brought the previously underacknowledged contradictions between the public and private in science into focus. The tentative and coded public discussions about homosexuality circumscribed the possibility of developing nonhomophobic policies. What was missing from psychiatry before the war was a full-fledged public determination to accept homosexuality, the lack of which contributed to the insidiousness of the ways screening enhanced discrimination.

The contradiction that the war brought to the surface was not only about psychiatrists' views of homosexuality, but also about the use of screening in general. The premise of screening out the unfit did not work in the way that Sullivan had hoped, because the judgment of who made a good soldier depended upon individualized examinations modeled after clinical practice. Psychiatrists before the war, particularly those who supported the new psychiatry, were not hesitant about expanding clinical insights to apply to an entire society. If anything, the expansion was considered both a professional opportunity for, and a social responsibility of, psychiatrists. But in the end, the direct application of a clinical approach to the mass screening of America's youth was not sustainable for practical and conceptual reasons. Sullivan expected psychiatrists to carry out short but intensive investigations of candidates' personalities, but this approach was not realistic either at state institutions or in the mass screening. Sullivan was certainly aware of this problem, even before he became directly involved in the design of the screening system. In 1940, for instance, he acknowledged that attention to individual patients was not possible at state institutions: "You don't get information unless you play with the patient, and in the state hospital you don't have time to play with the patient. . . . I don't know what to do."[81] He understood that the method he used in clinical practice was not feasible at large-scale institutions. In wartime screening, however, he promoted the same method. Although aware of its limitations, the method was the single tool he had in hand. But in the end, the method designed in small institutions was difficult to scale up, not least because the larger scale illuminated moral issues in a public arena—issues kept within the confines of the private.

The failure of the screening system brought about significant consequences for different groups of minorities. For homosexual men and women, it bolstered a prejudice that they were "unfit" soldiers and thus must be kept out of the army. To be sure, a number of them entered and served the military successfully. Even before the close of the war, psychiatrists began to publish findings about homosexual soldiers who were skilled and well educated and "made credible records for themselves." Their contributions were not limited to those normally related to military duty. Some homosexual men, for instance, volunteered to take up female roles in the army's recreational stage shows, offering rare occasions of relief for their comrades. That homosexual men and women were good soldiers was an unpronounced, but nevertheless recognized, fact in numerous units. Not surprisingly, then, the screening out of homosexual individuals was enforced only with great inconsistency. Some examiners were homosexual men who did not see the point of eliminating fully competent men, while others simply did not have time in interviews to do anything beyond asking a few formulaic questions. Indeed, in a 1945 study, psychiatrists C. C. Fry and E. G. Rostow revealed that among 183 men whom they had known to be homosexual, only 29 were screened out because of their "homosexual proclivities," while an additional 14 were discharged after induction. As many as 118 of the men served in the army successfully.[82]

Nonetheless, the army continued to state publicly that homosexual soldiers did unquestionable harm to their "normal" counterparts based on a belief "that homosexuality constituted an undesirable trait of character." This rigid stance, which lacked any basis, drew critique from a few psychiatrists, including Menninger. Taking note of the unfairness of dishonorable discharge, Menninger in 1948 recommended that homosexual soldiers be discharged with honor if they had not committed a sexual offence. But he also suggested that the effort of homosexual soldiers who felt mistreated and appealed for a reassessment of their status of discharge might go unrewarded: "It may well be for these men to recognize . . . that the odds are against them; prejudice still exits!" Moreover, Menninger did not question the rule to eliminate homosexual personnel from the army altogether. "Homosexuals . . . have immature personalities which make them . . . grossly pathological. Like any sick person, they deserve understanding instead of condemnation." The pathological model, as well as the model of protection, remained strong. These models made it difficult for homosexuals and sympathetic scientists alike to make strides for equality in public.[83]

In sharp contrast, the disproportionately large elimination of black soldiers from military service, as well as segregated training camps and combat units, caused instant public outrage among African American leaders. These critics, including those from national organizations such as the National Association for the Advancement of Colored People (NAACP) and local African American medical societies, cited racism as causing damage to the

morale among black soldiers. Their critique drew on a well-established public discourse against racism that intellectuals had created before the war.
Already in the 1920s and 1930s it was not unusual for liberal scientists to
extend their agenda of inclusion to racial minorities; such an extension was
a respectable, even popular subject of science. To be sure, scientific liberalism did not prevent the unjust screening system and racial segregation in
the army. But unlike the critique against heterosexism that had not occupied
a place in the public discussion of science, a critique of racism had taken
root broadly in scientific thinking by the beginning of the war. As a result,
when war mobilization brought to the surface gross racism, critics were able
to address how it contradicted the American ideal of equality. In fact, a number of African American soldiers were not hesitant in voicing their frustration about the hypocrisy of fighting the war against racial injustice with the
segregated armed forces. In their minds, such practice went directly against
the foundation of democracy. The public scrutiny of racism that scientists
had carried out before the war began to integrate racial enlightenment into
American democratic values, which all were expected to observe. Thus as
early as 1943, a gradual integration of U.S. troops began. This was partly
prompted by the practical problems that segregation brought about—the
damage to African American soldiers' morale, the gross miscommunication
between the races that hurt the smooth operation of the military, and the
increasing demand for more soldiers. Nonetheless it is striking that black
and white observers alike could address racial discrimination as an unjust
practice along the way.[84] This was not the case with sexual minorities,
because there was no preexisting tie between the critique against heterosexism and the support of democracy. Consequently, the policy of exclusion
continued for homosexual men and women who aspired to serve the nation
in uniform. It is revealing that when homosexual men and women began to
create homophile grassroots organizations such as the Mattachine Society in
the 1950s, they set their goal to disseminate the idea of sexual minorities as
something comparable to African Americans.' In public and political arenas,
the status of sexual minorities was seen as being far behind that of racial
and ethnic groups.[85]

The continuing failure of psychiatric screening was so apparent that it
was almost abandoned by the military during the Vietnam War, but Sullivan
did not survive to see Vietnam. In his mind, the project to make the United
States a healthier society continued to be vital. He devoted his remaining life
after World War II to extending this project all over the world. However, his
effort here did not produce the result he wanted, either. His contribution to
postwar peace projects, including the United Nations Educational, Scientific,
and Cultural Organization (UNESCO) and the World Federation for Mental
Health, generated favorable responses from a few liberals and intellectuals.

But most Americans were eager to return to normalcy and enjoy their nation's economic prosperity, while the rest of the world was occupied with recovering from the damage of the war. American idealism, which Sullivan and his fellow medical and social scientists had cultivated in a small circle, was not popular. Their failed effort to bring private practice and public policy-making together would have a lingering effect in postwar years.

6

"One-Man" Liberalism Goes to the World

As the United States entered the postwar era, the role that scientists were expected to play in the nation's effort to construct an image as a leader of nations took on a new face. In addition to the apparent need to both "assist" and "collaborate" with former enemies, there was an emerging international forum for American scientists to meet and converse with leaders from both Western and non-Western countries. For a number of scientists who participated in this forum, this meant testing the water to work with "others" as equals, not as subjects of their intellectual inquiries, so as to create organizations that promoted science, education, health (physical, psychological, and social), and peace in the postwar international community. Harry Stack Sullivan, Ruth Fulton Benedict, Margaret Mead, and Lawrence K. Frank, among others, occupied important places in the United States' engagement in this assignment.

Historians have illuminated certain cultural limitations that circumscribed the U.S. approach to postwar international relationships in general—for example, Naoko Shibusawa has argued that "paternalistic liberalism" dominated Americans' relationship to occupied Japan, while Frank Costigliola has shown how U.S. political leaders applied gendered, often pathologizing language to not only the Soviet Union but also Western allies like French and West Germany in the Cold War era. So it is not surprising that scientists' commitment to international collaborations in the 1940s, too, revealed a marked lack of equality between "us" and "others." What is striking, however, is that much of the thinking that drove scientists' conflicted approach to homosexuality before the war shaped, both metaphorically and practically, America's postwar foreign relationship. Some of the key terms that scientists had used in their prewar discussion of homosexuality—"immature," "effeminate," in need of complete "reeducation"—were rampantly applied in their thinking about and imagining of foreign nations. This became possible because of the transformation of medical and social scientific thinking after the war, which rested on a fresh emphasis of the "danger" of "immature" persons in general, and homosexual persons in particular, within the context of the nation's effort to restore and rebuild American families. Homosexuality became everyone's problem, not something confined to a small number of the "afflicted," making the concept easily applicable to any group considered suspect. To be sure, there were no internationally shared policies regarding homosexuality established in the 1940s, so it cannot be argued that the paternalistic language applied to homosexuality created a specific program against it. Nevertheless, it is important to note that this particular language permeated American scientists' relationship with their foreign counterparts, helping to create an unarticulated, and yet powerful, assumption that differences between "us" and "others" were "natural [and] immutable," or a sign of the inferior, "true nature" of foreigners, something that had already been scientifically proved.[1]

In addition to being a source of these problematic metaphors, the science of homosexuality contributed, in Sullivan's case, to the making of a "one-man" liberalism that prevailed in conferences and programs at the World Health Organization (WHO), the World Federation for Mental Health (WFMH), and UNESCO, three major organizations that sought to foster scientific collaboration internationally after the war. In this "one-man" liberalism that excluded opinions of "others" in practice behind the proclaimed ideal of inclusion, the gap between "public" and "private" practices of science loomed large. Specifically, there emerged connections between the inner-circle culture that flourished before the war and scientists' postwar approach to international programs. Scientific practices that valued and, indeed, relied on their separation from outsiders had an unmistakable impact on the exclusion of "others" in U.S. foreign relations. Despite the fact that some American scientists sought out the inclusion of differences, their approaches failed to change the view held by their foreign counterparts that the United States was not interested in opinions of the less powerful. Now, victory in hand, Americans were more self-confident of their policies, and this, combined with the inner-circle culture that Sullivan and others brought to the international stage, significantly shaped the U.S. contribution to postwar reconstruction. When "public" metaphors that infantilized and pathologized homosexuality were combined with "private" practices of exclusion, it can be seen as nothing less than a disaster for U.S. foreign relationships. This process in which scientists formulated international programs illuminates the fundamental limit of American liberalism of the era—the limitation that was significantly shaped by the prewar scientists' conflicted approach to homosexuality: one approach for public, another for private. At this point, an alternative—a comprehensive examination of subjectivity of both "us" and "others"—articulated by the life history group, had lost its force. The declining engagement of scientists with subjectivity in science became the foundation of what was seen as authentic science and, at the same time, helped create the terms for a difficult and yet decisively public battle for the equality of sexual minorities in the following decades.

Schisms and Compartmentalization

In the summer of 1939, at the age of forty-seven, a few months before he began his work for the Selective Service, Sullivan decided to close his clinic in New York City, ending his career as a practitioner. He continued to teach at branches of the Washington School of Psychiatry in Washington, DC, and New York City, and he supervised psychiatrists at Chestnut Lodge Hospital, a psychoanalytically oriented private mental hospital in Rockville, Maryland. Indeed, most of his articles published after his death were based on the lectures and seminars he offered at the school and the hospital, facilitated by the fact that he had a number of students eager to record his words for posthumous publication. But he never returned to practice, a notable decision for a man viewed as a clinical genius and with a deep attachment to people with troubled minds. In his last decade of life, Sullivan engaged himself in the nation at war, and then in international conferences to establish a new "order" in the postwar world. In psychiatric and psychoanalytic communities, he remained a respected, if mysterious, figure, while in his personal life, he seems increasingly to have been isolated, with no one to really comfort him. James Inscoe was with him, but there was severe tension between them, especially as Sullivan's health began to deteriorate in the mid-1940s.

To leave New York City and abandon his clinical practice certainly was a turning point for Sullivan, but perhaps not necessarily a difficult decision to make. By the end of the 1930s, he had several reasons to do so. In February 1939, Edward Sapir, a longtime collaborator and one of his closest friends, died, ending Sullivan's regular visits to New Haven. Moreover, there was an increasing tension among psychiatrists and psychoanalysts in the New York area, and it became difficult to continue a collegial relationship with his colleagues, as he had done in the first half of the 1930s. Indeed, New York City was the center of political schisms in psychoanalysis in the late 1930s and early 1940s, arising from disagreements about what counted as authentic psychoanalysis. After Karen Horney published *The Neurotic Personality of Our Time*, in 1937, which focused on social and cultural factors in mental illness and sharply departed from orthodox psychoanalysis, which prioritized psychosexual conditions as the root cause of neuroses, she became exceedingly isolated in the New York Psychoanalytic Society. Her isolation amid harsh criticism from her peers became so extreme by the end of the 1930s that her students could not pass exams in training institutions associated with the society. The society regarded her students as "not doing psychoanalysis" and eventually deprived her of her status of training analyst and demoted her to a lecturer.[2] In turn, she left the society in 1941 to establish the Society for the Advancement of Psychoanalysis and its training institute, the American Institute for Psychoanalysis.[3] Clara Thompson and William V. Silverberg joined her, while the equally sympathetic Erich Fromm and Sullivan became the institute's honorary members.

Around the same time, Lucile Dooley, a psychoanalyst with whom Sullivan founded the Washington School of Psychiatry, resigned from the school and the William Alanson White Psychiatric Foundation, most likely because she could not stand Sullivan and his associates' dissent from the orthodoxy.[4] Despite the spirit of "freedom" the members of Horney's institute claimed to uphold, however, it soon had a schism of its own, because of what Thompson called "the power struggle" between its members. In 1943, for instance, Horney took away Fromm's status as a training analyst, because they believed he was "damaging the Institute" with his popularity.[5] The fact that he did not have a medical degree was deemed problematic as well. Siding against them, Sullivan resigned from his position as an honorary member. Thomson, too, left along with Fromm, and established the New York branch of the Washington school (which in 1946 changed its name to the William Alanson White Institute of Psychiatry).[6] This made some of Sullivan's colleagues at the school, especially those in Washington, DC, such as Dooley, feel at odds with the orthodoxy, often inadvertently. Although most of the institutional splits happened in the 1940s, there is no doubt that the partisan politics in psychoanalysis in the late 1930s contributed to Sullivan's frustration with his less than amicable intellectual life in New York City.[7]

It seems that Sullivan's clinical practice in the 1930s offered him little gratification as well. Most of his patients—both those within and without his inner circle—belonged to the urban middle class, whose population had mild problems, not severe psychoses. Despite his earlier belief that he could prevent psychoses by treating neuroses, Sullivan often found his patients' illness difficult to cure at its core. In his eyes, his patients' materialistic lifestyle was a problem in itself—an observation shared by many of his colleagues who practiced in the metropolis—and he could be harsh in his accusations. He argued, for instance, that "petty fancy living" or a set of "practically meaningless routines," frequently found in his patients, made it difficult for them to get out of such a pattern of life and to make meaningful connections with others.[8] Ironically, psychoanalysts themselves were ensconced in the urban upper middle class, which exposed them to what their profession defined as neurosis-generating circumstances unique to that class. Sullivan himself eagerly pursued material comfort. Both in 1938 and 1939, he was in financial crisis, mostly because of his extravagant spending.[9] In 1938, with the possibility of personal bankruptcy on the horizon, he asked his well-to-do friends to help him. Instead of making what people would consider a sober effort to reconstruct his finances, however, he continued to spend freely. Once he bought a "handful" of opals to show off to the friends who had just loaned him money, as one of these friends bitterly recalled later.[10] Such obsession with privilege seemed to be relatively unchecked in his social life, just as he became a "god"-like figure among his professional associates.

In fact, it is probably not an exaggeration to describe Sullivan around this time as a godlike figure in his profession. Because of several schisms that took place in the early 1940s, people who worked with him at the Washington school and Chestnut Lodge were already willing followers—or so Sullivan expected. Certainly, many of his students were delighted to have such a well-known psychiatrist as a mentor. They saw him as an intense, charismatic teacher, and they remembered him as a sharp thinker, if not the most lucid speaker. Students also found Sullivan intimidating. Mabel Black Cohen, a participant in the Chestnut seminars between 1942 and 1946 and a student in one of his classes at the Washington school, recalled her impression of Sullivan as follows:

> The reactions to S[ullivan] were quite varied. Some people were quite frightened of him, and were never comfortable with him at all; others, like myself, started out scared to death, but lost some of the fear in the process of learning from him. And he had a tendency to pick out favorites. . . . [They] became very impressed by him. . . . A number of kids in the seminar started to over-identify with him and started to talking [sic] like he . . . did. . . . His bearing, manner, charisma, set up a hero-worshipping situation with people who needed a hero, not a word, a gesture on his part. . . . [It was] just that that was the nature of the relationship. . . . The built-up reputation with which he came to the Lodge—which he maintained so brilliantly contributed [to this relationship].[11]

Cohen found Sullivan not unapproachable, but this appears to have been because she felt that he liked her all right.[12] There were others who never felt comfortable around Sullivan. As Hilde Bruch, another student of his from this era, remembered, he had a reputation for being "very outspoken with people he didn't like," and students were afraid that as a teacher he might be as harsh as he was with colleagues he despised.[13] Such fear certainly drove some students away from Sullivan's classes.[14] Those who stayed were either his favorites or students who still wished to learn from him despite their fear. This created an environment in which communication was largely unilateral—from the teacher to his students. Ruth Moulton, yet another student, thought that he seemed to have "too much dignity and sarcas[m]," which "kept people from attacking" him. Like Cohen, Moulton thought that his students "worshipped him," resulting in a coterie known as "the control group." No criticism against him was allowed and all his words and gestures were supposed to be appreciated.[15] Although it is possible that such descriptions were exaggerated, this was the way Sullivan's teaching impressed some of his students.

His colleagues around this time were not so different from his students when it came to mixing their deference with fear. The writer Lloyd Frankenberg, then an attendant at Chestnut Lodge (he was a conscientious objector during the war and was assigned to his attendant's position in a work camp in Maryland, in late 1944, at the recommendation of psychoanalyst Janet McKenzie Rioch), recalled that Sullivan was the hospital's "chief theoretician and presiding deity." He was not accessible to the hospital's support staff, and it took Frankenberg "several weeks" to "have a glimpse of 'God.'" Although Frankenberg wished to receive Sullivan's analysis, he soon learned that "God only analyzes the other analysts." "It's a bit Kafka-like," Frankenberg wrote in his memoir, "with us in the village, incommunicado except for cryptic messages from the Castle."[16] Like his inner circle in the 1930s, then, Sullivan's followers were a small and selective group who did not offer much criticism of their teacher. There are some significant differences between the 1930s and 1940s, however. For one, there was less embracing of cultural refinement in the inner circle of the 1940s. In the 1930s, there was an unmistakable sense that people in the circle thought that they were smart, sophisticated urbanites. They were friends, having good times over good food and drinks. In contrast, people's memories from the 1940s seem less excited and even stifled. It is difficult to detect anything fun or unironic from their memories of the time.

Another crucial difference between the 1930s and 1940s was the extent to which the inner-circle culture permeated Sullivan's life. In the earlier decade, Sullivan had a vibrant connection to interdisciplinary scholars who did not belong to his inner circle. Indeed, the "public" science that he pursued with these scholars was in contrast with—not an extension of—the "private" science that he nurtured only among selected individuals. But a decade later, his circle of followers included most of his professional associates; it was a circle around which Sullivan's life revolved. To be sure, the years when he engaged in wartime policy-making were a notable exception. But even the psychiatric screening failed largely because of the incompatibility between clinical practice and policy-making, suggesting that Sullivan did not have a strategy for bringing insights based on small-group discussions to large-scale public programs. The inner-circle culture had much to do with this unsuccessful connection, and the same culture contributed to the failure of his work for postwar international organizations as well. Despite his experience of working with the military and the government during the war, the culture of the profession Sullivan brought to his work for the WHO, WFMH, and UNESCO was selective, stifling, and unprepared for working through disagreements.

Sullivan's personal life also followed this pattern of withdrawal to a small circle of followers, indicating that the profession's tendency for compartmentalization had ramifications in domestic scenes as much as it did on the international stage. Although it is difficult to argue that his relationship with James Inscoe had an immediate impact on his public, professional life, it reveals the deterioration of Sullivan's ability to communicate with others, which in turn circumscribed his work for international organizations. Unlike what occurred in his years in New York City, Sullivan did not socialize much in the 1940s. Many people whom he had befriended in the 1930s—Karen Horney, Erich Fromm, Clifton Read, and John Vassos—were not part of his life by the mid-1940s.[17] When Sullivan fell ill in early 1945 with acute bacterial endocarditis but refused to go to a hospital, the caretaking fell almost solely on Jimmie's shoulders. Some of Sullivan's colleagues at Chestnut Lodge helped Jimmie at their house in Bethesda, but taking care of Sullivan turned out to be extremely difficult. The foremost problem was that there was a strange tension between Jimmie the caretaker and Harry the patient. Some who visited them at their home when Sullivan was ill commented on this tension. William V. Silverberg, for instance, recalled that Jimmie decorated his room on the second floor in blue green, the color Sullivan disliked the most. Sullivan was repelled by the color blue so much so that he could not even sit down on a blue chair.[18] Naturally, Silverberg believed that "by that time, HSS [Sullivan] was not climbing to the second floor" at all.[19] Moreover, when Lloyd Frankenberg was assisting Jimmie briefly to nurse Sullivan, he found himself eating all his meals with Jimmie, because "Dr. Sullivan always eats alone."[20]

The problem was not only that Harry and Jimmie were drifting apart; there was also the matter of deteriorating communication. While Sullivan was sick, Jimmie tried to be as quiet as possible, at his partner's request. But it created a peculiar atmosphere in the house. When Frankenberg agreed to assist Jimmie, Ray Pope, Frankenberg's supervisor, explained that there had been another attendant assigned to help Jimmie, but he could not stand the tension and had fled. Frankenberg reported:

"Jimmy has his own peculiarities," said Ray. "He's a nice boy—I say boy; he's in his thirties—but he is quite recessive. He shares with

Dr. Sullivan a dislike of asking for anything. You have to guess what they'd like. . . . Naturally it has to be excessively quiet there. . . . Jimmie tries to talk in whispers. Well, after three days of this the attendant just vanished. He turned up here eventually, having apparently gone on a bender in Washington. For a boy who doesn't normally drink, the experience must have been quite shattering."[21]

The tension that drove this teetotaler to a drinking binge was also stressful to the next assistant to Jimmie, David McK. Rioch—Sullivan's junior colleague at Chestnut Lodge. When Frankenberg came in to replace Rioch, Rioch looked "slightly distraught" and "greeted us [Pope and Frankenberg] . . . with a glance of relief." Soon, Frankenberg realized that the root of the tension was Jimmie and Harry's inability to talk directly and straightforwardly to each other. One day when Frankenberg was making Sullivan's bed, he found a memo from Sullivan to his doctor Edward Stieglitz that read: "Tell Jimmy, for sweet Jesus' sake, not to go tiptoeing around the outside of the house to get to the kitchen. Much more disturbing than if he strode straight through here." For Frankenberg, it was not surprising that Jimmie was anxious not to disturb the ailing Sullivan. But when Frankenberg read this note, he wondered if it was "too disturbing to Jimmy if Dr. Sullivan were to tell him in person." Thus, the tension seemed to arise between Jimmie, who was concerned about bothering Sullivan, and Sullivan, who was worried about hurting Jimmie—all this taking place between people who did not like to ask for anything directly. No wonder, then, that when Clara Thomson came to see Sullivan and asked why he and Jimmie did not ask straight out when they wanted something, they "both" said, "Oh, no!" as if it were the least probable thing in the world.[22] Apparently, Sullivan and Jimmie were incapable of getting out of the constraints they placed upon themselves; people who came to assist them, all of whom were Sullivan's followers, could not help them snap out of the strain either. Even those who perceived the problem, such as Frankenberg and Thompson, would not press their point. Such was etiquette in the inner-circle culture: it might not have caused Harry and Jimmie any strain, but it certainly increased difficulties.

Their partnership was further strained by Inscoe's increasing frustration with his status as a "boy" in Sullivan's household, suggesting the impact of persistent paternalism in their relationship. When Sullivan got well and resumed his lectures at Washington School of Psychiatry in late 1945, Jimmie occasionally accompanied him to Washington, DC, but did not to come to his lectures. As Frankenberg observed, Jimmie had "small patience with theory" and was not interested in Sullivan's intellectual activities. What Jimmie liked instead was to drive about the town with Frankenberg and call on friends. To Frankenberg's surprise, Jimmie became "voluble" with his friends, quite unlike his usual quiet self. Jimmie thought that his nursing of Sullivan was not recognized. Jimmie would tell his friends, "When you do it well, you have nothing to show for it." "The wives [to whom Jimmie talked] agree[d] with him that housework is the most tiresome on earth," Frankenberg recalled.[23] Such frustration on Jimmie's part existed in the 1930s, but seems to have intensified as his life with Sullivan reached its last quarter. Jimmie was a homemaker from the beginning of their partnership in 1928, and he continued to do the shopping, cooking, and cleaning to the end of Sullivan's life. Perhaps in part because of these domestic duties, Jimmie did not have a chance to pursue a career of his own, as he might have foreseen when he left his parents' home to live with Sullivan. Indeed, when Sullivan died, leaving almost no assets to Jimmie, Jimmie had to sell the Bethesda house and go to work, but had a hard time finding even a clerical job. The inequality between the partners persisted, damaging their ability to talk to each other. Although there are large differences in scale, a similar paternalistic dynamism, and resulting lack of open communication, influenced the scientific thinking about partnerships in both Americans' domestic life and international relationships. No doubt this thinking reflected a predominant concern that the war had a devastating effect on men, women, and American families.

From Clinical to Social Hygiene

Even as psychoanalysis developed schisms that generated small groups of followers, some of the instigators of these shifts aspired to further their profession's relevancy to broader sociocultural issues. Horney's book on neurosis was dismissed by orthodox Freudians precisely because of her sociological approach to psychiatric problems. Sullivan, despite his "seclusion" into an inner circle, continued to address the social implications of mental illness. Apparently, the wartime failure to apply clinical methods to mass screening had not impressed psychiatrists as a problem of fundamental incompatibility; rather, it was a wake-up call to further tailor their theories for social needs and problems. This sentiment was not unique to psychiatrists. Psychologists, sociologists, and anthropologists shared an urgent sense of responsibility—that scientists must help the nation to use victory in the war to reestablish social order and create promises of a better future. In their discussion, the dissociation of families, changing gender relationships, and "immature" personalities were of central concern.

The preoccupation of postwar medical and social scientists with families may seem ironic, given that their fields had explored meanings of modern, personal relationships outside traditional institutions and values most insistently before the war. But the wartime separation of families, especially the long-term separation of husbands from wives, became an instant subject of science as some of its problematic consequences seemed to become apparent after the war. The *American Journal of Sociology*, the *American Journal of Psychiatry*, and more specialized journals such as *Marriage and Family Living* were outlets for discussion of the problem of separated marriages. An insightful essay by sociologist John F. Cuber in 1943 illuminates the nature of scientists' concern about marriage and family. In Cuber's view, the problem lay in what he called "schizoid morality," developed during the war in the army. Being away from their "female companions," many men in the armed forces engaged in "'hedonistic' sexual satisfaction—homosexuality, autoeroticism, miscellaneous sex perversion [such as sexual relationships with 'the low type of women from whom prostitutes were made']" more frequently than they would have in civilian society. By resorting to these acts regularly for a prolonged time, soldiers developed a moral code that was either exclusive or disrespectful of women—a code that would jeopardize marital relationships when the war was over.[24]

Sociologist Henry Elkin, who himself served in the U.S. Army as a second lieutenant, agreed, arguing that "primitive" expressions of virility—those that were self-assertive and aggressive—persisted among men in the military. This was not simply because men were separated from a "feminine influence" that curtailed such expressions in ordinary times; it was also because "American culture [upholds] the ideal of virility . . . that often prevail in preadolescent gangs and play groups; e.g., lower-class 'toughness' as against upper-class 'sissy' effeteness." Elkin also observed how such virility contributed to homosexual attitudes and inclinations that were, though disguised, widespread in the army. To be sure, soldiers—including those whom Elkin considered to be "latent" homosexuals—might put pictures of "pin-up girls." But this was merely an affirmation of a male bond, whereby everyone's virility was implicated in this public display of female figures. Strikingly, Elkin pointed to elements of immaturity in both male homosexuality and men's disregard of femininity—a kind of femininity that helped men to tame and control their masculinity. On the one hand, homosexuality was something associated with a "childhood stage of emotional experience," a view in line with the scientific theories before the war. But unlike prewar scientists who viewed homosexual men as "effeminate," "civilized," and "sophisticated," Elkin saw homosexually inclined men as rough talking ("griping"), hard drinking, and virile, men who, by reducing the "image of ideal femininity [to] a bathing suit . . . [direct] the appreciation of femininity itself into the form of primitive erotic experience." This astute observation marked the emergence of a new "kind" of homosexual man in postwar scientific discourse. In addition to effeminate men who dominated scientists' discussion of homosexuality before the war, men who were the most typically

"American" and masculine occupied the forefront of scientific concern about male sexuality after the war.[25]

These "virile" males who harbored homosexuality, as well as "effeminate" homosexual men, were believed to pose a serious threat to postwar American families. In the 1930s, men who projected a "virile" image in same-sex relationships could be seen as superior to "effeminate" homosexual men; at least masculine homosexual men were not "true" homosexuals, because they were not biologically predisposed. Or masculine men were seen to be benign because, unlike "fairies," these men did not use their sexuality to manipulate others. In contrast, postwar masculinity—in particular, a kind of masculinity that insisted on excluding femininity unless the latter was objectified—was more troubling, as it undermined marriage and families. Wives who heard "sensational stories about the morals of men in service" might well begin to question their marital bond.[26] Husbands whose unconscious homosexual impulses were brought to the surface as a result of army life, which unduly encouraged "the dominant, aggressive quality" embedded in masculinity, would find it difficult to go back to stable, marital relationships.[27] Medical and social scientists responded to these grim prospects by stressing the responsibility of scientists and policy makers to offer solutions. For instance, after declaring that the "Western family is rapidly approaching its . . . violent crisis," sociologist Carle C. Zimmerman in 1946 warned that "even heterosexuality itself will be challenged" in this crisis. To counter this dangerous trend of "antifamilialism," he urged sociologists to "erect a much more sophisticated . . . family sociology" that made "family values" more acceptable to the public.[28] Although offering a different emphasis, Lawrence K. Frank shared this sense of crisis and responsibility with Zimmerman. In Frank's observation, good families were crucial for reconstructing a sound nation. If families were to be dissociated, all kinds of "human defeat," including crime, homosexuality, and mental illness, would flourish. Like Zimmerman, Frank suggested that scientists help create "agencies and programs" for improving family lives, be it health education, child hygiene, or home economics.[29]

There were many others who were equally assertive in offering prescriptions for postwar problems, but some did so with a specific focus on the role of sex in marital life. Positing that marriage and reproduction are "normal" and sure signs of "maturity," for instance, Nadina R. Kavinoky, a physician in California, claimed an urgent need to teach married couples about the crucial role of sex in their partnerships. Especially given the wartime separation of husbands from their wives, physicians "must [help Americans] make real to the soldier the possibility of a happy family life on his return," suggesting her fear that such possibility may not be visible if medicine did not intervene. Here again, the underlying concern was men's exposure to "immature" sexuality in the military and their possible inability to put it behind them even when the war ended. If these men could not become mature, they would fail not only in their marriages but also in their careers, posing a threat to the nation's economy. Kavinoky argued that medical professionals must offer more sex education programs , both from the psychological and physiological points of view.[30]

Putting a similar emphasis on sex education, sociologist Bernard N. Desenberg took a slightly different approach by offering a critique of "the conjugal bond [that] is too proper and too legitimate." His point was not that Americans needed to make sex life in marriage less proper; rather, it was that a certain prohibiting attitude toward sex must be changed. For instance, parents might offer sex education that stressed the significance of monogamous sex life in marriage. Such education, often focused on "don'ts," did not recognize sexual emotions and desires that children might experience well before marriage. As a result, young Americans often thought of sex as something that was "wrong" and "indecent"—something that needed to be kept in "silence." This, in turn, pushed youths, especially men, to the "sex pattern [that] stress[ed] forbidden and off-color objects" as a source of pleasure. When they were married, and when sex became a routine, its propriety could ruin sexual excitement and gratification. Frustrated, a husband might begin a "quest for the new and different [that] can lead to homosexual desires . . . searching for stimulating sensations." What American marriage needed disparately, then, was education that better linked pleasure, emotional bond, and sex in marriage.[31] Although they were not directly related to war experiences, the parallel between Desenberg's discussion and Kavinoky's is striking. Both seemed to be concerned about what Elkin and Cuber described as "schizoid" or "immature" sexuality that would not fit into heterosexual relationships in marriage. As the war caused problematic sexuality to be more prevailing—or more visible—among Americans, more emphasis needed to be placed on education that restored pleasure in sex within marriage. Without such education, virtually all could turn to homosexuality.

In the postwar scientific examinations of sexuality, then, the true danger did not lie in individuals who were self-identified sexual minorities; rather, it lay in those who might step inside the institution of marriage and damage it from within, especially by nullifying heterosexual sexual pleasure. Reflecting just such anxiety over the dissociation of American families, Harry Stack Sullivan in the Chestnut Lodge seminar offered a telling insight into homosexual men, particularly the role of those who were not overtly homosexual in behavior. His discussion deserves careful attention here, because it illuminates how his thinking was in line not only with scientific understanding of male homosexuality in the context of the heightened concern about marriage, but also with changing notions of masculinity and

femininity in postwar America. Sullivan called one group of covert homosexual men "unhappy homosexuals" who, when circumstances permitted,
created quasi son-mother relationships with sexually repressed women.
These men had had homosexual relationships in their preadolescence, were
aware of their homosexual inclination, and "continued a homosexual type
of discharge of lust," but "without being able to adjust their values so that
it is satisfactory"—that is, without being able to eliminate their feeling of
disgust about homosexuality. Dissatisfied, these men pursued a heterosexual relationship; but because such a relationship was not what these men
really desired, their relationships with women could not be normal. Indeed,
their relations were "not really intimate" sexually. These homosexual men
often acted childish, forcing their female partners into the role of a mother;
women who played such a role, because they were sexually repressed, were
willing to remain nonsexual with their husbands.[32] In this way, covert homosexual men, together with sexually uninterested women, invalidated sexual
pleasure in marriage.

Sullivan further pointed out that there were individuals who "dissociated" their homosexual tendencies even more fully than "unhappy
homosexuals." Such individuals had had "the experience of happiness
which [they] had in definite homosexual operations when [they were] . . .
preadolescent[s]," but expelled such experience from their consciousness.[33]
Oftentimes, these individuals were married and made reasonable adjustments to heterosexual life. But they often experienced terrible anxiety when
they met a person who had "many outstanding traits of the preadolescent
partner, so that the resemblance would . . . be . . . sufficient to provoke a
vivid recall of the early, highly satisfactory [homosexual] experience." They
might or might not act on their homosexual desire with such a person, but
in their consciousness, they would feel that such a person needed to be
avoided, often creating "unpleasant" relations with the person.[34] In sum, this
is a group of homosexual men whose relationships with men were unstable
because of their hidden homosexual inclinations. Their problem did not
remain in same-sex friendship. Frequently, their marital relations suffered
from inexplicable strain as well. Both "unhappy homosexuals" and men
who were not aware of their homosexuality, Sullivan argued, failed to reach
the preadolescent stage, and thus their homosexuality must be seen as "a
complex mental disorder" that fortified an "abnormal mental process." He
warned his Chestnut Lodge students against tolerating such homosexuality
in clinical practice, because doing so would only widen "a revolting difference between him [the homosexual] and good people."[35]

Both groups of homosexual men that Sullivan identified in the seminar
were dissimilar to the "feminine" homosexual men he had placed at the center of his discussion in the 1930s. Unlike effeminate men who did not pursue

heterosexual relationships, homosexual men in Sullivan's 1940s analysis were in relationships with women, frequently through the institution of marriage. Thus, issues of homosexuality in his discussion were not independent from American families—indeed, it might be at the core of marital bonds and problems, suggesting the continuing conformity of his public approach to homosexuality to mainstream scientific discourse. Not surprisingly, women who were in relationships with these men were unaware of the men's homosexual desires. The women were either oblivious (in the case of those who were married to homosexual men) or sexually imperfect themselves (in the case of those who were "repressed"). Women were helpless at best in their relationships with homosexual men or, at worst, helped nurture homosexuality by playing a motherlike role. Clearly, these relationships were far removed from what Cuber and Elkin upheld as an ideal heterosexual relationship, in which femininity helped masculinity to mature with its civility, refinement, and measuredness. As scientists began to see homosexual men as implicated in marriage, women's role in shaping men's homosexuality was more critically defined. It was precisely in this focus on women's role that the prewar connection between femininity and immaturity was redefined and rerooted in the postwar scientific thinking of homosexuality: women who were not aware of their relationships with others (a sign of immaturity) could foster men's homosexuality. The result—homosexual men who sneaked into marriage through these women who were unarticulate and not self-aware—constituted a medical and moral issue, because such men might do harm to the nation's fundamental institutions.

These arguments certainly set the stage for homosexual-generating mothers (and their close cousins schizophrenia-generating mothers), who influenced the medical discourse on homosexuality in the 1950s.[36] They also laid the groundwork for the government-led persecution of homosexual individuals who, because of their assumed pathological immaturity and instability, became the subject of political suspicion in Cold War America.[37] Scientists in the years immediately after World War II were eager to identify individuals who seemed to be a risk to familial, social, and political stability based on their mental and personal characteristics. The "latent" homosexual men like those who appeared in discussions by Cuber, Elkin, Desenberg, and Sullivan were certainly suspect; there were others who were equally dangerous and should not be ignored. Scientists' discussions of these individuals further illuminate the connection between the personal and the political in the postwar years—similar, in some ways, to the prewar understanding of mental problems in social contexts, but unique in its emphasis on the "risk" group's close relationship to political unrest. Sullivan was among those who offered insights into these dangerous populations, by asserting a new way of distinguishing "disintegrative" factors in society from "integrative" factors.

In his definition, individuals who had a limited, "simple" understanding of reality were "disintegrative." Naturally, the mentally deficient such as the "idiot, imbecile, moron, and borderline intellect" were not "integrative." The mentally disordered, too, were not "integrative." In contrast, those who were "the best informed and the most skillful among us," who could see "complex" realities of interpersonal relations, were "integrative" and thus should be placed in leadership positions. Between these two extremes were individuals who had reasonable "social intelligence"—individuals smart enough to understand and follow the guidance of leaders.[38]

Strikingly, this analysis, no doubt based on medical diagnostic standards, was easily transferred to Sullivan's observation of political instability:

> We . . . realize the extent to which . . . misdirection of effort can give . . . comfort to the enemy. . . . The "neutral" pacific folk, those devoted to . . . pacific appeasement and compromise, the doubters of our allied United Nations . . . all of these disintegrative phenomena become . . . more disturbingly evil. [So do] antisocial "groups," whether they be international cartels, unhappy circles of anarchists, or merely a couple of psychopaths solving everything in a barroom [become evil].[39]

It is not only the mentally disordered and deficient, but also political dissidents or dissenters who were "disintegrative." The association between mental illness, social disintegration, and political nonconformity was made just as seamlessly as the connection between women-hating homosexual men, the dissociation of families, and the decline in economic production. Moreover, Sullivan was not shy about using similar logic in his assessment of America's relation to foreign countries. It was his belief that the Western world, including "these United States," was the most "progress[ed]" in human history. Again, his reason was that citizens in Western society were better informed about reality, and thus Western leaders must "insure opportunity to save us, the people of the West, and to spare the rest of the world the dark age that would follow extinction of the West."[40] Clearly, Western society and the rest of the world were put into the categories of superior "leaders" and inferior "followers." Just as he categorized the mentally ill on the basis of their supposed ability to understand the realities of interpersonal relations, he divided the world into the comprehending and not so comprehending. His interpersonal theory of mental illness, along with theories of scientists such as Zimmerman and Frank who made an immediate association between sexual relationships and the institution of the family, offered a significant rationale for piecing together aberrant personal characteristics to constitute political liability. In postwar scientific discourse, then, "dubious" personal attributes such as homosexuality and a lack of understanding of reality became indistinguishable from nonmainstream (or anti-American) political beliefs both in national and international contexts. No doubt the Cold War persecution of homosexual persons as communists was in line with this reasoning that permeated the social and medical sciences in the late 1940s. Homosexual persons were communists not because of any political beliefs they had; it was because homosexuality itself was a dangerous sociopolitical trait that required no further explanation.

To a significant degree, this seamless connection between the sexual, personal, and political in postwar America was rooted in the developmental model of "immaturity" that had dominated interwar medical and social scientific thinking. Not surprisingly, sexism was predominant in this model—"immaturity" took the form of femininity—and remained strong in the scientific view of "disintegrative" factors. Thus, "immature" persons and nations were by definition unarticulate and not self-aware. But because of the emerging scientific concern about men who acted rough and were disrespectful of women—"latent" homosexual men, as some scientists called them—"disintegrative" persons after the war were not just effeminate. They might be individuals who looked normal; they might even be the most typical young American men, who were robust and full of energy. Because the war deprived them of appropriate exposure to femininity, these men could not tame and control their masculinity. Moreover, they could not pursue sexual pleasure in "decent" ways, challenging the very foundation of the marital bond. In turn, their wives might be either using these men to hide their own sexual incapacities or were unaware of their husbands' true needs—both a sign of psychosexual immaturity. Such concern about both men's and women's sexuality gone wrong, apparent in the postwar science of homosexuality, was intensified by the assumed link between sexual problems, deficient personalities, and political nonconformity. This augmented concern would soon find its outlet in the conferences that were instrumental in the creation of UNESCO, WHO, and the World Federation for Mental Health (WFMH). Building on the connection made with the government during the war, psychiatrists—psychoanalytically oriented psychiatrists in particular—solidified their influence not only in the private sector but also within the government bureaucracy in the second half of the 1940s. It was not such a big step for psychiatrists to bring the expanded professional network to the international mental health programs.

On the National and International Stage

Postwar psychiatry took a definite turn toward centralization, urging both regional and national organizations to further consolidate the connection with government agencies. In late 1945, for example, the William Alanson

White Psychiatric Foundation held a roundtable conference for the Technical Training of Personnel in the Reestablishment of a Peacetime Society program, designed for the promotion of psychiatric training nationwide. In this onetime conference, participants made a case for more collaboration between psychiatrists and the Veteran's Administration. Specifically, they recommended that the VA offer mental health professionals certified positions within the government.[41] These positions would ensure professional status and job security; encourage more people to pursue careers in the profession; and as a result, help the nation to stay healthy.[42] Such a grassroots effort facilitated the passage of the National Mental Health Act of 1946, which was aimed at the promotion of psychiatric research, education, and treatment through partnership with the government. The act led to the landmark establishment of the National Institute of Mental Health in 1949, further promoting collaboration among mental health professions via the federal government's support.[43]

These developments did not occur without critique. At one point in the course of discussion in the Peacetime Society program, for example, Samuel W. Hamilton, a Mental Hospital Advisor to the U.S. Public Health Service, questioned the broad application of psychiatry under a nationwide umbrella:

> I think without something approaching totalitarian control, we cannot tell people just to whom they are going to go . . . and it will be a pity when that thing is done . . . in the United States. . . . I think when we go to meddling with the qualifications other people shall have, . . . some day we are likely to be told quite sharply that we had better stay within what we are competent for.[44]

Hamilton was afraid that the expansion of psychiatry into every corner of life, particularly under government imposition, could be "totalitarian." His critique was well received by other conference participants, including Major General Brock Chisholm, the deputy minister of national health and welfare in Canada, who was soon to become the executive secretary of the Interim Commission of the WHO. This was not necessarily surprising, considering that the war, which had just ended, had raised serious doubts about the dire consequences of massive state control of individual freedom. Even those who had appointments with the government agencies, such as Hamilton and Chisholm, could see that the extended use of psychiatry had its risks.

Interestingly, Sullivan, who was also present at the conference and was soon to join Chisholm in an effort to create mental health program in the WHO, replied to Hamilton with strong words of disagreement, foreshadowing some of the problems that would soon arise from of the U.S. effort of

centralization on the international stage: "I cannot . . . agree . . . with everything Dr. Hamilton has said. . . . I must say I think it is truly the ingenuity of
. . . [the] Devil's advocate that finds in this effort of this conference a move
to prescribe to unrelated people our ideas of what they should do."[45]

Sullivan's response grew from his belief that medical problems such
as immature personalities would have national and international ramifications.[46] Such an adamant—and uncritical—belief in the use of clinical
insights in public programs was incompatible with the difficult questions
implicit in Hamilton's and Chisholm's responses: how would scientists create standards to put people into the categories of "leaders" and "followers,"
when people's backgrounds are diverse? What role should American scientists play in creating, implementing, and exercising these standards, without
appearing totalitarian? How would scientists' responsibilities fit into the
democratic ideals that the United States claimed to have pursued in its war
effort? On the one hand, psychiatrists felt obliged to "diagnose" the mentally sick and the sociopolitically disintegrating. On the other, there was an
emerging awareness that American leadership might appear nonegalitarian
at best and totalitarian at worst in the postwar international community.

These were the challenges Sullivan and some U.S. scientists failed to
respond to—or even recognize—throughout their work for UNESCO programs
and the International Preparatory Commission for the International Congress on Mental Health (IPC), which led to the establishment of the WFMH
in 1948 and the mental health program of the WHO in 1949.[47] Their blind-
ness to these concerns had bleak consequences, no less than the failure of
implementing the nondiscriminatory Selective Service screening standard
for homosexual individuals. What the U.S. representatives did (and did not
do), of course, was not a single cause of what some described as "bewilder-
ing" failure of these international programs. But their approach to UNESCO
and the IPC played a part; in the end, it was U.S. scientists who led the planning and implementing of these programs. In particular, Sullivan's approach
mirrored the culture and discourse of the scientific communities of which
he had been a part. Following his steps, especially with a focus on his gendered language and his pronounced trust in science, illuminates how certain
components of the prewar culture—components nurtured in the tension
between "public" and "private" sciences of homosexuality—shaped American leadership and its relationship with "others" after the war. Ultimately, it
was the limits of liberalism in science that failed to include the subjectivity
of both leaders among "us," that is, scientists, and "others."

Sullivan's interest in international organizations intensified in 1945,
after the conference for the Peacetime Society program. Soon, in his 1946
article "The Cultural Revolution to End War," he laid out what he considered
to be psychiatrists' responsibilities internationally. Following his earlier

concept of well-informed "leaders" who corrected "disintegrative" elements in society, he argued that psychiatrists from Western societies must work together to "identify the human factors which have repeatedly eventuated in wars [and] . . . political factors operating in . . . aggregations." Once these dangerous factors were corrected, wars would become "unnecessary for *mature* people" (italics in original). To begin with, the war happened because "there have never been enough mature people in the right places," and thus, the most important thing was to prohibit immature people from taking charge. His message was clear: psychiatrists should regulate "aggressive," "angry," and "immature" people who were "like children . . . who failed to develop human potentialities," while making sure that "quiet," "calm," "intelligent," and "mature" people were placed in leadership positions. It is psychiatrists themselves who should be leaders—not only by identifying immature people, but also by guiding them with mature insights.[48] At the same time as drawing on the prewar psychiatric theory of personality development, his discussion of maturity and immaturity clearly reflected the postwar era's new concern about masculinity, and male sexuality in particular. Immature men, and by extension, immature peoples and countries, exhibited violent, uncontrollable behaviors.

Moreover, reflecting the profession's increasing association with the state, Sullivan made a case that psychiatric leaders worked within a government agency, not "private philanthropy," by which he meant sporadic actions of individual psychiatrists.[49] In international politics, a "mighty garrison state" would play the role of the government agency. He had no doubt that such a state would be appreciated by all who were intelligent, both "leaders" and "followers":

> I think that the peoples of the world would be less hesitant to become subjects of a world government eternally vigilant to maintain overwhelming destructive force, ready instantly to use every sanction and to destroy any who would again provoke war, *if it were evident to the thoughtful among them* that . . . this mighty garrison state which would exercise sovereignty over every person in the world was to be but a temporary precaution to protect the helpless while men of good will would be working out a fully civilized way of life for the people of the earth. It is from the custodians of knowledge and those skilled in human techniques that the evidence of this benevolent probability must come. (Italics in original.)[50]

Clearly, in his belief, a "fully civilized way of life" should be applied all over the world. The "men of good will," equipped with an ability to understand human relations, would be the carriers of that way of life. These guardians of the garrison state would possess destructive power, but it would not be a problem because they were knowledgeable and skillful scientists. He stressed this connection between science and an appropriate leadership again in 1946, in his support for the newborn weapon of mass destruction:

> The bomb that fell on Hiroshima punctuated history. The man whose wisdom and foresight . . . made that bomb had dealt with human destiny with fully human competence. The gods of local certainties, of local moralities, of local loyalty . . . of hate and prejudice and the intolerance of others passed into history.[51]

Unlike Margaret Mead, who had been involved in national mobilization during the war but nevertheless became an immediate critic of America's use of atomic bombs in 1945, Sullivan never reversed his support—and, indeed, admiration—of science. Clearly, "science" in his discourse continued to expand in terms of both the range of fields it included and its areas of application. This sort of trust in science was what a number of intellectuals of the time questioned, because in many ways, the horror of modern warfare originated in science and its products. But in Sullivan's rhetoric, U.S. scientists were exempt from the risk of causing horrific destruction. He emphasized how they had insights that "stem[med] from traditions which emphasize the . . . dignity of human beings" and had the best chance to show an example of "interpersonal intimacy" to the rest of the world.[52] In his view, it was "we," American scientists, "who must do the lion's share *of the work*" (italics in original), because "no other part of the world has anything like our . . . expanding interests beyond the traditional disciplinary frontiers, new frames of reference born of our unique history of freedom."[53] Even the "work" of mass destruction exemplified intimacy, compassion, and altruism, as long as it was done by U.S. scientists. Amid this unlimited trust in American science, the subjectivity of those who died from the bomb, as well as those who survived, was nonexistent. In the 1930s, a similar dynamism had shaped Sullivan's private practices; now it helped formulate U.S. leadership in the world.

Sullivan's rhetoric also illuminated his vision of the combination of masculine and feminine characteristics in American leadership—scientific leadership in particular. These leaders were "civilized," "benevolent," and caring of others: they were not dictators who ruled by violence. They were equipped with science, but their intelligence and gravitas did not dissuade them from taking bold action if need be. Indeed, it was the "wisdom" and "foresight" of scientists that prompted them to use weapons. Destruction was a result not of unconstrained impulses, but of measured and calculated insights. With this breed of leadership, American scientists would be able to take up the "lion's share." Thanks to their tradition of freedom, they were, and would be able to become, pathbreakers—experts who would open up "frontiers." Here, one does not detect the possibility for uncontrollable male aggression that concerned scientists such as Cuber and Elkin. Instead, masculine leadership—a kind of leadership that tirelessly shifted through the unfamiliar in order to forcefully eliminate local small-mindedness—was made more collected and sympathetic by femininity. It was precisely this synthesis that made U.S. leadership humane, strong, and legitimate.

There was no doubt that science was a ideal arena in which to complete this synthesis, because its image, values, and practices included both traditionally masculine characteristics such as boldness, curiosity, and objectivity, and such newly emphasized feminine virtues as quietude, thoughtfulness, and benevolence. In this combination, dubious characteristics such as men's uncontrolled aggression and women's lack of awareness disappeared. What predominated instead was leadership that united intellectual sophistication and cultural refinement, something that had been articulated in the private science of homosexuality in the prewar years, but only peripherally in public scientific discourse. It seems as if certain desirable images of homosexual men became swiftly public as homosexuality became everyone's problem—the problem of an ill-balanced combination of gender-specific characteristics—after the war. Certainly, this does not mean that Sullivan claimed publicly that U.S. leadership should be modeled after the image of homosexual men articulated in the inner-circle culture before the war. Nevertheless, certain characteristics of "virile" homosexual men that he upheld among his followers—smart and cultured, and at the same time, not "effeminate" at all—seemed to be carried over to what he presented as an ideal leader in the world that had been scarred by aggression. As an American scientist blessed with well-balanced male and female virtues, Sullivan was no longer concerned if his subjectivity as a homosexual man might be publicly exposed. Unlike his clinical practice in the 1920s that explored better acceptance of homosexuality, Sullivan's work in the 1940s lost both subjective and scientific links to homosexual individuals as social minorities.

Sullivan brought this particular kind of "world-wide," scientific leadership that hinged on both masculinity and femininity to the preparatory meeting of the IPC congress, which met in August 1948 in Roffey Park, Sussex, England. The congress's first task was to recommend the establishment of the WFMH on the basis of the "constructive counsel of the world's psychiatrists, social scientist, educators, social workers, and others concerned."[54] Around the same time, Sullivan had become involved in two projects related to UNESCO: the Tension Project and the Seminar on Childhood Education; conferences related to these efforts were held in June 1948 in Paris, and in August 1948 in Podebrady, Czechoslovakia, respectively. The Tension Project involved eight scholars from Brazil, France, Hungary, Norway, the United

Kingdom, and the United States: Gordon W. Allport (psychology), Gilberto Freyre (sociology), Georges Gurvitch (sociology), Max Horkheimer (philosophy), Arne Naess (philosophy), John Rickman (psychology), Alexander Szalai (sociology), and Sullivan (psychiatry).[55] In their eleven-day conference, these participants prepared a statement on the "causes of nationalistic aggression and the conditions necessary for international understanding."[56] Not surprisingly, subjects such as "ignorance, anxiety, and aggressiveness" and "power 'vacuum' and inter-group tension" were highlighted as potential areas of interest, reflecting scientists' concern about what seemed to be a lack of an access to facts and "rational" leadership in some countries. Moreover, the statement made frequent use of the concept of "patterns of culture" in order to suggest that some of them might "predispose" people to aggression when exposed to deprivation. This was an extended use of Ruth Benedict's idea in the 1930s—not surprisingly so, because she had helped American representatives to prepare a memorandum presented at the conference. Here, the role of scientists resembled Sullivan's image of American leaders who integrated masculine determination with feminine refinement: it was to provide nations predisposed to "qualities . . . unfavorable to peaceful relations with foreign groups" with guidance to "re-educate" themselves, so that "violent hostility" would be eliminated. This role combined intellectual solidness—traditionally a masculine characteristic—with a benign, nurturing influence, so as to take charge of dangerously out-of-control impulses.[57] Sullivan was gratified by the conference's achievement, particularly because he believed that it confirmed the usefulness of "full freedom for questions and the discussion of opposing . . . views [such as] Marxist in contrast to 'capitalistic'" views.[58]

But such projection of open-mindedness and willing inclusion of differences was more difficult to maintain in the IPC congress, revealing that people whom American scientists deemed uncomprehending and in need of reeducation were not all that happy about that designation. Unlike the UNESCO conference, which consisted of a small group of scientists, the IPC congress brought together twenty-three conferees from ten countries (seven from the United Kingdom; seven from the United States; two from Holland; and one each from Brazil, Canada, Ireland, France, Italy, Sweden, and Switzerland). Preceding the IPC, preparatory commissions had been created in twenty-seven countries. Each commission consisted of a substantial number of professionals, bringing the total number of individuals who contributed to the IPC either directly or indirectly to about five thousand.[59] The conferees' responsibility was to examine the reports of the preparatory commissions, and to prepare a statement about possible approaches to improve mental health worldwide, which was to be discussed in the congress.

The conference began in a collegial atmosphere, but the majority of the conferees concluded, at the end of two weeks, that the conference was a failure and the statement useless. Writing anonymously in the week following the conference, some referred to what one of the conferees called an "occasional discomfort":

> [Conferee] A: [There was] a . . . tension between the Chairman [Lawrence K. Frank] and another member . . . who was often exasperating in his slow verbosity, consuming much precious time when there was all too little to spare.[60]

> [Conferee] B: [The conference was] a leaderless group . . . the initial enthusiasm rapidly turning into bewilderment. . . . Gang formation took place. Figures strong enough to gather some members around themselves . . . formed points of crystallization. This was particularly evident around one figure whose chief significance for the group was negative: criticism of the chairman. . . . [His group] assumed characteristics of the true gang: it isolated itself in an aura of secrecy, it even separated from the rest of the members by disappearing a whole day, and came back after a prolonged absence surrounded by tales of great deeds done.[61]

Similar critiques were evident among other participants' reflections as well. One conferee commented ironically, "No arrangement was made to record the process of group formation and tensions at work. Such a document might have been more valuable than the IPC Statement itself."[62] Another believed it was unfortunate that "hardly any attempt [was] made to integrate individual personalities so as to secure smooth functioning . . . this is a rather sad criticism as it was . . . composed of experts in the science of human relations."[63] Yet another conferee pointed out that at the end of the conference, an editor was selected from the group that conferee B called a "gang" and exercised considerable influence on the drafting of the statement. The frustration about this one-man editorship was intense. One participant felt that the conference was "*almost unsuccessful*" because of "too much editorial responsibility given to *one man*, and at the same time insufficient clarification of [the] duties of that one man" (italics in original).[64] Another recalled that the there was much "confusion at the election of one single editor with full powers—in contradiction of the very principle of IPC."[65]

In the group of twenty-three representatives, this much dissatisfaction was difficult to ignore. As Sullivan admitted, "the target-person" in these critiques was Sullivan himself. In an attempt to defend himself, he claimed that

Frank and he had had a good working relationship.[66] He also claimed that he had nothing to do with the appointment of an editor. But the conferees' frustration was undeniable, and Sullivan's role in its accumulation paramount. He attempted to re-create the culture he had developed in his clinical practice and continued to nurture in a small group of his followers. He was a charismatic leader in such a group, in which members were expected to know when to remain "incommunicado." Thus, even as he proclaimed "full freedom" for questions and disagreements, the inner-circle culture and practices that it had nurtured seeped out to shape the foreign perception of U.S. leadership.

The actions of Sullivan and his colleagues were also an extension of his paternalistic view of well-informed, comprehending "leaders" and less informed "followers" who could not understand "facts." For participants who did not belong to Sullivan's group, this seemed incomprehensible and utterly self-centered. Oftentimes, such self-centeredness was seen as an imposition of Western values on non-Western conferees. As one member observed, Sullivan's group did not include participants from non-English-speaking countries.[67] These participants "understood English fairly well" particularly when they talked with one person, but found it difficult to "take intelligent part in the discussions" in the IPC sessions. As a result, these members "became inhibited" in the course of the conference.[68] When Sullivan's group took action, most of conferees from non-English-speaking countries "could not determine their position."[69] Those who had the "best command of language . . . formed a closed group which dominated the discussion." Clearly, skill at verbal communication created privileged access to information, and thus an uneven influence on the course of discussion. When Sullivan failed to see this imbalance and took a group of English-speaking conferees to one side, many conferees felt further frustrated. Almost all agreed that the conference was "limited" or "imbalanced" in terms of representation. One member said that it was a defect of the conference that it allowed the "glaring overweight of Western European culture."[70] Another felt disappointed because its statement did "not include, even under a separate heading, any minority opinions, or opinions of circles far removed from Western conceptions, traditional but at the same time evolved. . . . [The conference was] the least 'world-wide.'"[71] All the approaches Sullivan supported in the 1940s—the division between "leaders" and "followers" based on the "mature" understanding of "facts," and the inner-circle tactic of exclusion—seem to have generated massive frustration in the midst of attempted communication between cultures, languages, and politics.

Other representatives of the United States, including Lawrence Frank and Margaret Mead, were clearly frustrated by Sullivan's paternalistic, one-man approach, but they could not stop him from doing damage to others' image of the United States. Frank, for instance, was appalled by how Sullivan "acted like a spoiled child . . . [or] a lone wolf" and how he "was a fly in the ointment" who was preoccupied with being "the most powerful and prestigious." But Frank as a chairman did not choose to criticize Sullivan in front of others, when it might have been the only way to restore the broken trust. Mead was equally annoyed by Sullivan, particularly because he "started out attacking me and baiting me in every conceivable way" and "behaved as if he was being nasty to a previous sweetheart" as soon as the meeting started. This, as Mead speculated, was because Sullivan believed that she was allied with his opponents. She also recalled how, after Sullivan disappeared from the site with his followers to "wreck the conference," he was "sitting in the middle of the room in a big chair drinking his seventeenth Scotch" to hear Mead's presentation of the commissions' reports. She felt that her presentation was able to alleviate some of his doubt about her; nevertheless, her effort did not override the frustration that ran through the participants' reflections. At a crucial moment in the making of American leadership, Sullivan's one-man show seemed to overshadow even the best intentions to do it in other ways.

In the aftermath, Sullivan insisted that most "comments from members of the IPC explicitly expressed satisfaction with the outcome, and I know that most of the members who did not file final criticism were pleased." Such a characterization simply does not gibe with the flood of criticism. To be sure, it is noteworthy that he published all these critical comments in his own journal, *Psychiatry*; at least he was fair enough to make them audible. And yet after reading the critiques, Sullivan simply concluded that the overall response was positive. In the end, his secretive group finalized the statement, which was to serve as a blueprint of the WFMH. The statement and the WFMH itself supported the concept of "world citizenship" and the need to cultivate "progressive acceptance" of the concept all over the globe.[72] The statement also upheld the notion of "common human aspiration" for mental health, which should tie all the nations together, including Western and non-Western countries.[73] It even came with a cautionary note that "adequate and appropriate living with others . . . is not to be achieved by imposing or indoctrinating." Nothing was more ironic than these statements, considering the way in which they were created. The subjectivity of "others"—even when explicitly expressed—did not seem to matter, while the subjectivity of "us," the scientists, was exempt from any qualification.

In the next international conference he attended in 1948, Sullivan again made use of the problematic model of mature "leaders" and immature "followers," this time with a specific focus on children's patterns of development. During the five-week UNESCO seminar "Childhood Education toward World-Mindedness," in Czechoslovakia, Sullivan presented a paper titled

"Psychiatry, Education, and the UNESCO 'Tensions Project.'" In this presentation, he first explained different stages of personality development and emphasized the significance of education at each phase to "[raise] socially desirable people."[74] Then he suggested that UNESCO help create educational programs that ensured normal personality growth, including one that would correct the "preponderance of female teachers . . . [that] impose[d] undue restrictions in healthy self-expressions for the majority of school children." Using an article by Canadian psychiatrist Gordon Stephens, Sullivan complained how "too many attractive, mature women teachers, rich with teaching experience, marry and are replaced by less experienced teachers." What was lacking in schools, then, was female teachers who embodied a fully realized femininity and adulthood. Instead of benefiting from these desirable teachers, schoolchildren, especially boys in urban districts, were "over-exposed" to inexperienced, and supposedly immature, woman figures. This, combined with the lack of "opportunities of useful contacts with [their] father," would put children's development at risk.[75] In addition to being based on the assumption that boys were the primary subjects of education, this argument resonated with the view that true "maturity" must be based on the integration of feminine and masculine characteristics. Also implicit in this approach was the view that, if lacking sufficient exposure to and internalization of femininity, male children might not develop heterosexuality. Such risk must be eliminated by efforts of scientists of "goodwill and sound judgment," Sullivan argued, reiterating the role of scientists as thoughtful observers of human growth.

Although in less gendered language, Ruth Benedict, another U.S. participant of the seminar, shared this almost unreserved belief in science. To be sure, drawing upon the tradition of relativism, she stressed the fallacy of a "centuries old . . . attitude" that had urged Americans to claim that "other nations must accept the virtues and practices with which they [Americans] are familiar." An alternative attitude was that of social scientists, who studied "national differences . . . down into such fundamental things as the way we bring up our children." Her belief was that scientific studies had shown that there were no superior and inferior races. Indeed, the arrogance of racism "defies what is scientifically known of human races."[76] Just as apparent as her relativism and belief in equality, however, is a lack of recognition that the social sciences were a Western tradition. Opposing racism, Benedict relied on science and its presumed ability to make unbiased observations about difference. In turn, scientific studies would offer better methods of educating children, so that children could become adults mindful of peace. What was missing from this reasoning was the recognition that science, broadly considered, was a source of the assumption that human differences were immutable, even if these differences were culturally constructed.

Human diversity might have its origin in different child rearing and life histories, but nevertheless these placed peoples at different points on the spectrum between maturity and immaturity. Ultimately, this limited sense of science in its contexts—particularly what it meant for American scientists to go into countries of "aggressors" to study patterns of education—made it difficult for Benedict's ideas to bear fruit in international encounters.

The frustration that flooded the IPC's non-U.S. participants' comments indicates that "others" were attentive to the lack of equality implicit in America's leadership. Not only conceptually but also in their tactics American scientists effectively turned away from disagreement and diversity. In this process of exclusion, the distinction between "leaders" and "followers" was confirmed in significantly gendered language. Because it called for both feminine and masculine characteristics for American scientists to claim their "mature" leadership, it naturally followed that nations that seemed disproportionately feminine or masculine—too appeasing or aggressive—were placed in the category of "immaturity." Not surprisingly, the U.S. postwar relationship with "difficult allies"—countries that disagreed with aspects of American policies—were frequently described in language that assumed that these allies were "in some way diminished from the norm of healthy heterosexual male."[77] Thus, the most problematic of the allies, Soviet Union, appeared to U.S. diplomats as too driven, aggressive, and "monstrously . . . hypermasculine."[78] In contrast, France's effort to ameliorate the Cold War was seen as a sign of the nation's "out-of-control femininity."[79] Asian countries generally fell into this category of too much femininity. India, in part because of its long history of "servility" in the colonial era, was believed to be a country where "the majority of . . . men had been deprived of their manliness and their virility"; in fact, they seemed "inclined to homosexuality or . . . sexual renunciation."[80] Notably, the imbalance in gender was immediately linked to homosexuality, suggesting the crucial place that sexual "immaturity" occupied in shaping gender-biased international relationships.

The former enemies, Japan and Germany in particular, drew even more elaborately gendered and sexualized metaphors. Although both countries' aggression during the war was frequently depicted as masculinity gone out of control, Americans' understanding was that this loss of control was not the nature of masculinity per se (as it was defined by American masculinity); rather, these men's masculinity was not true masculinity to begin with. For example, unlike American masculinity, which was deprived of opportunities to mature because of the war, Japanese men's masculinity had always been immature, a view that had its roots in nineteenth-century Orientalism, which "feminized Japan as a dainty 'land of fans and flowers' and 'a realized fairyland.'" Not only in their culture, but also in their appearance, the Japanese in general seemed younger—their skin less hairy and their height shorter than that of Westerners. Not surprisingly, then, what might be called the "homosexualization" of Japan began right after the war. Some even claimed a greater percentage of homosexuality in the Japanese armed forces, so as to reiterate the country's need to nurture genuine masculinity—under U.S. guidance, of course.[81] Regarding Germany, Americans took a different, but equally sagacious, route to a much needed reconciliation under U.S. leadership. While Americans' prewar image of Germans was predominantly based on Nazis soldiers and thus was oriented around men, the postwar image relied heavily upon German women with whom GIs associated during the occupation period—women who lost their husbands and partners, women who were deprived of means and eager to pursue romantic relationships with Americans.[82] This overly "effeminized" image of Germans made it easier for the United States to see them as children in need of assistance, not angry and uncontrollable enemies.

Americans felt free to manipulate these gendered images not because their domestic gender relationships were stable; indeed, Americans' masculinity, femininity, and sexuality were questioned and largely redefined after the war. But at least the United States was able to uphold scientific leadership, which incorporated both male and female virtues, allowing U.S. scientists to rise above troubled identities elsewhere. This theoretically and metaphorically assumed advantage was put into practice at the UNESCO programs and the IPC, quite effectively so because of the inner-circle tactic. Instead of helping the different and the silenced to flourish, as it often did before the war, the inner-circle tactic used by scientists in the crucial postwar years worked to eliminate the fewer and the powerless. The leaders were not only tough and smart, but also sophisticated and benevolent. In the end, there was no need for anyone else to be on the stage, because the big brothers got it all.

What Happened to Subjectivity?

The science of homosexuality, along with the medical and social sciences that shaped it, continued to diffuse in the 1940s. In one sense, this change was an expansion from a field of science that concerned itself primarily with a small group of the "afflicted" to a source of wide-ranging, albeit gendered, observations that offered useful concepts for Americans to sort out what constituted the normal and the healthy. Moreover, as highlighted in Sullivan's career, the science of homosexuality took a definite turn from private to public—first, tentatively and gingerly during the war, then willingly and forcefully afterward. This was in part because he did not practice clinically in the 1940s: his life and career no longer included one-on-one relationships with patients, severing opportunities for him to explore the scientific and the subjective in private. More important, the science of homosexuality became "public" because it was not about a select small group of people anymore; it was about the problem of heterosexuality gone out of balance. What vanished in this change was the subjectivity of both scientists and sexual minorities that made the field unique, compelling, and problematic. To be sure, the subjectivity of scientists who were sexual minorities, in the 1920s and 1930s, was kept separate from their public discourse. The science of homosexuality in public morphed into a critique of racism and sexism, which did not disclose too much subjectivity of scientists and sexual minorities. But the connection between scientists' subjectivity—sexual subjectivity in particular—and their interest in homosexuality continued to be alive in their private practices. When homosexuality became a public-policy issue during the war, this particular kind of science, bound up in Sullivan's case with his identity as a gay man, made a distinct attempt to make itself heard so as to counter homophobia. While this was an unsuccessful effort domestically, the science of homosexuality helped scientists to assert leadership that all were expected to follow once it was brought to international scenes. Here, the science of homosexuality exercised a tactical and metaphorical influence, never presenting itself as immediately related to sexual minorities; nor were its insights presented as related to scientists. Scientists as individuals who might have a subjective, as well as scientific, commitment to their studies became less relevant or legitimate.

There are signs that such an erosion of the awareness of subjectivity—both scientists' and their subjects'—was felt as a loss by both Sullivan and Benedict, who had shared their excitement about the "life history" method and "participant observations" in the 1930s. Sullivan, for one, made a notable comment after coming back from the IPC, which suggested his desire to continue to include the personal and the subjective in science. His belief was that international, interdisciplinary conferences could be facilitated if "each representative shall have made known in an opening statement the aspect of his life history relevant to his participation; such as general and particularly significant experience."[83] He considered such telling of life histories as helping conferees understand each other and as facilitating the identification of common goals. He did not seem concerned about the possibility that the disclosure of personal information might complicate, rather than assist, communication. In this way, as in other contexts, Sullivan's belief in the highly personalized method was naive as well as genuine.

Benedict in 1947, too, offered what she admitted to be a "heretical statement" about anthropology, when she made a speech as lame duck president of the American Anthropological Association. Contrary to a common claim that anthropology was the scientific study of culture—a claim she herself would make in the UNESCO conference—Benedict argued that anthropological questions were similar to those posed by the humanities. But this was not meant to reflect regret; rather, she commended "the great tradition of the humanities . . . distinguished by command of vast detail . . . and the sensitivities it has . . . fostered to the quality of men's minds and emotions." The humanities can illuminate an individual case by showing "*what is*, [by] seeing that it happened and must have happened" (italics in original), Benedict reminded her audience, citing literary critic A. C. Bradley. Because of such careful attention to specifics, the humanities managed to resist simplistic "explanations." Such resistance was seen in the life history method in anthropology as well, but most life history materials were wasted in an increased disciplinary attempt for generalizations:

> Many life histories have been collected. . . . Very little, however, has been done . . . with [them]. . . . The nature of the life-history material made this largely inevitable, . . . for it is a time-consuming and repetitious way of obtaining straight ethnography, and if that is all they are to be used for, any field worker knows how to obtain such data more economically.

Benedict's point, of course, was that life histories were not supposed to be used to collect ethnographical data. If anthropologists were to make life histories "count in anthropological . . . understanding," they had "only one recourse: we must be . . . able to study them according to the best tradition of the humanities."[84]

Both Benedict's and Sullivan's recalling of life history—a method to examine subjectivity in science—highlights the end of an era in which science's relationship to subjectivity was largely in flux. When scientists marched onto the national and international stage, there was no room for life histories of the performers, such as those that Sullivan recommended (his proposal was not taken seriously). Benedict called for a return to the humanities, but when she went to the UNESCO conference her role was to encompass the use of science in preventing aggression. Here, the image of American leaders relied upon measured understanding of "facts," making it difficult for the reasonable frustration of others with America's condescension to be reckoned. In the end, a significant part of the problem was attitude, practice, and culture. The demise of an attempt to grasp subjectivity in science had domestic ramifications as well. For one, the decline was followed by increased intervention into the rights of sexual minorities in the 1950s, most notably through President Dwight D. Eisenhower's executive order 10450 in 1953 that allowed the government to fire its employees based on their presumed homosexuality. Such a denial of civil rights was in part based on a medical claim that homosexual persons were immature and incapable of self-control, posing a risk to national security. What separated

this medical science—a kind of science on which the rampant, public persecution of sexual minorities in the 1950s relied—from the science of homosexuality in the 1920s and 1930s was a diminished appreciation of the fact
that the subject of scientific study, in this case sexuality, was inseparable
from a person as a whole. A considerable number of medical theories on
homosexuality published between 1952 and 1973—when homosexuality was
a formal entry in the register of diseases in the APA's *Diagnostic and Statistical Manual*—assumed that homosexuality was an entity that needed to be
treated actively. Indeed, those who supported this assumption, many of
them psychoanalytically oriented psychiatrists, were assertive in proposing
therapies to change homosexuality into heterosexuality. Edmund Bergler,
Irbing Bieber, and Charles Socarides, all trained psychoanalysts, contributed
to devising a range of conversion therapies. Although their views were not
necessarily representative of the era's psychiatric approach to homosexuality—for instance, psychiatrists who were called upon by the government to
advise on the elimination of "sexual perverts" from federal agencies were
generally sympathetic to the plight of homosexual persons—the contrast
between medical scientists before the war and those who became influential
after the conflict remains striking.[85] Those in the earlier period examined
the stigmatization of homosexuality in a critical light, in part because, for
both doctors and patients, homosexuality was part of their life histories, not
a factor that could be separated and transformed. As Benedict proclaimed,
the understanding of "what is," not its manipulation, was the purpose of
science, and ultimately, the goal of the era's liberalism. In contrast, postwar
medicine turned to an objectification of homosexuality, or what Benedict
called "straight ethnography," which can be observed independently from
its environment in the eyes of both examiners and examinees. No longer
was it an ingredient of a person's life that, inevitably, was part of a whole.

In response to this increased effort to "treat" homosexuality, sexual
minorities of the 1960s and 1970s used a tactic that was strikingly dissimilar
to that used in the 1920s and 1930s. In the earlier decades, the approach that
sexual minorities took to a better acceptance was deeply intertwined with
the medical and social sciences. This was not only because these were the
fields that had much to say about the subject of homosexuality; in science,
sexual minorities were able to find allies who were willing to know who they
were and what they wanted. To be sure, these scientists' published articles
might discuss homosexuality as social or medical abnormality. Nevertheless,
in their private practices, they might understand that many sexual minorities were, indeed, as varied as any group of people. They might even think
that sexual minorities deserved special recognition as uniquely talented
individuals. Without doubt, such recognition had its own risks; in Sullivan's
practice, it became by the 1930s bound up with exploitation rather than

empowerment. Even so, science's attempt to grasp subjectivity, because it was considered to be the most important subject of groundbreaking, exciting, and authentic scientific studies, created a possibility for the nonstigmatizing exploration of sexual experiences. Sullivan's practice did not have to become problematic; if his exploration of subjectivity had been more open and thorough, it could have created a truly therapeutic community for sexual minorities. His exploration of subjectivity, both his and his patients,' did not go far enough to accomplish this, but some patients certainly recognized the potential. It was the science community of the interwar years that nurtured the potential; it is not surprising, then, that many sexual minorities sought out comfort and inspiration in their alliance with science, if largely in private.

This did not apply to the mainstream relationship between sexual minorities and scientists after the war. In response to ever assertive medical interventions, sexual minorities began to claim their rights for health, well-being, and acceptance in a decisively "public" forum. No longer did a patient rely on one on one conversations with a psychiatrist that might help him or her gain self-acceptance. To be sure, there were scientists such as Alfred C. Kinsey and Evelyn Hooker who nurtured personal relationships with sexual minorities. But the purpose of these relationships was to claim the normality and health of sexual minorities in public, not to comfort them in private. Sexual minorities literally went public—by breaking out on to the street in the Stonewall uprising or by demanding an invitation to present panels on homosexuality at APA meetings—sometimes in collaboration with sympathetic scientists. In this activism, there emerged a tactic modeled after the African American civil rights movement. As gay activist Gary Alinder proclaimed at the 1970 APA convention, psychiatrists who defined homosexuality as an illness were fundamentally flawed because "if [they] talked about black people the way [they talk] about homosexuals, [they] would be drawn and quartered and would deserve it." In the light of this declaration, it was clear that science was an oppressor who must be marked as such. More important, the assault must take place in public, because it was to follow the preceding activism, which had been decidedly public. The demise of subjectivity in science in general and within the science of homosexuality in particular opened a way toward both gains and setbacks after the war, first in the rise of conversion therapies, and then in the determination of sexual minorities and their allies in science to pursue equality largely in public, no longer in private. Private practices, as scientists embraced them in the 1920s and 1930s, had significantly less place and relevancy in postwar American liberalism. Not only the science of homosexuality, but also the gay rights movement, was determined to be public.

NOTES

ABBREVIATIONS USED IN THE NOTES

Archives and Papers

MSA	Michael Stuart Allen papers in possession of Michael Stuart Allen, San Francisco
HSP	Helen Swick Perry papers in possession of Stewart E. Perry, Cambridge, Massachusetts
LC	Margaret Mead papers, Manuscript Division, Library of Congress, Washington, DC
RC	Ralph Crowley papers, Courtesy of Oskar Diethelm Library, DeWitt Wallace Institute for the History of Psychiatry, Weill Cornell Medical College, New York City, New York
SEP	Sheppard and Enoch Pratt Hospital, Department of Medical Record, Baltimore, Maryland
VC	Ruth Fulton Benedict papers, Archives and Special Collections Library, Vassar College, Poughkeepsie, New York
WAWI	William Alanson White Institute archive, New York City, New York
WSP	Washington School of Psychiatry archive, Courtesy of Washington School of Psychiatry, Washington, DC

Journals

AJP	*American Journal of Psychiatry*
AJS	*American Journal of Sociology*
AA	*American Anthropologist*
MH	*Mental Hygiene*
PQ	*Psychiatric Quarterly*
PSY	*Psychiatry*

Individuals and Institutions

MM	Margaret Mead
RFB	Ruth Fulton Benedict
WAWPF	William Alanson White Psychiatric Foundation

INTRODUCTION

1. "A Sharply Divided Washington Supreme Court Upholds State's Ban on Same-Sex Marriage," *New York Times* (July 27, 2006): A-18.

2. On the rise of urban communities of sexual minorities and their increased visibility, see George Chauncey, *Gay New York: Gender, Urban Culture, and the Making of the Gay Male World, 1890–1940* (New York: Basic Books, 1994); Nan Alamilla Boyd, *Wide Open Town: A History of Queer San Francisco to 1965* (Berkeley: University of California Press, 2003); Roderick A. Ferguson, *Aberrations in Black: Toward a Queer of Color Critique* (Minneapolis: University of Minnesota Press, 2004); Daniel Hurewitz, *Bohemian Los Angeles and the Making of Modern Politics* (Berkeley: University of California Press, 2007). On the transformation of gender relationships, sexual expressions, and culture in the 1920s and 1930s, see Warren Susman, *Culture as History: The Transformation of American Society in the Twentieth Century* (New York: Pantheon Books, 1984); Beth L. Bailey, *From Front Porch to Back Seat: Courtship in Twentieth-Century America* (Baltimore: Johns Hopkins University Press, 1988); Regina G. Kunzel, *Fallen Women, Problem Girls: Unmarried Mothers and the Professionalization of Social Work, 1890–1945* (New Haven: Yale University Press, 1993); Kevin White, *The First Sexual Revolution: The Emergence of Male Heterosexuality in Modern America* (New York: New York University Press, 1993); Ruth M. Alexander, *The "Girl Problem," Female Sexual Delinquency in New York, 1900–1930* (Ithaca: Cornell University Press, 1995). On the state-led persecution of sexual minorities in the 1950s, see David K. Johnson, *The Lavender Scare: The Cold War Persecution of Gays and Lesbians in the Federal Government* (Chicago: University of Chicago Press, 2004); Margot Canaday, *The Straight State: Sexuality and Citizenship in Twentieth-Century America* (Princeton: Princeton University Press, 2009).

3. Chauncey, *Gay New York*, chap. 12.

4. John D'Emilio and Estelle B. Freedman, *Intimate Matters: A History of Sexuality in America*, 2d ed. (Chicago: University of Chicago Press, 1988).

5. Ronald Bayer, *Homosexuality and American Psychiatry: The Politics of Diagnosis* (New York: Basic Books, 1981); Allan Bérubé, *Coming Out under Fire: The History of Gay Men and Women in World War Two* (New York: Free Press, 1990); Lucy Bland and Laura L. Doan, *Sexology in Culture: Labeling Bodies and Desires* (Chicago: University of Chicago Press, 1998); Jennifer Terry, *An American Obsession: Science, Medicine, and Homosexuality in Modern Society* (Chicago: University of Chicago Press, 1999); Henry L. Minton, *Departing from Deviance: A History of Homosexual Rights and Emancipatory Science in America* (Chicago: University of Chicago Press, 2002); Vernon A. Rosario, *Homosexuality and Science: A Guide to Debate* (Santa Barbara, CA: ABC-CLIO, 2002).

6. The scholarship that has highlighted the contrast between liberals and conservatives includes John D'Emilio, *Sexual Politics, Sexual Communities: The Making of a Sexual Minority in the United States, 1940–1970* (Chicago: University of Chicago Press, 1983); Kenneth Lewes, *The Psychoanalytic Theory of Male Homosexuality* (New York: Simon and Schuster, 1988); Byrne R. S. Fone, *A Road to Stonewall: Male Homosexuality and Homophobia in English and American Literature, 1750–1969* (New York: Twayne, 1995); Gary L. Atkins, *Gay Seattle: Stories of Exile and Belonging* (Seattle: University of Washington Press, 2003). Some examples of the scholarship that has offered a more nuanced picture of scientists are Bert Hansen, "American Physicians' Earliest Writings about Homosexuals, 1880–1900," *Milbank Quarterly* 67.Supplement 1

(1989): 92–108; Erin G. Carlston, "'A Finer Differentiation': Female Homosexuality and the American Medical Community, 1926–1940," in *Science and Homosexualities*, ed. Vernon Rosario (New York: Routledge, 1997), 177–196.

7. The one-on-one format does not make interactions between a doctor and a patient "private" in some absolute sense. But doctors, students, and patients involved in the specific one-on-one sessions I examine were aware of the fact that their interactions were protected from outside scrutiny. Thus the format allowed them to discuss certain issues such as homosexual experiences that they refrained from talking during group sessions.

8. On Sullivan's interpersonal theory, its relation to the social sciences, or both, see Patrick Mullahy, *The Contributions of Harry Stack Sullivan: A Symposium on Interpersonal Theory in Psychiatry and Social Sciences* (New York: Hermitage Press, 1952); Dorothy R. Blitsten, *The Social Theory of Harry Stack Sullivan* (New York: William-Frederick Press, 1953); Charles S. Johnson, "Harry Stack Sullivan, Social Scientist," in Harry Stack Sullivan, *The Fusion of Psychiatry and Social Science* (New York: W. W. Norton, 1964), xxxiii–xxxv; Helen Swick Perry, *Psychiatrist of America: The Life of Harry Stack Sullivan* (Cambridge: Belknap Press of Harvard University Press, 1982); David Mck. Rioch, "Recollections of Harry Stack Sullivan and of the Development of His Interpersonal Psychiatry," *Psychiatry (PSY)* 48 (1985): 141–157; Kenneth L. Chatelaine, "Harry Stack Sullivan," in *Portraits of Pioneers in Psychology*, ed. Gregory A. Kimble et al. (Hillsdale, NJ: Lawrence Erlbaum Associates, 1991), 325–340; F. Barton Evans III, *Harry Stack Sullivan: Interpersonal Theory and Psychotherapy* (New York: Routledge, 1996).

9. On the history of the "life history" method and its makers, broadly defined, see L. L. Langness and Gelya Frank, *Lives: An Anthropological Approach to Biography* (Novato, CA: Chandler & Sharp, 1981); Martin Bulmer, *The Chicago School of Sociology: Institutionalization, Diversity, and the Rise of Sociological Research* (Chicago: University of Chicago Press, 1984); George W. Stocking Jr., ed. *Malinowski, Rivers, Benedict and Others: Culture and Personality* (Madison: University of Wisconsin Press, 1986); Richard Handler, "Boasian Anthropology and the Critique of American Culture," *American Quarterly* 42 (June 1990): 252–273; Luigi Tomasi ed., *The Tradition of the Chicago School of Sociology* (Surrey: Ashgate, 1998); Philip Manning, *Freud and American Sociology* (Malden, MA: Polity Press, 2005).

10. Dorothy Ross, *The Origins of America Social Science* (New York: Cambridge University Press, 1991).

11. On the orthodox Freudians' approach to homosexuality, see Sigmund Freud, *Three Essays on the Theory of Sexuality* (1905; New York: Basic Books, 1962); Sigmund Freud, "Certain Neurotic Mechanism in Jealousy, Paranoia, and Homosexuality," *International Journal of Psycho-analysis* 4 (January–April 1923): 1–10; Theodore R. Robie, "The Investigation of the Oedipus and Homosexual Complexes in Schizophrenia," *Psychiatric Quarterly (PQ)* 1 (1927): 231–241, 468–484; Paul Schilder, "On Homosexuality," *Psychoanalytic Review* 16 (1929): 377–389; Douglas Bryan, "Bisexuality," *International Journal of Psycho-analysis* 11 (1930): 150–166. On American Freudians' understanding of homosexuality, see Henry Abelove, "Freud, Male Homosexuality, and the Americans," *Dissent* 33 (1986): 59–69; Lewes, *The Psychoanalytic Theory*. On Americanization of Freudian psychoanalysis in general, see John C. Burnham, "From Avant-Garde to Specialism: Psychoanalysis in America," *Journal of the History of Behavioral Science* 15, no. 2 (1979): 128–134; Russell Jacoby,

The Repression of Psychoanalysis: Otto Fenichel and the Political Freudians (Chicago: University of Chicago Press, 1983).

12. On the relative lack of sources about sexuality, see Jonathan Katz, *Gay American History: Lesbians and Gay Men in the U.S.A.* (New York: Crowell, 1976); Estelle B. Freedman and John D'Emilio, "Problems Encountered in Writing the History of Sexuality: Sources, Theory and Interpretation," *Journal of Sex Research* 27 (November 1990): 481–495; John Wrathall, "Provenance as Text: Reading the Silence around Sexuality in Manuscript Collections," *Journal of American History* 79, no. 1 (1992): 165–178; Estelle B. Freedman, "'The Burning of Letters Continues': Elusive Identities and the Historical Construction of Sexuality," in *Modern American Queer History*, ed. Allida M. Black (Philadelphia: Temple University Press, 2001), 51–68. Some examples of the scholarship that has addressed the contested place of subjectivity (of scholars and their subjects) in history are Samuel H. Barton and Carl Pletsch, eds., *Introspection in Biography: The Biographer's Quest for Self-Awareness* (Hillsdale, NJ: Analytic Press, 1985); "Self and Subject: A Roundtable Discussion," *Journal of American History* 89 (June 2002): 17–65; "AHR Roundtable: Historians and Biography," *American Historical Review* 114 (June 2009): 587–661.

13. "Sullivan, James (James Inscoe Sullivan's letter to Helen Swick Perry, October 12, 1971)," HSP.

14. Margaret Mead, *An Anthropologist at Work* (Boston: Houghton Mifflin, 1959).

15. Ruth Fulton Benedict (RFB) to Margaret Mead (MM), November 13, 1931, Box S5, Folder 6, LC; RFB to MM, June 4, 1936, Box S5, Folder 8, LC.

16. Arthur Harry Chapman, *Harry Stack Sullivan: His Life and His Work* (New York: G. P. Putman's Sons, 1976), 62; Kenneth L. Chatelaine, *The Formative Years: Harry Stack Sullivan* (Washington, DC: University Press of America, 1981), 34; Kenneth L. Chatelaine, "Harry Stack Sullivan: The Real Sullivan and What Sullivan Really Said, Founder of Interpersonal Psychiatry, an Introduction to His Life and Theoretical Contributions" (unpublished), 35; "Gill, Tom (interview with Tom Gill, August 9, 1963)," HSP. The recent scholarship has been more candid about Sullivan's homosexuality. See Jon Harned, "Harry Stack Sullivan and the Gay Psychoanalysis," *American Imago* 55, no. 3 (1988): 299–317; Michael Stuart Allen, "Sullivan's Closet: A Reappraisal of Harry Stack Sullivan's Life and His Pioneering Role in American Psychiatry," *Journal of Homosexuality* 29, no. 1 (1995): 1–20; Michael Stuart Allen, "The Island of Dr. Sullivan," *The Gay and Lesbian Review* 7, no. 1 (Winter 2000): 16–19; Bert Hansen, "Public Careers and Private Sexuality: Some Gay and Lesbian Lives in the History of Medicine and Public Health," *American Journal of Public Health* 92, no. 1 (January 2002): 36–44; Peter Hegarty, "Was He Queer . . . or Just Irish? Reading the Life of Harry Stack Sullivan," *Lesbian and Gay Psychology Review* 5 (2004): 103–108; Mark J. Blechner, "The Gay Harry Stack Sullivan: The Interactions Between His Life, Clinical Work, and Theory," *Contemporary Psychoanalysis* 41, no. 1 (January 2005): 1–19; Mark J. Blechner, *Sex Changes: Transformation in Society and Psychoanalysis* (New York: Routledge, 2009).

17. Hilary Lapsley, *Margaret Mead and Ruth Benedict: The Kinship of Women* (Amherst: University of Massachusetts Press, 1999); Lois W. Banner, *Intertwined Lives: Margaret Mead, Ruth Benedict, and Their Circle* (New York: Knopf, 2003); Julia Liss, "Review (of *Intertwined Lives*)," *Journal of American History* 91, no. 3 (2004): 1068–1069; Henrika Kuklick, "Review (of *Intertwined Lives*)," *Pacific Historical Review* 74 (August 2005): 471–473.

18. The difficulty of understanding sexual minorities and gender-atypical individuals in Native American communities is illuminated by a series of studies that relied on anthropological studies of the past, rather than primary, oral historical records taken directly from the informants. See Sue-Ellen Jacobs, "Berdache: A Brief Review of the Literature," *Colorado Anthropologist* 1 (1968): 25–40; Donald G. Forgey, "The Institution of Berdache among the North American Plains Indians," *Journal of Sex Research* 11 (1975): 1–15; Harriet Whitehead, "The Bow and the Burden Strap: A New Look at Institutionalized Homosexuality in Native North America," in *Sexual Meanings, the Cultural Construction of Gender and Sexuality*, ed. Sherry Ortner and Harriet Whitehead (Cambridge: Cambridge University Press, 1981), 80–115; Charles Callender and Lee M. Kochems, "The North American Berdache," *Current Anthropology* 24 (August–October 1983): 443–470; Evelyn Blackwood, "Sexuality and Gender in Certain Native American Tribes: The Case of Cross-Gender Females," *Signs* 10 (Autumn 1984): 27–42; Jonathan Goldberg, "Sodomy in the New World: Anthropologies Old and New," *Social Text* 29 (1991): 46–56; Walter L. Williams, "Being Gay and Doing Research on Homosexuality in Non-Western Cultures," *Journal of Sex Research* 30 (May 1993): 115–120; Kath Weston, *Long Slow Burn: Sexuality and Social Science* (New York: Routledge, 1998), 154–155; Anjali Arondekar, "Without a Trace: Sexuality and the Colonial Archive," *Journal of the History of Sexuality* 14 (January 2005): 10–27.

19. On the use of clinical records in reconstructing medical practices, see Robert Coles, *The Call of Stories* (Boston: Houghton Mifflin, 1989), 1–3; Guenter B. Risse and John Harley Warner, "Reconstructing Clinical Activities: Patient Records in Medical History," *Social History of Medicine* 5 (1992): 183–205; Nancy M. P. King and Ann Folwell Stanford, "Patient Stories, Doctor Stories, and True Stories: a Cautionary Reading," *Literature and Medicine* 11 (fall 1992): 185–199; John Harley Warner, "The Use of Patient Records by Historians: Patterns, Possibilities and Perplexities," *Health and History: Bulletin of the Australian Society for the History of Medicine* 1 (1999): 101–111.

20. On the expansion of Sigmund Freud's psychoanalysis in America, see Philip Cushman, *Constructing the Self, Constructing America: A Cultural History of Psychotherapy* (Reading, MA: Addison-Wesley, 1995); Nathan G. Hale Jr., *The Rise and Crisis of Psychoanalysis in the United States: Freud and the Americans, 1917–1985* (New York: Oxford University Press, 1995); Ely Zaretsky, *Secrets of the Soul: A Social and Cultural History of Psychoanalysis* (New York: Vintage Books, 2005). On the mental hygiene movement, see Gerald N. Grob, *Mental Illness and American Society, 1875–1940* (Princeton: Princeton University Press, 1983).

21. There are, of course, limits to the use of "gays," "lesbians," and "sexual minorities" in this book. When I do not have evidence of a clear tie between the past and "gays," "lesbians," or "sexual minorities" today, I use "homosexual individuals," "homosexual men and women," and "people who had same-sex sexual relationships, experiences, or feelings" to refer to people whom scientists described as "homosexuals." Moreover, when I find it necessary to stress a scientist's sense of alienation as someone scientifically defined as a "homosexual," I use the term instead of a "gay," "lesbian," or "sexual minority," even though I refer to the same scientist as a "gay scientist" or "lesbian scientist" elsewhere. Ironically, "gay" in the recent usage of English (especially among young Americans) carries negative connotations such as "wrong," "uncool," and "annoying," while "homosexual" seems to strike many as neutrally descriptive. My effort to avoid inap-

propriate language may prove at least partially futile; our means to eliminate prejudicial language is as much bound up with our particular historical time as a prejudice itself.

22. Kathy Rudy, "Radical Feminism, Lesbian Separatism, and Queer Theory," *Feminist Studies* 27 (Spring 2001): 191–222; Julian Carter, "On Mother-Love: History, Queer Theory, and Nonlesbian Identity," *Journal of the History of Sexuality* 14 (January 2005): 107–138.

CHAPTER 1   A MAN, A DOCTOR, AND HIS PATIENTS

1. On Sullivan's career in the 1920s, see, Clarence G. Schulz, "Sullivan's Clinical Contribution during the Sheppard-Pratt Era: 1923–1930," *PSY* 41 (1978): 117–128; David McKenzie Rioch, "Recollections of Harry Stack Sullivan and of the Development of His Interpersonal Theory," *PSY* 48 (May 1985): 141–167; Robert W. Gibson, "The Application of Psychoanalytic Principles to the Hospitalized Patient," in *Psychoanalysis and Psychosis*, ed. Ann-Louis Silver (Madison: International University Press, 1989), 183–205.

2. On Sullivan's clinical practice involving physical contact, see Kenneth L. Chatelaine, *The Formative Years: Harry Stack Sullivan* (Washington, DC: University Press of America, 1981); Michael Stuart Allen, "Sullivan's Closet: A Reappraisal of Harry Stack Sullivan's Life and His Pioneering Role in American Psychiatry," *Journal of Homosexuality* 29, no. 1 (1995): 1–20; Bert Hansen, "Public Careers and Private Sexuality: Some Gay and Lesbian Lives in the History of Medicine and Public Health," *American Journal of Public Health* 92 (January 2002): 36–44; Mark J. Blechner, "The Gay Harry Stack Sullivan: The Interactions between His Life, Clinical Work, and Theory," *Contemporary Psychoanalysis* 41 (January 2005): 1–19; Peter Hegarty, "Harry Stack Sullivan and His Chums: Archive Fever in American Psychiatry?" *History of the Human Sciences* 18, no. 3 (2005): 35–53.

3. On the new psychiatry, see Gerald N. Grob, *Mental Illness and American Society, 1875–1940* (Princeton: Princeton University Press, 1983); Lawrence J. Friedman, "The Demise of Asylum," *Reviews in American History* 12 (1984): 241–247; Lawrence J. Friedman, "In Retrospect: Gerald Grob's The State and the Mentally Ill; A Turning Point in the Study of the American Mental Hospital," *Reviews in American History* 18 (1990): 292–310; Gerald N. Grob, *The Mad Among Us: A History of the Care of America's Mentally Ill* (New York: Free Press, 1994); Elizabeth Lunbeck, *The Psychiatric Persuasion: Knowledge, Gender, and Power in Modern America* (Princeton: Princeton University Press, 1994).

4. Sylvia B. Sutton, *Crossroads in Psychiatry: A History of the McLean Hospital* (Washington, DC: American Psychiatric Press, 1986); Lawrence J. Friedman, *Menninger: The Family and the Clinic* (New York: Knopf, 1990); Lunbeck, *Psychiatric Persuasion*; Gail A. Hornstein, *To Redeem One Person Is to Redeem the World: The Life of Frieda Fromm-Reichmann* (New York: Free Press, 2002).

5. The information about Sheppard-Pratt in this paragraph is from Bliss Forbush and Byron Forbush, *Gatehouse: The Evolution of the Sheppard and Enoch Pratt* (Philadelphia: Lippincott, 1971), chap. 2.

6. On American psychoanalysis in the 1910s and 1920s, see John C. Burnham, "From Avant-Garde to Specialism: Psychoanalysis in America," *Journal of the History of Behavioral Science* 15, no. 2 (1979): 128–134; Nathan G. Hale Jr., "Freud's Reich, the

Psychiatric Establishment, and Founding of the American Psychoanalytic Association: Professional Styles in Conflict," *Journal of the History of the Behavioral Sciences* 15 (April 1979): 135–141; Ann-Louis Silver, "Psychoanalysis and Psychosis: Players and History in the United States," *Psychoanalysis and History* 4, no. 1 (2002): 45–66.

7. The following discussion is based on an analysis of the 1,696 clinical files at Sheppard and Enoch Pratt Hospital, June 1922 to April 1930, serial number from 4326 to 6377. The total 1,696 does not include 187 files that I could not locate at Sheppard-Pratt, 40 files whose contents were mostly missing, and 128 files whose contents were not accessible because they were transferred to newer files due to readmission.

8. Clinical record, Nos. 5662, 5729, SEP.

9. Clinical record, Nos. 6117, 6156, SEP.

10. Clinical record, No. 5983, SEP. See also Nos. 5023 (4995, 6106), 5533, 5921 (4420), 5950, and 6146 for similar expressions of patients' appreciation the hospital.

11. Clinical record, Nos. 5085 (5696), 5716, SEP.

12. David Rothman, *The Discovery of the Asylum: Social Order and Disorder in the New Republic* (Boston: Little, Brown, 1971); Andrew Scull, *Social Order/Mental Disorder: Anglo-American Psychiatry in Historical Perspective* (London: Routledge, 1989).

13. Franz Alexander and Sheldon Selesnick, *The History of Psychiatry: An Evaluation of Psychiatric Thought and Practice from Prehistoric Times to the Present* (New York: Harper and Row, 1966); Lawrence Kolb and Leon Roizin, *The First Psychiatric Institute: How Research and Education Changed Practice* (Washington, DC: American Psychiatric Press, 1993).

14. Clinical record, No. 6182, SEP.

15. Clinical record, No. 6117, SEP.

16. Clinical record, No. 5983, SEP. See also Nos. 6156, 6182.

17. On critical interpretation of medical records, see Larry R. Churchill and Sandra W. Churchill, "Storytelling in Medical Arenas: The Art of Self-Determination," *Literature and Medicine* 1 (1982): 73–79; Rita Charon, "To Build a Case: Medical Histories as Traditions in Conflict," *Literature and Medicine* 11 (Spring 1992): 115–132.

18. A doctor held a brief interview with a patient soon after admission, which was recorded in the first three parts. The interview aimed to uncover the patient's general attitude. At that time, the patient was asked for family and personal histories as well. Frequently, family members were invited to offer these histories. In interviews, a doctor assessed a patient's personality (bright, cheerful, talkative), medical history (physical and mental), delivery condition, educational history, sexual development (history of sexual relation and masturbation), occupational history, and onset of symptoms. Physical and mental examinations followed, so as to identify existing symptoms such as fever, headache, muscle pain, delusion, and hallucination. Clinical observations were made daily during the first week of hospitalization and, after that, once a week. Usually they included four or five sentences describing patients' activities such as their participation in occupational classes.

19. From 1926 to 1930, conferences began with the presentation of personal and family histories, physical and mental examinations, and clinical observations by a doctor in charge of a patient. Several other doctors were present, and one of them, usually an assistant physician, started the interview. Then, senior doctors joined in the

conversation, and finally, Sullivan. The length of the interview varied, from about twenty minutes to an hour. When it was over, the patient left the room, and the doctors discussed diagnoses and prognoses. Sullivan made the final decision.

20. When doctors found a prognosis favorable, they kept a patient for another month or so for occupational therapy, recreational activities, and brief interviews on a regular basis. Then they held a second conference to review the patient's progress.

21. These numbers concern the files that include transcriptions of special interviews. Special interviews whose transcriptions are missing are not included.

22. See footnote seven for further information about these 1,696 files. It is most likely that more than twenty-two patients had a special interview with Sullivan. Some files that did not include a record of a special interview contained a comment such as "the patient has been interviewed by Dr. Sullivan." Clinical records, Nos. 6106, 5898, and 5921, SEP.

23. See, for example, clinical record, Nos. 5950, 5999, 6141, and 6156, SEP.

24. Chatelaine, *The Formative Years*, 455.

25. Clinical record, No. 5716, SEP. See also No. 5983 for a similar comment.

26. Clinical record, No. 5716, SEP.

27. Clinical record, No. 5541, SEP.

28. Clinical record, No. 5373, SEP.

29. Clinical record, No. 5533, SEP.

30. Clinical record, No. 5625, SEP.

31. Clinical record, No. 5371, SEP.

32. Clinical record, No. 5541, SEP.

33. Clinical record, No. 5426, SEP.

34. Quotation from clinical record, No. 5625, SEP.

35. Harry Stack Sullivan, "Peculiarity of Thought in Schizophrenia," in Henry Stack Sullivan, *Schizophrenia as a Human Process* (New York: W. W. Norton, 1962), 26–99 (originally published in *AJP* 82 [1925]: 21–86, 26–99, 93).

36. Clinical record, No. 6106, SEP.

37. Sullivan, "Peculiarity of Thought," 95.

38. This was a departure from Freudian understanding of sexuality, based on the specific experiences of a modern family rather than the abstract theory of the Oedipus complex.

39. Clinical record, No. 5983, SEP.

40. Clinical record, No. 6102, SEP.

41. Clinical record, No. 5392, SEP.

42. Clinical record, No. 5950, SEP. On the contemporary understanding of psychopathic personality, see George E. Partridge, "A Study of 50 Cases of Psychopathic Personality," *AJP* 84 (1927–1928): 953–973; George E. Partridge, "Psychotic Reaction in the Psychopath," *AJP* 85 (1928–1929): 493–518.

43. A. A. Brill, "Homoeroticism and Paranoia," *AJP* 13 (1934): 957–974; George S. Sprague, "Varieties of Homosexual Manifestations," *AJP* 92 (1935): 143–154; James Page and John Warkentin, "Masculinity and Paranoia," *Journal of Abnormal and Social Psychology* 33 (1938): 527–531.

44. Clinical record, No. 5907, SEP.

45. Harry Stack Sullivan, "Schizophrenia: Its Conservative and Malignant Features," in Sullivan, *Schizophrenia as a Human Process* (originally published in *AJP* 81 [1924]: 77–91), 7–22, 18.

46. William Alanson White, "Some Considerations Bearing on the Diagnosis and Treatment of Dementia Praecox," *AJP* 1, no. 2 (1921): 193–198; Charles E. Gibbs, "Relation of Puberty to Behavior and Personality in Patients with Dementia Praecox," *AJP* 3, no. 1 (1923): 121–129; Nolan D. C. Lewis, "Mechanisms in Certain Cases of Prolonged Schizophrenia," *AJP* 9, no. 3 (1929): 543–552; William Malamud and Wilbur R. Miller, "Psychotherapy in the Schizophrenias," *AJP* 11, no. 3 (1931): 457–480.

47. Harry Stack Sullivan, "Tentative Criteria of Malignancy in Schizophrenia," in Sullivan, *Schizophrenia as a Human Process* (originally published in *AJP* 84 [1927]: 759–782), 158–183, 179–180.

48. Sullivan, "Peculiarity of Thought," 94–95.

49. See note 3.

50. Clinical record, No. 5586, SEP.

51. Clinical record, No. 5428, SEP.

52. Clinical record, No. 5428, SEP.

53. Clinical record, No. 5428, SEP.

54. Chatelaine, *The Formative Years*, 455.

55. Bernard Robbins papers, Folder 9, Section 1, Bernard Robbins Institute, Boston University, Boston. Courtesy of Robert S. Cohen (deceased) and Ben Harris (University of New Hampshire).

56. William Alanson White, *Outline of Psychiatry* (New York: Journal of Nervous and Mental Disease, 1909), 220.

57. Clinical record, No. 5428, SEP.

58. Clinical record, No. 5426, SEP.

59. Clinical record, No. 5426, SEP.

60. Chatelaine, *The Formative Years*, 455.

61. Clinical record, No. 5428, SEP.

62. As discussed earlier, Sullivan had fourteen special interviews with seven patients in 1926, and with thirteen patients in 1927. There are two patients before 1926 whose files include records of special interviews, while two patient files from the period 1928–1929 include such records.

63. William W. Elgin, "Harry Stack Sullivan, as I Remember Him (May 13, 1964)," HSP.

64. Clinical record, No. 6146, SEP. The ellipses are mine.

65. Helen Swick Perry, *Psychiatrist of America: The Life of Harry Stack Sullivan* (Cambridge: Belknap Press of Harvard University Press, 1982), 209.

66. "Sapir, Philip and Jean (interview with Jean Sapir, August 17, 1972)," HSP.

67. Allen, "Sullivan's Closet"; "Interview with Helen Swick Perry (September 23, 1987)," MSA.

68. "Letters from James Inscoe Sullivan to Ralph M. Crowley, M.D., from July 28, 1971 to March 27, 1976," Box 2, Series I, Folder 2, RC.

69. "Letter from James Inscoe to Ralph M. Crowley, M.D. (March 10, 1976)," Box 2, Series I, Folder 2, RC.

70. Such disguise of homosexual relationships was not uncommon. See George Chauncey, *Gay New York: Gender, Urban Culture, and the Making of the Gay Male World 1890–1940* (New York: Basic Books, 1994), 43–44, 107, 273–278; John Loughery, *The Other Side of Silence: Men's Lives and Gay Identities—a Twentieth-Century History* (New York: Henry Holt, 1998), 69–73.

71. "Letter from James Inscoe to Ralph M. Crowley, M.D. (March 21, 1976)," Box 2, Series I, Folder 2, RC. J. Ruthwin Evans, an attendant at Sheppard-Pratt from 1926 to 1953, told Perry that Jimmie was never a patient at the hospital.

72. Perry, *Psychiatrist of America*, 209.

73. Chatelaine, "Harry Stack Sullivan: The Real Sullivan and What Sullivan Really Said," 12; F. Barton Evans III, *Harry Stack Sullivan: Interpersonal Theory and Psychotherapy* (New York: Routledge, 1996), 41.

74. Perry, *Psychiatrist of America*, 319.

75. The conflict between subjectivity and science can be also found in the lives of the first generation of sexologists. See, for example, Hubert Kennedy, "Karl Heinrich Ulrichs, First Theorist of Homosexuality," in *Science and Homosexualities*, ed. Vernon Rosario (New York: Routledge, 1997), 26–45; James D. Steakley, "Per Scientiam ad Justitiam Magnus Hirschfeld and the Sexual Politics of Innate Homosexuality," in *Science and Homosexualities*, ed. Rosario, 133–154. On Gay and Painter, see Henry L. Minton, *Departing from Deviance: A History of Homosexual Rights and Emancipatory Science in America* (Chicago: University of Chicago Press, 2002). On Kinsey, see James H. Jones, *Alfred C. Kinsey: A Public/Private Life* (New York: W. W. Norton, 1999); Jonathan Gathorne-Hardy, *Sex the Measure of All Things: A Life of Alfred C. Kinsey* (Bloomington: Indiana University Press, 2000). On Mead and Benedict, see Hilary Lapsley, *Margaret Mead and Ruth Benedict: The Kinship of Women* (Amherst: University of Massachusetts Press, 1999); Lois W. Banner, *Intertwined Lives: Margaret Mead, Ruth Benedict, and Their Circle* (New York: Knopf, 2003).

CHAPTER 2   ILLNESS WITHIN A HOSPITAL AND WITHOUT

1. Clinical record, No. 5371, SEP.

2. Paula S. Fass, *The Damned and the Beautiful: American Youth in the 1920's* (New York: Oxford University Press, 1977); Beth L. Bailey, *From Front Porch to Back Seat: Courtship in Twentieth-Century America* (Baltimore: Johns Hopkins University Press, 1988) offer useful overviews of the change in American youth culture during the 1920s. On the transformation of sexual and gender relationships, see V. F. Calverton and S. D. Schmalhausen ed., *Sex in Civilization* (London: Allen and Unwin, 1930); Peter N. Sterns, "Men, Boys, and Anger in American Society, 1860–1940," in *Manliness and Morality: Middle-Class Masculinity in Britain and America*, ed. J. A. Mangan and James Walvin (Manchester: Manchester University Press, 1987); Carroll Smith-Rosenberg, "Discourses of Sexuality and Subjectivity: The New Women, 1870–1936," in *Hidden from History: Reclaiming the Gay and Lesbian Past*, ed. Martin Bauml Duberman, Martha Vicinus, and George Chauncey Jr. (New York: Nal Books, 1989), 264–280. On the changing meaning of religion, see George Marsden, *Fundamentalism and American Culture* (New York: Oxford University Press, 1980). John Bodnar, *The Transplanted: A History of Immigrants in Urban America* (Bloomington: Indiana University Press, 1985); and James R. Grossman, *Land of Hope: Chicago, Black Southerners, and the Great*

Migration (Chicago: University of Chicago Press, 1989) offer excellent discussions of racial and ethnic migration.

3. Kevin White, *The First Sexual Revolution: The Emergence of Male Heterosexuality in Modern America* (New York: New York University Press, 1993); Gail Bederman, *Manliness and Civilization: A Cultural History of Gender and Race in the United States, 1880–1917* (Chicago: University of Chicago Press, 1995); Angus McLaren, *The Trial of Masculinity: Policing Sexual Boundaries, 1870–1930* (Chicago: University of Chicago Press, 1997).

4. Freddy Mortier, Willem Colen, and Frank Simon, "Inner-Scientific Reconstructions in the Discourse on Masturbation (1740–1950)," *Paedagogica Historica* 30, no. 3 (1994): 817–848; Jean Stengers and Anne van Neck, *Masturbation: The History of a Great Terror* (New York: Macmillan, 2001); Thomas Walter Laqueur, *Solitary Sex: A Cultural History of Masturbation* (New York: Zone Books, 2003).

5. Clinical record, No. 5428, SEP.

6. Clinical record, No. 5620, SEP.

7. Clinical record, No. 5898, SEP.

8. Clinical record, No. 6194, SEP.

9. Clinical record, No. 4495, SEP.

10. Clinical record, No. 5533, SEP.

11. Clinical record, No. 5426, SEP.

12. Barbara Sicherman, "The Paradox of Prudence: Mental Health in the Gilded Age," *Journal of American History* 62, no. 4 (1976): 890–912; George Chauncey, "Christian Brotherhood or Sexual Perversion? Homosexual Identities and the Construction of Sexual Boundaries in the World War I Era," *Journal of Social History* 19 (1985): 189–212; Ely Zaretsky, *Secrets of the Soul: A Social and Cultural History of Psychoanalysis* (New York: Vintage Books, 2005), 183–184.

13. Clinical record, No. 5538, SEP.

14. Clinical record, No. 6032, SEP.

15. Clinical record, No. 5586, SEP.

16. Clinical record, No. 6119, SEP.

17. Clinical record, No. 5428, SEP.

18. Clinical record, No. 5533, SEP.

19. Lesley A. Hall, *Hidden Anxieties: Male Sexuality, 1900–1950* (Cambridge, MA: Policy Press, 1991); Richard Collier, *Masculinity, Law, and the Family* (London: Routledge, 1995).

20. Clinical record, No. 6117, SEP.

21. Roy Lubove, *The Professional Altruist: The Emergence of Social Work as a Career, 1880–1930* (Cambridge: Harvard University Press, 1965); Burton J. Bledstein, *The Culture of Professionalism: The Middle Class and the Development of Higher Education in America* (New York: W. W. Norton, 1976); Lynn D. Gordon, *Gender and Higher Education in the Progressive Era* (New Haven: Yale University Press, 1990); Ellen Fitzpatrick, *Endless Crusade: Women Social Scientists and Progressive Reform* (New York: Oxford University Press, 1990).

22. Clinical record, No. 4995, SEP.

23. Clinical record, No. 5639, SEP.

24. Pete Daniel, *Standing at the Crossroads: Southern Life since 1900* (New York: Hill and Wang, 1986); Edward Ayers, *The Promise of the New South* (New York: Oxford Uni-

versity Press, 1992); William Link, *The Paradox of Southern Progressivism* (Chapel Hill: University of North Carolina Press, 1992); Grace Hale, *Making Whiteness: The Culture of Segregation in the South* (New York: Pantheon Books, 1998); Glenda Gilmore, *Defying Dixie: The Radical Roots of Civil Rights* (New York: W. W. Norton, 2008).

25. Clinical record, No. 6156, SEP.

26. Clinical record, No. 6032, SEP.

27. Olivier Zunz, *The Changing Face of Inequality: Urbanization, Industrial Development, and Immigrants in Detroit, 1880–1920* (Chicago: University of Chicago Press, 1982); Bodnar, *The Transplanted*; Matthew Frye Jacobson, *Whiteness of a Different Color: European Immigrants and the Alchemy of Race* (Cambridge: Harvard University Press, 1998).

28. Clinical record, No. 6141, SEP.

29. Clinical record, No. 5950, SEP.

30. Clinical record, No. 6004, SEP.

31. Clinical record, No. 5999, SEP.

32. Clinical record, No. 6156, SEP.

33. For example, Sullivan called a fifteen-year-old schizophrenic patient by his first name throughout the patient's stay at Sheppard Pratt, both in special interviews and conferences. See clinical record, No. 5570, SEP.

34. Clinical record, No. 4995, SEP.

35. Clinical record, No. 6141, SEP.

36. Clinical record, Nos. 5426, 5533, and 5586, SEP.

37. Harry Stack Sullivan, "The Common Field of Research and Clinical Psychiatry," in Sullivan, *Schizophrenia as a Human Process* (originally published in *PQ* 1 [1927]: 276–291), 140–156, 151.

38. Clinical record, No. 5662, SEP.

39. Clinical record, No. 5729, SEP.

40. Clinical record, No. 5729, SEP.

41. Clinical record, No. 6182, SEP.

42. Clinical record, No. 6141, SEP.

43. Clinical record, No. 6224, SEP.

44. Clinical record, No. 5662, SEP.

45. Clinical record, No. 6106, SEP.

46. Clinical record, No. 5585, SEP.

47. Bliss Forbush and Byron Forbush, *Gatehouse: The Evolution of the Sheppard and Enoch Pratt* (Philadelphia: Lippincott, 1971), chap. 7.

48. Clinical record, No. 5373, SEP.

49. Clinical record, No. 5373, SEP.

50. Clinical record, No. 5428, SEP.

51. Clinical record, No. 5533, SEP.

52. Clinical record, No. 5533, SEP.

53. Clinical record, No. 6032, SEP.

54. Bernard Robbins papers, Folder 9, Section 1, Bernard Robbins Institute, Boston University, Boston.

55. Clinical record, No. 6236, SEP.

56. Clinical record, No. 5613, SEP.

57. Clinical record, No. 5786, SEP.

58. Clinical record, No. 4995, SEP.

59. Kenneth L. Chatelaine, *The Formative Years: Harry Stack Sullivan* (Washington, DC: University Press of America, 1981), 452.

60. Clinical record, No. 5889, SEP.

61. Forbush and Forbush, *Gatehouse*, chap. 8. Chapman wrote this to the hospital board.

62. Clifton Read, "Harry Stack Sullivan: A Remembrance (undated)," MSA, 20.

CHAPTER 3   LIFE HISTORY FOR SCIENCE AND SUBJECTIVITY

1. Warren Susman, *Culture as History: The Transformation of American Society in the Twentieth Century* (New York: Pantheon Books, 1984); Jackson Lears, *No Place of Grace: Antimodernism and the Transformation of American Culture, 1880–1920* (Chicago: University of Chicago Press, 1981); Richard Hander, *Critics against Culture: Anthropological Observers of Mass Society* (Madison: University of Wisconsin Press, 2005).

2. Historians have written monographs about these intellectuals. See Rolf Linder, *The Reportage of Urban Culture: Robert Park and the Chicago School* (Cambridge: Cambridge University Press, 1996), trans. Adrian Morris Jeremy Gaines and Martin Chalmers; Regina Darnell, *Edward Sapir: Linguist, Anthropologist, Humanist* (Berkeley: University of California Press, 1990); Patrick J. Gilpin, *Charles S. Johnson: Leadership beyond the Veil in the Age of Jim Crow* (New York: State University of New York Press, 2003); William Ascher, *Revitalizing Political Psychology: the Legacy of Harold D. Lasswell* (Mahwah, NJ: Lawrence Erlbaum, 2005); Nancy Lutkehaus, *Margaret Mead: the Making of an American Icon* (Princeton: Princeton University Press, 2008); Hilary Lapsley, *Margaret Mead and Ruth Benedict: The Kinship of Women* (Amherst: University of Massachusetts Press, 1999); Lois W. Banner, *Intertwined Lives: Margaret Mead, Ruth Benedict, and Their Circle* (New York: Knopf, 2003); Judith S. Modell, *Ruth Benedict: Patterns of Life* (Philadelphia: University of Pennsylvania Press, 1983); Virginia Heyer Young, *Ruth Benedict: Beyond Relativity, Beyond Pattern* (Lincoln: University of Nebraska Press, 2005).

3. John Dollard, *Criteria for the Life History: With Analysis of Six Notable Documents* (New York: Peter Smith, 1935), iv.

4. On psychiatrists' frustration with the neglect of psychiatric education at medical schools, see APA, "Proceedings: Report of the Committee on Medical Services," *AJP* 84 (1927): 316–321; *AJP* 85 (1928): 363–369; *AJP* 86 (1929): 417–423.

5. Gerald N. Grob, *Mental Illness and American Society, 1875–1940* (Princeton: Princeton University Press, 1983); Joel Braslow, *Mental Ills and Bodily Cures: Psychiatric Treatment in the First Half of the Twentieth Century* (Berkeley: University of California Press, 1997); Jack Pressman, *Last Resort: Psychosurgery and the Limits of Medicine* (New York: Cambridge University Press, 1998). On the making of the national survey system, see APA, "Proceedings: Report of the Committee on Statistics," *AJP* 83 (1926): 366–367; *AJP* 84 (1927): 325–327; *AJP* 85 (1928): 370–372; Horatio M. Pollock, "Progress and Present Status of Statistics of Mental Disease," *Mental Hygiene (MH)* 11 (1927): 156–161; Horatio M. Pollock, "Better Statistics of Mental Disease," *MH* 12

(1928): 81–84. For the increase in the number of inpatients at mental hospitals, see, for example, U.S. Bureau of the Census, *Patients in Hospitals for Mental Disease* (Washington, DC: Department of Commerce, 1926, 1933, 1935).

6. Clara Thompson and Patrick Mullahy, *Psychoanalysis: Evolution and Development* (New York: Hermitage House, 1950); Franz Alexander and Sheldon Selesnick, *The History of Psychiatry: An Evaluation of Psychiatric Thought and Practice from Prehistoric Times to the Present* (New York: Harper & Row, 1966); Raymond E. Fancher, *Psychiatric Psychology: The Development of Freud's Thought* (New York: W. W. Norton, 1973).

7. Nathan G. Hale Jr., *The Rise and Crisis of Psychoanalysis in the United States: Freud and the Americans, 1917–1985* (New York: Oxford University Press, 1995), 141–156, 161–166.

8. On Adolf Meyer, see Saul Feierstein, "Adolf Meyer: Life and Work" (PhD diss., University of Zurich, 1965); Theodore Lidz, "Adolf Meyer and the Development of American Psychiatry," *AJP* 123 (September 1966): 320–332; Pressman, *Last Resort*, chap. I.

9. John C. Burnham, "Psychiatry, Psychology and the Progressive Movement," *American Quarterly* 12 (1960): 457–465; Grob, *Mental Illness*, 145, 120–122, 160–166; Elizabeth Lunbeck, *The Psychiatric Persuasion: Knowledge, Gender, and Power in Modern America* (Princeton: Princeton University Press, 1994), 20–24, 177–181.

10. Dollard, *Criteria for the Life History*, 26.

11. Ibid., 5.

12. Ronald L. Howard, Louis Th. Van Leeuwen, and John Mogey ed., *A Social History of American Family Sociology, 1865–1940* (Westport, CT: Greenwood Press, 1981); Martin Bulmer, *The Chicago School of Sociology: Institutionalization, Diversity, and the Rise of Sociological Research* (Chicago: University of Chicago Press, 1984); Robert C. Bannister, *Sociology and Scientism: The American Quest for Objectivity, 1880–1940* (Chapel Hill: University of North Carolina Press, 1987); Dorothy Ross, *The Origin of American Social Sciences* (New York: Cambridge University Press, 1991); Philip Manning, *Freud and American Sociology* (Malden, MA: Polity Press, 2005).

13. APA, *Proceedings: First Colloquium on Personality Investigation* (Ann Arbor, MI: UMI, 1929), 5–6.

14. Kimball Young, "Topical Summaries of Current Personality Studies," *American Journal of Sociology (AJS)* 32, no. 6 (1927): 953–971, cited in Manning, *Freud and American Sociology*, 27.

15. Edward Sapir, "The Contribution of Psychiatry to and Understanding of Behavior in Society," *AJS* 42 (1937): 862–869, 863, 870.

16. Margaret Mead, "More Comprehensive Field Methods," *American Anthropologist (AA)* 35, no. I (1935): 1–15, 7, 9, 15.

17. Florence R. Kluckhohn, "The Participant-Observer Technique in Small Communities," *AJS* 46, no. 3 (1940): 331–343, 337.

18. On the development of Freud-influenced anthropology, see William C. Manson, *The Psychodynamics of Culture: Abram Kardiner and Neo-Freudian Anthropology* (New York: Greenwood Press, 1988); William C. Manson, "Abram Kardiner and the Neo-Freudian Alternative in Culture and Personality," in *Malinowski*, ed. Stocking, 72–94.

19. APA, *Proceedings: First Colloquium*, front page; APA, "Proceedings: Report of the Council Meeting, June 3," *AJP* 84 (1927): 353–354. On the establishment and early

activities of the Committee on Relations with Social Sciences, see APA, "Proceedings: Report of Committee on Relations with Social Sciences," *AJP* 84 (1927): 298–299; *AJP* 85 (1928): 378–380.

20. Robert E. Park, *The Principles of Human Behavior*, Studies in Social Science Series, vol. 6 (Chicago: Zalaz, 1915); Thomas D. Eliot, "A Psychoanalytic Interpretation of Group Formation and Behavior," *AJS* 26, no. 3 (1920): 333–352, 335. For a discussion of how these social scientists modified Freud's theory to make it into their "homegrown version of psychoanalysis," see Manning, *Freud and American Sociology*, 19–27.

21. Banner, *Intertwined Lives*, 184.

22. Elton Mayo, "Psychiatry and Sociology in Relation to Social Disorganization," *AJS* 42, no. 6 (1937): 825–831, 829–830.

23. Sander L. Gilman, *Difference and Pathology: Stereotypes of Sexuality, Race, and Madness* (Ithaca: Cornell University Press, 1985), chap. 9.

24. Read Bain, "Sociology and Psychoanalysis," *American Sociological Review* 1, no. 2 (1936): 203–316, 208–212.

25. On anthropological fascination with "primitive" cultures and their sense that these cultures need preservation, see Frank Speck, "Ethical Attributes of the Labrador Indians," *AA* 35 (October–December 1933): 559–594; Margaret Mead, *The Changing Culture of an Indian Tribe* (New York: Columbia University Press, 1932), chap. 10.

26. On Lawrence K. Frank's role in the Laura Spelman Rockefeller Memorial Foundation and the Social Science Research Council (organized by the foundation in 1923), see Donald Fisher, *Fundamental Development of the Social Sciences: Rockefeller Philanthropy and the United States Social Science Research Council* (Ann Arbor: University of Michigan Press, 1993); Dennis Bryson, "Lawrence K. Frank, Knowledge, and the Production of the 'Social,'" *Poetics Today* 19, no. 3 (1998): 401–421.

27. APA, *Proceedings: Second Colloquium on Personality Investigation* (Ann Arbor, MI: UMI, 1930), 80.

28. Ibid., 80–82.

29. Sapir, "The Contribution of Psychiatry," 862.

30. APA, *Proceedings: First Colloquium*, 60–61, 70–74; APA, *Proceedings: Second Colloquium*, 137–138, 140.

31. Harold Lasswell papers, Folders 782 and 783, Box 56, 1928, Manuscript and Archives, Yale University Library, New Haven.

32. APA, *Proceedings: Second Colloquium*, 52–53.

33. Ibid., 53–54.

34. Clinical record, No. 5999, SEP.

35. Sullivan's critique of Lasswell's book can be found in Harry Stack Sullivan, "Book Review," *AJP* 87 (1930): 363–364. See also "Report of the Committee on Relation with the Social Science," *AJP* 87 (1930): 323–324, which characterized Lasswell's book as one of the committee's accomplishments.

36. On Freud's continuing impact on sociologists, see Ernest Burgess, "The Influence of Sigmund Freud upon Sociology in the United States," *AJP* 45, no. 3 (1939): 356–374; Bulmer, *The Chicago School of Sociology*, chap. 6. On social scientists' discussion of life history in the 1930s, see Walter C. Reckless and Lowell S. Selling, "A Sociological and Psychiatric Interview Compared," *American Journal of Orthopsychiatry*

7 (1937): 532–539; Dorwin Cartwright and John R. P. French Jr., "The Reliability of Life-History Studies," *Character and Personality: An International Psychological Quarterly* 8, no. 2 (1939): 110–119.

37. Allison Davis and John Dollard, *Children of Bondage: The Personality Development of Negro Youth in the Urban South* (Washington, DC: American Council of Education, 1940), xii.

38. Benedict taught at the Washington School of Psychiatry as the school's fellow. See letters between the school's officials and Benedict (from March 13, 1945 to February 26, 1946) in VC.

39. The journal remained interdisciplinary throughout Sullivan's lifetime. In 1947, he reviewed 350 items that had appeared in the journal in its first decade of publication and found that the 197 authors of these items included, apart from mental health professionals, 19 sociologists, 13 anthropologists, 7 political scientists, 6 educators, 4 social workers, 3 lawyers, 2 philosophers, and 2 historians. See Harry Stack Sullivan, "Ten Years of Psychiatry: A Statement by the Editor," *PSY* 10 (1947): 433–435.

40. Alfred H. Stanton and Morris S. Schwartz, *The Mental Hospital: A Study of Institutional Participation in Psychiatric Illness and Treatment* (New York: Basic Books, 1954). See also their preliminary research, "The Management of a Type of Institutional Participation in Mental Hospital," *PSY* 12 (1949): 13–26, supported by a "grant made to the Washington School of Psychiatry by the Division of Mental Hygiene U.S. Public Health Service" (13). Also it is noteworthy that there was a conference in 1934, and again in 1947, on interdisciplinary collaboration in the study of culture and personality. These conferences were outgrowths of the personality colloquia and were attended by anthropologists, psychologists, and psychiatrists. The papers presented at the 1947 conference were published in S. Stansfeld Sargent and Marian W. Smith, eds., *Culture and Personality: Defining Our Terms* (New York: Viking Fund, 1949).

41. Harry Stack Sullivan, "The Onset of Schizophrenia," in Sullivan, *Schizophrenia as a Human Process* (originally published in *AJP* 84 [1927]: 105–134): 104–136, 104, 108–109; Harry Stack Sullivan, "Discussion (for Louis A. Lurie, "The Relation of Endocrinopathic States to Conduct Disorders of Children")," *AJP* 86 (1929): 305.

42. Harry Stack Sullivan, "Projected Book: Psychopathology of Youth (circa 1926)," WSP, 22. See also Sullivan, "Projected Book: Dynamics of the Mind: Prolegomena to Psychopathology (circa 1926)," WSP, 31.

43. Sullivan, "Projected Book: Dynamics of the Mind," 28.

44. Harry Stack Sullivan, "Discussion (for Lawson G. Lowrey, "The Study of Personality")," *AJP* 86 (1929): 700–702, 702; Harry Stack Sullivan, "Speech to Physicians (1931)," WSP, 7.

45. See, for example, Harry Stack Sullivan, "Discussion (for Erich Lindemann and William Malamud, 'Experimental Analysis of the Psychopathological Effects of Intoxicating Drugs')," *AJP* 90 (1934): 879–881.

46. Henry Stack Sullivan, *Personal Psychopathology: Early Formulations* (New York: W. W. Norton, 1972; written between 1929 and 1933), 2, 10–11, 29. Further page references to this work appear parenthetically in the text.

47. "Sapir, Jean and Philip (interview with Jean Sapir, the wife of Edward Sapir, August 17, 1972)," HSP. See also Helen Swick Perry, *Psychiatrist of America: The Life of Harry Stack Sullivan* (Cambridge: Belknap Press of Harvard University Press, 1982), 335.

48. On Sullivan's participation in the seminar, see Charles S. Johnson, "Sullivan's Contribution to Sociology," in *The Contributions of Harry Stack Sullivan: A Symposium on Interpersonal Theory in Psychiatry and Social Sciences*, ed. Patrick Mullahy (New York: Hermitage House, 1952), 215–216; Robert Cassidy, *Margaret Mead: A Voice for the Century* (New York: University Books, 1982), 44; Banner, *Intertwined Lives*, 288.

49. Dollard, *Criteria for the Life History*; Davis and Dollard, *Children of Bondage*; John Dollard, *Caste and Class in a Southern Town* (New York: Harper and Brothers, 1937).

50. Records of the Institute of Human Relations, RU 483, Folder 134, Box 14, 1930–1932, Manuscript and Archives, Yale University Library, New Haven.

51. Perry, *Psychiatrist of America*, 357–358. For Powdermaker's account of Sullivan's influence on her thinking, see Hortense Powdermaker, *Stranger and Friend: The Way of an Anthropologist* (New York: W. W. Norton, 1966), 134–135.

52. Harry Stack Sullivan, "Editorial Note: The William Alanson White Psychiatric Foundation," *PSY* 1 (1938 [originally published as Harry Stack Sullivan, "The William Alanson White Psychiatric Foundation: A Note," *AJP* 93 (1937): 1456–1459]): 135–140, 137.

53. Harry Stack Sullivan, "Memorandum on a Psychiatric Reconnaissance," in Charles S. Johnson, *Growing Up in the Black Belt: Negro Youth in the Rural South* (Washington, DC: American Council of Education, 1941), 328–333; Harry Stack Sullivan, "Discussion of the Case of Warren Wall," in E. Franklin Frazier, *Negro Youth at the Crossways: Their Personality Development in the Middle States* (Washington, DC: American Council of Education, 1940), 228–234. During his work in Mississippi in 1939, Sullivan was hosted by the poet William Percy. Accounts of their collaboration can be found in Anne C. Rose, "Putting the South on the Psychological Map: The Impact of Region and Race on the Human Sciences during the 1930s," *Journal of Southern History* 71, no. 2 (2005): 321–356, 321–322; Bertram Wyatt-Brown, *The House of Percy: Honor, Melancholy, and Imagination in a Southern Family* (New York: Oxford University Press, 1994), 296.

54. Sullivan, "Discussion of the Case of Warren Wall," 233.

55. Sullivan, "Memorandum on a Psychiatric Reconnaissance," 330.

56. Sullivan also admitted that he "could not bridge the cultural gap" with plantation workers, and that he had "many pseudo-conversations" that disguised, rather than revealed, the interviewees' feelings. It took him a while to realize that the conversations were pseudo, because "the Negro seem[ed] to have a notably great capacity for sensing by intuition interpersonal reality" and thus did not make it easy for Sullivan to see that they were not revealing themselves to the white interviewer. Without doubt, Sullivan was impressed with sensibility toward interactions he often observed among his African American informants. See Sullivan, "Memorandum on a Psychiatric Reconnaissance," 332.

57. Sullivan, "Discussion of the Case of Warren Wall," 230.

58. See, for example, Walter F. Robie, *The Art of Love* (London: Medical Research Society, 1925); G. V. Hamilton, *A Research in Marriage* (New York: Albert and Charles Boni, 1929); Winifred V. Richmond, "Sex Problems of Adolescence," *Journal of Educational Sociology* 8, no. 6 (1935): 333–341.

59. Rose, "Putting the South," 323, 337. On social scientists' interests in "others" within, see Roger A. Salerno, *Sociology Noir: Studies at the University of Chicago in Loneliness, Marginality, and Deviance, 1915–1935* (Jefferson, NC: McFarland, 2007).

60. Sullivan, "Discussion of the Case of Warren Wall," 234. As apparent in his writing, he was openly critical of an "archaic" white Puritanism, particularly its teaching that "sex without issue was Sin." See Henry Stack Sullivan, "Cultural Stress and Adolescent Crisis," in Sullivan, *Schizophrenia as Human Process* (originally published as "Male Adolescence," in Sullivan, *Personal Psychopathology*, 182–244), 321–351.

61. Dollard noted the possibility that African Americans, have "much freer psychiatric capacity to utilize" sexual opportunities, even as it stressed the impact of caste on the preconception that African American women are more seductive, accessible, and sexually gratifying. See Dollard, *Caste and Class*, 136–137, 172.

62. Sullivan, "Discussion of the Case of Warren Wall," 233–234.

63. Correspondence between Charles S. Johnson and Harry S. Sullivan in Records of the Institute of Human Relations, Folder 134, Box 13, 1938–1940, Special Collections/Archives, John Hope and Aurelia E. Franklin Library, Fisk University, Nashville.

64. Rose, "Putting the South," 338.

65. Sullivan often expressed his support for the mental hygiene movement during the 1920s and 1930s. In 1926, he noted, "The great work being done in Child Guidance will presently show how much we may hope to accomplish." See Harry Stack Sullivan, "The Pursuit of Sanity: Essay on Mental Hygiene (1926)," WSP, 9. See also Harry Stack Sullivan, "Mental Hygiene and the Modern World," *Modern World* 1 (1927): 153–157; Harry Stack Sullivan, "Application of the Principles of Mental Hygiene to the Practice of Medicine (April 7, 1938)," WSP; Harry Stack Sullivan, "What Is This Psychiatry? (October 5, 1938)" WSP; Harry Stack Sullivan, "Formal Discussion: Summary and Critique," in *Mental Health*, ed. F. R. Moulton and P. O. Komora (Lancaster, PA: The Science House, 1939), 276–278. In the late 1930s, Sullivan was an active participant in regional mental hygiene programs. See "Clippings, 1937–1941" ("Extension of Mental Hygiene Activities Seen Health Move," *Grand Rapid Herald* [April 22, 1939] and "Dr. Sullivan to Lead Mental Health Program," *Sunday Star* [Washington, DC: May 14, 1939]), WSP.

66. This emphasis on the curability of illness was apparent elsewhere in Sullivan's writings. See, for example, Sullivan, "Tentative Criteria"; Harry Stack Sullivan, "Environmental Factors in Etiology and Course Under Treatment of Schizophrenia," *Medical Journal and Record* 133 (1931): 19–22; Harry Stack Sullivan, "The Modified Psychoanalytic Treatment of Schizophrenia," *AJP* 88 (1931): 519–540.

67. On the psychiatric view of schizophrenia as the most serious mental illness needing attention from social and medical reformers, see Horatio M. Pollock, "Dementia Praecox as a Social Problem," *MH* 3 (1919): 575–579; Edith M. Furbush, "The Social Significance of Dementia Praecox," *MH* 6 (1922): 288–299; Nolan D. C. Lewis, *Research in Dementia Praecox: Past Attainments, Present Trends and Future Possibilities* (New York: NCMH, 1936).

68. Frankwood E. Williams, "Psychiatry and Its Relation to the Teaching of Medicine," *AJP* 85 (1928): 689–700.

69. Harry Stack Sullivan, "A Note on Implications of Psychiatry, the Study of Interpersonal Relations, for Investigations in the Social Sciences," in Harry Stack Sullivan, *The Fusion of Psychiatry and Social Science* (New York: W. W. Norton, 1964, originally published in *AJS* 42 [1937]: 848–461): 15–29, 15. *The Fusion* is a collection of papers written between 1934 and 1949.

70. Sullivan, "A Note on Implications," 25; Harry Stack Sullivan, "A Note on Formulating the Relationship of the Individual and the Group," *AJS* 44 (1939): 932–937.

71. Harry Stack Sullivan, "Psychiatry," *Encyclopaedia of the Social Sciences* 1 (1934): 7–12; Harry Stack Sullivan, "The Data of Psychiatry," in Sullivan, *The Fusion* (originally published in *PSY* 1 [1938]: 121–134): 32–55, 48; Harry Stack Sullivan, "Discussion: Section Meeting on Culture and Personality," *American Journal of Orthopsychiatry* 8 (1938): 608–609; Harry Stack Sullivan, "The Support of Psychiatric Research and Teaching," *PSY* 2 (1939): 273–279, 279.

72. Harry Stack Sullivan, "Notes on Investigation, Therapy, and Education in Psychiatry and Its Relation to Schizophrenia," *PSY* 4 (1941): 271–280, 274. See also "Proceedings: First Conference, Committee on Training Fellowship, National Research Council (December 21, 1935)," WSP.

73. Harry Stack Sullivan, "Training of the General Medical Student in Psychiatry," *American Journal of Orthopsychiatry* 1 (1931): 371–379, 373, 377.

74. William G. Rothstein, *American Medical Schools and the Practice of Medicine: A History* (New York: Oxford University Press, 1987), 134–138; John S. Haller Jr., *Medical Protestants: The Eclectics in American Medicine, 1925–1939* (Carbondale: Southern Illinois University Press, 1994), chap. 8. Sullivan himself sometimes was pessimistic about the prospect of making psychiatry a science. See, for example, Sullivan, "Discussion: Section Meeting," 609. Concerning reasons for his pessimism, see Harry Stack Sullivan, "Discussion (for Erich Lindemann and Jacob E. Finesinger, "The Effect of Adrenalin and Mecholyl in States of Anxiety in Psychoneurotic Patients")," *AJP* 95 (1938): 366–367, in which he argued "too many things are lumped in [a] term" in psychiatry, causing "enormous difficulties . . . [for scientists] . . . to say something very simple and dependable about human personality."

75. The Commission on Medical Education, *Medical Education: Final Report of the Commission on Medical Education* (New York: Office of the Director of Study, 1932); D. T. Davis, "Review: Medical Education," *Journal of Higher Education* 4, no. 6 (1933): 333–335; Marion E. Rannells, "The Psychiatric Social Worker's Technique in Meeting Resistance," *MH* 11, no. 1 (1927): 78–128; Grace F. Marcus, "How Case-Work Training May Be Adapted to Meet the Workers' Personal Problems," *MH* 11, no. 3 (1927): 449–459.

76. Sullivan, "William Alanson White Psychiatric Foundation."

77. Harry Stack Sullivan, "The Washington School of Psychiatry," *PSY* 1 (1938): 140–141.

78. William Alanson White Psychiatric Foundation, "Bulletin: Washington School of Psychiatry," *PSY* 2 (1939): 473(I)–477(V), 476(IV).

79. Douglas Noble, "The History of Washington Psychoanalytic Society and the Washington Psychoanalytic Institute (June 26, 1968)," HSP, 31.

80. White was the first coeditor of the eclectic journal *Psychoanalytic Review*, established in 1913.

81. Lawrence J. Friedman, *Menninger: The Family and the Clinic* (New York: Knopf, 1990); Karen Horney, *Neurotic Personality of Our Time* (New York: W. W. Norton, 1937); Clara Thompson, "The History of the William Alanson White Institute, March 15, 1955 (unpublished speech given at the William Alanson White Institute)," WAWI; Ralph M. Crowley and Maurice R. Green, "Revolution within Psychoanalysis: A History of the William Alanson White Institute (undated)," WAWI.

82. Harry Stack Sullivan, "This Journal," *PSY* 1 (1938): 141–143, 141.

83. Edward Sapir, Harold D. Lasswell, and Harry Stack Sullivan, "The Institute for Ethnic Psychiatry (circa mid-1930s)," WSP.

84. Rose, "Putting the South," 346–349.

85. See Harry Stack Sullivan, "Politics in State Hospital Systems," *AJP* 84 (1928): 1075–1077. He claimed that state institutions were hopeless, because "uninformed" and "untrained henchmen [superintendents]" dominated these institutions. He praised, in contrast, the recent development of an "institute for psychiatric research" in New York, and suggested that similar institutes be established nationwide.

86. U.S. Bureau of the Census, *Patients in Hospitals for Mental Disease.*

87. Margaret J. Rioch, "Fifty Years at the Washington School of Psychiatry," *PSY* 49 (1986): 33–44; "Hadley, Ernest and Agnes (interview with Agnes Hadley, September 25, 1968)," HSP. See also Perry, *Psychiatrist of America*, 329.

88. Gerald N. Grob, *The Mad among Us: A History of the Care of America's Mentally Ill* (New York: Free Press, 1994), chap. 9; Edward Shorter, *A History of Psychiatry: From the Era of the Asylum to the Age of Prozac* (New York: John Wiley and Sons, 1997), 246–281.

CHAPTER 4   HOMOSEXUALITY: THE STEPCHILD OF INTERWAR LIBERALISM

1. Sander L. Gilman, *Difference and Pathology: Stereotypes of Sexuality, Race, and Madness* (Ithaca: Cornell University Press, 1985), chap. 10.

2. On the interaction between whiteness, heterosexuality, and Western-centralism, see Julian Carter, "Normality, Whiteness, Authorship: Evolutionary Sexology and the Primitive Pervert," in *Science and Homosexualities*, ed. Vernon Rosario (New York: Routledge, 1997), 155–176; Julian Carter, *The Heart of Whiteness: Normal Sexuality and Race in America, 1880–1940* (Durham: Duke University Press, 2007). Regina G. Kunzel, "Situating Sex: Prison Sexual Culture in the Mid-Twentieth-Century United States," *GLQ: A Journal of Lesbian and Gay Studies* 8 (2003): 253–270, offers an excellent analysis of the interconnection between race, sexuality, and civilization.

3. This was in part because of Freudians' effort to normalize the topic of sex. See, for example, Havelock Ellis, "Freud's Influence on the Changed Attitude toward Sex," *AJP* 45 (November 1939): 309–317, 310, 317; E. Van Norman Emery, "Revising Our Attitudes toward Sex," *MH* 11 (1927): 324–338; Lawrence K. Frank, "Preparation for Marriage in the High School Program," *Living* 1 (January 1939): 9–12, which stressed the need to discuss sexual issues with frankness, especially with youth. Theodore Newcomb, "Recent Changes in Attitudes toward Sex and Marriage," *American Sociological Review* 2 (October 1937): 659–667, offers a different take on the issue, suggesting the gap between the "sexual excess of the 1920s" and youth's conservative views of premarital sex and divorce in the 1930s.

4. Ernest R. Groves, "Mental Hygiene in the College and the University," *Social Forces* 8 (September 1929) 37–50, 41, 47. Such approval of coeducational institutions was not universally shared. See Paul Popenoe, "Mate Selection," *American Sociological Review* 2 (October 1937): 735–743, which claimed four college education does "more harm than good [to women], so far as the development of [their] personality is concerned" (742).

5. Winifred V. Richmond, "Sex Problems of Adolescence," *Journal of Educational Sociology* 8, no. 6 (1935): 335–336.

6. Lowell S. Selling, "The Pseudo Family," *AJS* 37 (September 1931): 247–253. Such critique of "true" homosexual individuals was reflected upon state regulations that required the sterilization of "sexual pervert," those "afflicted with degenerate sexual tendencies," or those who committed "crime against nature." In 1930, there were eleven states that had such regulation. See Frederick W. Brown, "Eugenic Sterilization in the United States, Its Present Status," *Annals of the American Academy of Political and Social Science* 149 (May 1930): 22–35.

7. On medical understanding of homosexuality in the 1920s and 1930s, see Karin A. Martin, "Gender and Sexuality: Medical Opinion on Homosexuality," *Gender and Society* 7 (June 1993): 246–260; Erin G. Carlston, "A Finer Differentiation: Female Homosexuality and the American Medical Community, 1926–1940," in *Science and Homosexualities*, ed. Vernon Rosario (New York: Routledge, 1997), 177–196; Jennifer Terry, *An American Obsession: Science, Medicine, and Homosexuality in Modern Society* (Chicago: University of Chicago Press, 1999).

8. John F. W. Meagher, "Homosexuality: Its Psychological and Psychopathological Significance," *Urologic and Cutaneous Review* 33 (1929): 505–518, 506, 508; John R. Ernst, "Dementia Praecox Complexes," *Medical Journal and Record* 128 (1928): 381–386, 384; Aaron Rosanoff, "Human Sexuality, Normal and Abnormal," *Urologic and Cutaneous Review* 33 (1929): 523–530, 527; George W. Henry, "Social Factors in the Case Histories of One Hundred Underprivileged Homosexuals," *MH* 22 (October 1938): 591–611. For the connection between homosexuality and schizophrenia, see also Aaron Rosanoff, "A Theory of Chaotic Sexuality," *AJP* 92 (1935): 35–41. Not all physicians of the era were in support of favorable characteristics of homosexuality. See, for example, C. B. Horton and Eric Kent Clarke, "Transvestism or Eonism: Discussion, with Report of Two Cases," *AJP* 10 (1931): 1025–1030, which asserted that the authors could not confirm Havelock Ellis's view that transvestism tended to occur among the educated, refined, sensitive, and reserved. George S. Snyderman and William Josephs also claimed that homosexual persons were often found among "bohemians," groups of eccentric "freaks and psychopaths" who failed to adjust to social norms. George S. Snyderman and William Josephs, "Bohemia: The Underworld of Art," *Social Forces* 18 (December 1939): 187–199. Moreover, George W. Henry was not simply in support of homosexuality. See George W. Henry and Hugh M. Galbraith, "Constitutional Factors in Homosexuality," *AJP* 13, no. 6 (1934): 1249–1267, in which the authors argued the "appreciation of the bisexual nature of all humans . . . [caused] the increase in homosexual adjustments" and thus "western civilization has imposed even greater burdens upon those who established homes and reproduce" (1249).

9. Donald M. Hamilton, "Some Aspects of Homosexuality in Relation to Total Personality Development," *PQ* 13 (1939): 229–244, 229–230, 233–234; Abraham L. Wolbarst, "Sexual Perversions; Their Medial and Social Implications," *Medical Journal and Record* 134 (1931): 5–9; 62–65, 8, 65. See also Harry Benjamin, "An Echo of and an Addendum to 'For the Sake of Morality,'" *Medical Journal and Record* 134 (1931): 118–120, which claimed that homosexuality was based on constitutional factors; thus it should not be punished by law. On the other hand, there were those who disagreed with the constitutional basis of homosexuality, although not necessarily to support antihomosexual regulations. See, for instance, Joseph Wortis, "A Note on the Body Build of the Male Homosexual," *AJP* 93 (1937): 1121–1125; Joseph Wortis, "Intersexuality and Effeminacy in the Male Homosexual," *American Journal of Orthopsychiatry* 10 (1940): 567–570. Kenneth M. Walker, *Male Disorders of Sex* (New York: W. W. Norton, 1932) includes a discussion of the endocrine and surgical

treatment of homosexuality, suggesting that, even among constitutional theorists, there was no consensus about the malleability of homosexuality.

10. Richard Handler, "Boasian Anthropology and the Critique of American Culture," *American Quarterly* 42, no. 2 (June 1990): 252–273; Rudi C. Bleys, *The Geography of Perversion: Male-to-Male Sexual Behavior outside the West and the Ethnographic Imagination, 1750–1918* (New York: New York University Press, 1995), chaps. 4 and 5. Wilson D. Wallis, in "The Prejudice of Men," *AJS* 34 (March 1929): 804–821, suggested that anthropologists were aware of the human inclination to "consider [their own] culture superior to all others" (804), and of the fact that American scientists were not exempt from this inclination. For a similar discussion, see V. F. Calverton, "The Compulsive Basis of Social Thought: All Illustrated by the Varying Doctrines as to the Origins of Marriage and Family," *AJS* 36 (March 1931): 689–734; A. H. Maslow, "The Comparative Approach to Social Behavior," *Social Forces* 15 (May 1937): 487–490.

11. For critical discussion of anthropological studies of homosexuality, see Charles Callender and Lee M. Kochems, "The North American Berdache," *Current Anthropology* 24 (August–October 1983): 443–470; Evelyn Blackwood, ed., *Anthropology and Homosexual Behavior* (New York: The Haworth Press, 1986); Robert Fulton and Steven W. Anderson, "The Amerindian 'Man-Women': Gender, Liminality, and Cultural Continuity," *Current Anthropology* 33 (December 1992): 603–610. On anthropologists' problematic use of the concepts of gender and sexuality, see Mary McIntosh, "The Homosexual Role," *Social Problems* 16 (Autumn 1968): 182–192; David Greenberg, "Why Was the Berdache Ridiculed?" in *Anthropology and Homosexual Behavior*, ed. Evelyn Blackwood (New York: The Haworth Press, 1986), 179–189; Sabine Lang, *Men as Women, Women as Men, Changing Gender in Native Cultures*, trans. John L Vantine (Austin: University of Texas Press, 1998).

12. W. W. Hill, "The Status of the Hermaphrodite and Transvestite in Navaho Culture," *AA* 37.2-I (April–June 1935): 273–279; George Devereux, "Institutionalized Homosexuality of the Mohave Indians," *Human Biology* 9, no. 4 (1937): 498–527, 516; George Devereux, "The Social and Cultural Implications of Incest among the Mohave Indians," *PQ* 8 (1939): 510–533; John Gillin, "Personality in Preliterate Societies," *American Sociological Review* 4 (October 1939): 681–702.

13. Robert H. Lowie, *Primitive Religion* (New York: Boni and Liveright, 1924), 181; J. W. Layard, "Sharmanism: An Analysis Based on Comparison with the Flying Tricksters of Malekula," *Journal of the Royal Anthropological Institute of Great Britain and Ireland* 60 (July–December 1930): 525–550, 542; W. W. Hill, "Note on the Pima Berdache," *AA* 40 (April–June 1938): 338–340, 340; Devereux, "Social and Cultural Implications," 514. See also Leslie Spier, "Kalamath Ethnography," in *University of California Publications in American Archaeology and Ethnology*, ed. A. L. Kroeber and Robert H. Lowie (Berkeley: University of California Press, 1930), 51.

14. Elsie Clews Parsons, "The Aversion to Anomalies," *Journal of Philosophy, Psychology, and Scientific Methods* 12 (April 15, 1915): 212–219, 219; Elsie Clews Parsons, "The Zuni La'mama," *AA* 18 (October–December 1916): 521–528; Elsie Clews Parsons, *Social Freedom: A Study of the Conflicts between Social Classifications and Personality* (New York: G. P. Putnam's Sons, 1915); Oscar Lewis, "Manly-Hearted Women among the North Piegan," *AA* 43, no. 2-I (April–June 1941): 173–187, 184. On Parsons's stance on issues of homosexuality, see Lois W. Banner, *Intertwined Lives: Margaret Mead, Ruth Benedict, and Their Circle* (New York: Knopf, 2003), 146–151.

15. Ruth F. Benedict, "Anthropology and the Abnormal," *Journal of General Psychology* 10 (1934): 64, 75. See also Ruth F. Benedict, *Patterns of Culture* (Boston: Houghton Mifflin, 1934); Ruth F. Benedict, "Sex in Primitive Society," *American Journal of Orthopsychiatry* 9 (1939): 570–575.

16. Banner, *Intertwined Lives*, 366.

17. Harry Stack Sullivan, "Psychopathological Histories: Comments on Their Preparation and Summary (October 14, 1925)," WSP; Harry Stack Sullivan, "Sociogenesis of Homosexual Behavior (December 27, 1929)," WSP.

18. Harry Stack Sullivan, "Georgetown University Lectures (1939)," WSP, 16–18. See also Sullivan, "Psychopathological Histories," 17; Harry Stack Sullivan, *Clinical Studies in Psychiatry* (New York: W. W. Norton, 1956 [edited lectures originally given at Chestnut Lodge Hospital, between 1942 and 1946]), 142, 157, 163–164, 169–177.

19. William V. Silverberg, "The Personal Basis and Social Significance of Passive Male Homosexuality," *PSY* 1 (1938): 41–53, 51.

20. "Roth Moulton Interview (December 15, 1987)," MSA; "Harry Biele (December 9, 1988)," MSA. The author's telephone conversation with J. William Silverberg, the son of William V. Silverberg, on October 20, 2007.

21. Sapir's statement is striking also given the forbearing attitude toward Native Americans' male-to-male "friendship" he had shown in the personality colloquium a decade earlier. Sapir's attitude toward same-sex intimacy in "primitive" societies was not translated into a similarly accepting view of homosexuality in "civilized" America.

22. Edward Sapir, "Observations on the Sex Problem in America," *AJP* 85 (1928): 510–532, 529. See also Edward Sapir, "The Discipline of Sex," *Child Study* (March 1930): 170–173, 187–188.

23. Hilary Lapsley, *Margaret Mead and Ruth Benedict: The Kinship of Women* (Amherst: University of Massachusetts Press, 1999), 98–100.

24. On Sapir's views on sex in general, see Richard Handler, *Critics against Culture: Anthropological Observers of Mass Society* (Madison: University of Wisconsin Press, 2005), chaps. 4 and 5.

25. Banner, *Intertwined Lives*, 334.

26. Ibid., 358–359.

27. MM to RFB, March 29, 1933, Box R7, Folder 13, LC.

28. Ibid.

29. Banner, *Intertwined Lives*, 354–357.

30. RFB to MM, April 6, 1937, Box S5, Folder 8, LC; MM to RFB, August 3, 1939, Box S5, Folder 9, LC.

31. RFB to MM, November 4, 1932, Box S5, Folder 7, LC.

32. RFB to MM, September 18, 1932, Box S5, Folder 6, LC.

33. RFB to MM, July 6, 1937, Box S5, Folder 8, LC.

34. RFB to MM, July 24, 1937, Box S5, Folder 8, LC.

35. RFB to MM, May 24, 1931, Box S5, Folder 6, LC.

36. RFB to MM, July 6, 1937, Box S5, Folder 8, LC.

37. RFB to MM, December 15, 1932, Box S5, Folder 7, LC.

38. MM to RFB, undated, 1934, Box S5, Folder 7, LC.

39. RFB to MM, February 14, 1936, Box S5, Folder 8, LC.

40. RFB to MM, August 3, 1938, Box S5, Folder 9, LC.

41. "Blitsten, Dorothy (interview with Dorothy Blitsten, March 17, 1971)," HSP; "Ellison, Ralph (interview with Ralph Ellison, May [undated] 1970)," HSP. See also Helen Swick Perry, *Psychiatrist of America: The Life of Harry Stack Sullivan* (Cambridge: Belknap Press of Harvard University Press, 1982), 348–350.

42. "Clippings, 1937–1941," WSP.

43. "Mullahy, Patrick (letter from Patrick Mullahy to Helen Swick Perry, August 7, 1965)," HSP. See also Perry, *Psychiatrist of America*, 352.

44. Nathan G. Hale, *The Rise and Crisis of Psychoanalysis in the United States: Freud and the Americans, 1917–1985* (New York: Oxford University Press, 1995), 95.

45. From a file for Helen Swick Perry interviewee who requested anonymity.

46. "Will, Otto (interview with Otto Allen Will, April 10, 1973)," HSP.

47. Indeed, Sullivan in 1942 claimed that he was "among the four or five best paid psychiatrists in New York." See Perry, *Psychiatrist of America*, 350. See also Hale, *The Rise and Crisis*, 159.

48. Thompson, "The History," 9; Perry, *Psychiatrist of America*, 354–355.

49. Thompson was then a student of Sandor Ferenczi and had just been elected the first president of the Washington-Baltimore Psychoanalytic Society. Silverberg also was a European-trained psychoanalyst, a student of Franz Alexander. Karen Horney was Karl Abraham's student at the Berlin Psychoanalytic Institute and was a training analyst at the New York Psychoanalytic Institute, organized in 1931. Erich Fromm had had his training with Wilhelm Wittenberg and Hanna Sachs at the Berlin Psychoanalytic Institute before he came to the United States in 1934.

50. This was not news to people who had known Sullivan. William Elgin, an attendant at Sheppard-Pratt in the late 1920s, observed that Sullivan was "difficult to deal with" because he "was known to have strong likes and dislikes and was entirely unpredictable in his relationships with most people." See William Elgin, "Harry Stack Sullivan, as I Remember Him (unpublished memoir, May 13, 1964)," HSP. Similarly, Ernest Schachtel, Sullivan's psychoanalyst friend in New York, recalled that he had been confused when he had received a "nasty letter" from Sullivan. Schachtel was attempting to publish his paper in the journal *Politics*, and Sullivan "took a great offense at this" for reasons Schachtel never understood. See "New York Colleagues, Moulton, Schachtel (interview with Ernest Schachtel, April 16, 1970)," HSP.

51. "Frank, Lawrence K. (interview with Lawrence K. Frank in November 6, 1962)," HSP.

52. "Bullard, Dexter and Ann (interview with Dexter and Ann Bullard in February 1971)," HSP. See also, "Gill, Tom (interview with Tom Gill, August 9, 1963)," HSP.

53. "Harry Biele (interview with Harry Biele, December 9, 1988)," MSA.

54. Perry, *Psychiatrist of America*, chap. 24.

55. Philip, the son of the Sapirs, remembered how Harry and Jimmie occupied a room together when they were at the Sapirs,' and how Philip felt "ill at ease" because "when it was time to go to dinner, he did not know whether to go and knock on their door, or was he supposed to wait for them." See "Sapir, Philip and Jean (interview with Philip Sapir, March [date unspecified], 1971)," HSP.

56. "Silverberg, William V. (interview with William V. Silverberg, May 15, 1962)," HSP.

57. The following discussion of Sullivan and Clifton Read is based on Clifton Read, "Harry Stack Sullivan: A Remembrance (undated)," MSA.

58. "Bourke-White, Margaret (interview with John Vassos and Margaret Bourke-White, September 15, 1964)," HSP.

59. Studies have shown that sexual contacts between therapists and patients are not unusual, although they have also indicated that such contacts decreased after the 1979 revision of the *Ethical Principles of Psychologists* that defined "sexual intimacies with clients" as "unethical." See, for example, Ann W. Burgess and Carol H. Hartman, eds., *Sexual Exploitation of Patients by Health Professionals* (New York: Praeger, 1986). See also Charles Clay Dahlberg, "Sexual Contact between Patient and Therapist," *Contemporary Psychoanalysis* 5 (1970): 107–124, which includes a case of a male patient who considered himself as an "unsuccessful homosexual." The patient claimed that his male therapist "occasionally touched him," arguing that "there is a need for it in order to help him overcome his dislike for being touched." For a reference to sexual relations involving male therapists and male patients, see Jacqueline Bouhoutsos et al., "Sexual Intimacy between Psychotherapists and Patients," *Professional Psychology: Research and Practice* 14, no. 2 (1983): 185–196.

60. From a file for Helen Swick Perry interviewee who requested anonymity.

61. From a file for Helen Swick Perry interviewee who requested anonymity.

62. "Sapir, Philip and Jean (interview with Philip Sapir, March [date unspecified], 1971)," HSP.

63. There is no further evidence for Sullivan's relationship to Mullahy. But we know that Mullahy remained a determined supporter of Sullivan. Mullahy thought that Sullivan was "lovable," his personality was "remarkable," and he was "genius." Mullahy became a Sullivan researcher, published as many as five books on Sullivan, and edited a book of collected papers on Sullivan. See Patrick Mullahy, *A Study of Interpersonal Relations: New Contributions to Psychiatry* (New York: Hermitage Press, 1949); Clara Thomson and Patrick Mullahy, *Psychoanalysis: Evolution and Development* (New York: Hermitage House, 1950); Patrick Mullahy, *The Contributions of Harry Stack Sullivan: A Symposium on Interpersonal Theory in Psychiatry and Social Sciences* (New York: Hermitage Press, 1952); Patrick Mullahy, *Psychoanalysis and Interpersonal Psychiatry: The Contributions of Harry Stack Sullivan* (New York: Science House, 1970); Patrick Mullahy, *The Beginnings of Modern American Psychiatry: The Ideas of Harry Stack Sullivan* (Boston: Houghton Mifflin, 1970); Patrick Mullahy, *Interpersonal Psychiatry* (New York: Medical & Scientific Books, 1983).

64. "Interview with Philip Sapir (June 16, 1989)," MSA.

65. Ibid.

66. Ibid.

67. On the particular vulnerability of patients under psychotherapeutic treatment, see William H. Masters,, Virginia E. Johnson, and Robert C. Kolodny, eds., *Ethical Issues in Sex Therapy and Research* (Boston: Little, Brown, 1977), 158–159, where Judd Marmor, one of the authors in the volume, argues that "psychotherapeutic relationship [places] a special emphasis . . . on the therapeutic necessity for the patient to set aside his or her . . . defenses and to open himself or herself completely to the presumably benign and constructive influence of a therapist's professional skill."

68. "Will, Otto (interview with Otto Will, April 10, 1973)," HSP.

69. "Interview with Benjamin Weininger, M.D. (December 1, 1987)," MSA.

70. Michael Stuart Allen, "Sullivan's Closet: A Reappraisal of Harry Stack Sullivan's Life and His Pioneering Role in American Psychiatry," *Journal of Homosexuality* 29, no. 1 (1995): 3.

71. Ibid.

72. "Will, Otto (interview with Otto Will, April 10, 1973)," HSP.

73. "Interview with Harry Biele, (December 4, 1988)," MSA.

74. In her personal conversation in March 2003 with the author, a former student of the Washington School of Psychiatry in the late 1940s claimed that her training analyst often urged her to have sex with him, so as to be more sexually "relaxed."

75. There is some evidence suggesting that Sullivan believed that his private practices in the 1930s offered an accepting environment for sexual minorities, as seen in his idea of "therapeutic community": "[We need] therapeutic communities . . . which have peculiar form, peculiar purpose, that definitely differ from . . . the American scene at large" (Harry Stack Sullivan, "Adequate Personnel for Mental Hospitals and Other Treatment Agencies [a transcript of his lecture given at Third Annual Spring Conference sponsored by the Michigan Society for Mental Hygiene, April 21, 1939]," WSP, 3). But it also needs to be noted that studies have shown that the overwhelming majority of patients who experienced sexual relationships with their therapists responded negatively. See Kenneth S. Pope, "Therapist-Patient Sex as Sex Abuse: Six Scientific, Professional, and Practical Dilemmas in Addressing Victimization and Rehabilitation," *Professional Psychology: Research and Practice* 21 (August 1990): 227–239.

76. "Interview with Philip Sapir (June 16, 1989)," MSA.

77. "Interview with Harry Biele (December 4, 1988)," MSA; "Sapir, Philip and Jean (interview with Jean Sapir, August 17, 1972)," HSP; "Interview with Jean Pearce (1988)," MSA; "Interview with Philip Sapir (June 16, 1989)," MSA; "Bruch, Hilde (interview with Hilde Bruch, September 20, 1973)," HSP; "Frankenthal, Kate (interview with Kate Frankenthal, April 16, 1970)," HSP; Perry, *Psychiatrist of America*, 346. It was not uncommon for long-term partnerships between older and younger men to take the form of relationship similar to guardians and wards. See George Chauncey, *Gay New York: Gender, Urban Culture, and the Making of the Gay Male World 1890–1940* (New York: Basic Books, 1994), 88.

78. "Sullivan, James (James Inscoe Sullivan's letter to Helen Swick Perry, October 12, 1971)," HSP. See also Perry, *Psychiatrist of America*, 304.

79. "Sullivan, James (James Inscoe Sullivan's letter to Helen Swick Perry, November 22, 1971)," HSP.

80. "Sullivan, James (James Inscoe Sullivan's letter to Helen Swick Perry, May 14, 1971)," HSP.

81. See Perry, *Psychiatrist of America*, 344.

82. "Sapir, Philip and Jean (interview with Jean Sapir, August 17, 1972)," HSP.

83. "Sullivan, James (James Inscoe Sullivan's letter to Helen Swick Perry, June [date unspecified], 1971)," HSP.

84. "Sapir, Philip and Jean (interview with Jean Sapir, August 17, 1972)," HSP; "Interview with Helen Swick Perry (September 23, 1987)," MSA. According to this friend, Sullivan apologized the next day for Jimmie's behavior.

85. Read, "Harry Stack Sullivan," 16.

86. "Interview with Philip Sapir (June 16, 1989)," MSA.

87. Allen, "Sullivan's Closet," 14. Jimmie's photos are located at WSP.

CHAPTER 5   THE MILITARY, PSYCHIATRY, AND "UNFIT" SOLDIERS

1. Virginia Yans-McLaughlin, "Science, Democracy, and Ethics: Mobilizing Culture and Personality for World War II," in *Malinowski*, ed. Stocking, 184–217.

2. Harry Stack Sullivan, "Selective Service Psychiatry," *PSY* 4 (1941): 440–464, 442.

3. William Claire Menninger, *Psychiatry in a Troubled World: Yesterday's War and Today's Challenge* (New York: Macmillan, 1949), chaps. 1, 2, and 19.

4. Sullivan, "Selective Service Psychiatry," 442–443.

5. Nathan G. Hale, *The Rise and Crisis of Psychoanalysis in the United States: Freud and the Americans, 1917–1985* (New York: Oxford University Press, 1995), 178.

6. Ben Shephard, *A War of Nerves: Soldiers and Psychiatrists in the Twentieth Century* (Cambridge: Harvard University Press, 2002), 198. See also Rebecca Schwartz Greene, "The Role of the Psychiatrist in World War II" (PhD diss., Columbia University, 1976), 111–113; Helen Swick Perry, *Psychiatrist of America: The Life of Harry Stack Sullivan* (Cambridge: Belknap Press of Harvard University Press, 1982), 404.

7. Some psychiatrists disagreed with the extended application of psychiatry. Gregory Zilboorg (an eminent New York practitioner), for example, insisted that "psychiatric conditions are altogether disorganizations within the personality of individual . . . [and] a community can no more have schizophrenia than it can have pneumonia. . . . Much damage is being done by loose thinking on the part of the general public in psychiatric terms." See "Scientists Disagree on Psychiatry as Applied to Politics: D.C. Speakers Maintain Large U.S. Groups Live in Mental Fog," *Evening Star* (Washington, DC, December 30, 1938).

8. Harry Stack Sullivan, "Address to the Annual Scientific Assembly of the Medical Society of the District of Columbia (1940)," WSP, 7.

9. Yans-McLaughlin, "Science, Democracy, and Ethics," 193–197; Ruth F. Benedict, "On Declaring War," *New Republic* 105 (September 1, 1941): 279–280, cited by Margaret M. Caffrey, *Ruth Benedict: Stranger in This Land* (Austin: University of Texas Press, 1989), 303.

10. Harry Stack Sullivan, "Psychiatry and the National Defense," *PSY* 3 (1940): 619–624, 619.

11. Harry Stack Sullivan, "Memorandum from the William Alanson White Psychiatric Foundation on the Utilization of Psychiatry in the Promotion of National Security," *PSY* 3 (1940): 483–491, 490–491.

12. Harry Stack Sullivan, "Responsibility," *PSY* 2 (1939): 599–602, 601–602.

13. Harry Stack Sullivan, "Security of the American Commonwealths," *PSY* 1 (1938): 419–420, 419. Also see Harry Stack Sullivan, "Propaganda and Censorship," *PSY* 3 (1940): 628–632, on his critique of Nazi leadership.

14. Hilary Lapsley, *Margaret Mead and Ruth Benedict: The Kinship of Women* (Amherst: University of Massachusetts Press, 1999), 288–291; Lois W. Banner, *Intertwined Lives: Margaret Mead, Ruth Benedict, and Their Circle* (New York: Knopf, 2003), 412–423. See also Ruth Benedict, "Race Prejudice in the United States" (radio address, Wash-

ington, DC, 1946) in Margaret Mead, *An Anthropologist at Work* (Boston: Houghton Mifflin, 1959), 358–360.

15. Leo H. Bartemeier, "Schizoid Personality and Schizophrenia," *War Medicine* 1 (September 1941): 675–681, 677.

16. Harry Stack Sullivan, "The William Alanson White Psychiatric Foundation Bulletin: A Minimum Psychiatric Inspection of Registrants," *PSY* 3 (1940): 625–627, 626. Here Sullivan was referring to low IQ. He argued that psychiatrists at medical advisory boards should arrange "a psychometric test" for "those who are deficient in intelligence" at local boards. What is noteworthy is that he listed low intelligence as one of the mental handicaps to be detected in screening. This shows how wartime psychiatric examiners blurred the distinction between mental retardation and mental illness, particularly during the early years of the war. Psychologists began to administer mental proficiency tests at army induction centers later in the war, but their standards varied from one induction center to another. See Steven A. Gelb, "'Mental Deficients' Fighting Fascism: The Unplanned Normalization of World War II," in *Mental Retardation in America*, ed. Steve Noll and James W. Trent Jr. (New York: New York University Press, 2004), 308–321.

17. U.S. Bureau of the Census, *Patients in Hospitals for Mental Illness* (Washington, DC: Department of Commerce) (1926), 42; (1933), 10; (1941), 1–2. The headline for this classification is "psychosis with mental deficiency" (as opposed to "mental defect and deficiency" in Sullivan's screening criteria), indicating that in civilian practice, psychiatrists made a clearer distinction between mental illness and low IQ than in wartime screening. However, even in civilian practice, the diagnostic standard of the 1940s was not as specific as the standard used after World War II. See Gerald N. Grob, "Origins of *DSM-I*: A Study in Appearance and Reality," *AJP* 148 (1991): 421–431.

18. Sullivan, "William Alanson White Psychiatric Foundation Bulletin," 626.

19. Sullivan was one of nine members of the committee. Other members were Gen. Frederick Osborn (chairman, CACSS), Lt. Col. Charles B. Spruit (general staff, Medical Corps, War Department/medical officer, Selective Service Headquarters), Winfred Overholser (St. Elizabeths Hospital), Martin Cooley (U.S. Veteran's Administration), Lt. Col. William C. Porter (Medical Corps, U.S. Army), Clarence Dykstra (director, Selective Service System, National Headquarters), Gen. Lewis B. Hershey (general staff, Selective Service System, National Headquarters), and Col. William H. Draper, Jr. (U.S. Public Health Service). See Sullivan, "Selective Service Psychiatry," 443; Harry Stack Sullivan, "Status of Medical Function [of Selective Service] (August 6, 1940)," WSP.

20. Harry Stack Sullivan, "A Seminar on Practical Psychiatric Diagnosis: Selective Service System," *PSY* 4 (1941): 265–283, 281.

21. Even at an earlier stage, the shortage of psychiatrists was apparent. There were 515 medical boards in 1940, but there were "only 173 Fellows or Members of the American Psychiatric Association . . . serving in this capacity. Some fifty boards have other physicians reported by the American Medical Association as qualified psychiatrists; nearly 200 physicians designated as psychiatrists who have little, if any . . . psychiatric background." This was a concern, because in Sullivan's plan, psychiatrists at medical boards were to "assist local board examiners in learning to know whom to refer [to a medical board as a doubtful case]." See

Harry Stack Sullivan, "Psychiatric Mobilization in the U.S.A.," *AJP* Supplement 97 (1940): 2–4, 2.

22. Sullivan, "Psychiatry and the National Defense," 619.

23. Ibid., 620.

24. Sullivan, "Seminar on Practical Psychiatric Diagnosis," 267.

25. Ibid., 268.

26. Ibid., 271–274.

27. Ibid., 267.

28. Henry Stack Sullivan, "Psychiatry and the National Defense," *PSY* 4 (1941): 201–217, 217. This article is different from the one with the same title in *PSY* 3 (1940): 619–624. See also Vernon A. Rosario, *Homosexuality and Science: A Guide to Debate* (Santa Barbara, CA: ABC-CLIO, 2002), 88–89; Bérubé, *Coming Out under Fire*, 12.

29. Sullivan, "William Alanson White Psychiatric Foundation Bulletin," 627.

30. George Chauncey, *Gay New York: Gender, Urban Culture, and the Making of the Gay Male World 1890–1940* (New York: Basic Books, 1994), 13–14.

31. The original criteria did not make it clear that homosexual men needed to be rejected. After mid-1941, homosexuality became specified as a cause of rejection and the criteria were revised accordingly. See Sullivan, "Selective Service Psychiatry," 451; Sullivan, "Seminar on Practical Psychiatric Diagnosis," 265–283, particularly 265. On the change of terms used in the army criteria, see Michaela Hampf, "'Dykes' or 'Whores': Sexuality and the Women's Army Corps in the United States during World War II," *Women's Studies International Forum* 27 (2004): 13–20.

32. Bérubé, *Coming Out under Fire*, 2.

33. Sullivan, "Seminar on Practical Psychiatric Diagnosis," 273–278.

34. Harry Stack Sullivan, "Psychiatric Aspect of Morale," *AJS* 47 (1941): 277–301, 298. See also Harry Stack Sullivan, "An Editorial: Selective Service Psychiatry," *PSY* 4 (1941): 118–120.

35. Indeed, Sullivan's belief in homosexual men's psychological fragility might have been his main reason to agree to screen out homosexual men. The irony is that a number of gays and lesbians found opportunities for sexual liaisons and friendships while they served in the army. See John D'Emilio and Estelle B. Freedman, *Intimate Matters: A History of Sexuality in America*, 2d ed. (Chicago: University of Chicago Press, 1988), 288–290; Arthur Dong, *Coming Out under Fire* (Los Angeles: Deep Focus Productions, 1994), documentary film.

36. Douglas A. Thom, "Schizoid and Related Personalities," *War Medicine* 1, no. 3 (1941): 410–417, 416.

37. "Interview with Harry Biele (December 4 1988)," MSA.

38. Henry Stack Sullivan, *Conceptions of Modern Psychiatry* (New York: W. W. Norton, 1953) (originally published in *PSY* 3 [1940]: 1–117), 41; Harry Stack Sullivan, *The Psychiatric Interview*, ed. Helen Swick Perry and Mary Ladd Gawel (New York: W. W. Norton, 1954; originally given as a series of lectures at the WSP in 1945–1946), 237–238.

39. Sullivan, "Selective Service Psychiatry," 461.

40. Henry Stack Sullivan, *Personal Psychopathology: Early Formulations* (New York: W. W. Norton, 1972; written between 1929 and 1933), 194–258.

41. Dexter Mean Bullard, "Selective Service Psychiatry: Schizoid and Related Personalities; Mood Disorders and Psychopathic Personalities," *PSY* 4, no. 2 (1941): 231–239, 235.

42. Bartemeier, "Schizoid Personality," 677.

43. "Proceedings: Seminar on Practical Psychiatric Diagnosis (Chicago, May 19, 1941)," WSP, 47–48.

44. Ibid., 48–49.

45. On the association between psychopathic personality and homosexuality, see Bullard, "Selective Service Psychiatry," 238.

46. "Proceedings: Selective Service Psychiatry (San Francisco, June 20, 1941 [evening session])," WSP, 8–9.

47. Bérubé, *Coming Out under Fire*, 15.

48. Isidore I. Weiss, "Homosexuality: With Special Reference to Military Prisoners," *PQ* 20 (1946): 485–523; Colin J. Williams and Martin S. Weinberg, *Homosexuals and the Military: A Study of Less than Honorable Discharge* (New York: Harper and Row, 1971); Bérubé, *Coming Out under Fire*, 8, 24, 128–148, 202.

49. The screening boards grouped candidates into three categories: I-A (acceptable for full duty), I-B (acceptable for limited duty), 4-F (not acceptable for any duty). Those who received 4-F because of psychiatric reasons (4-F was a broad category referring to rejection because of any health reasons) were divided into eight groups of mental handicaps defined by the medical circular. Some examiners further categorized rejectees with more specific diagnoses such as "feeble-minded," "Peeping Tom," and "sexual psychopaths." During 1941, "homosexuality" was not used as a group designation but described as an aspect of personality disorders. Psychiatrists could proclaim, for example, "psychotic personality with homosexual symptoms" as a reason for rejection. With such detailed description, rejected homosexual men could be stigmatized specifically as such when back in local communities. Sullivan, along with others, deemed these designations inappropriate precisely because of the risk of stigmatization. But the detailed descriptions persisted, and group designations such as "psychotic personality" became associated with homosexuality. See Sullivan, "Seminar on Practical Psychiatric Diagnosis"; Sullivan, "Selective Service Psychiatry." Ernest E. Hadley et al., "An Experiment in Military Selection," *PSY* 5 (1942): 371–402; Rosario, *Homosexuality and Science*, 92–94; Bérubé, *Coming Out under Fire*, 14–28.

50. Harry Stack Sullivan, "Psychiatric Selection," *PSY* 5 (1942): 102–105.

51. Ellen Dwyer, "Psychiatry and Race during World War II," *Journal of the History of Medicine and Allied Sciences* 61 (April 2006): 117–143, 125; Leonard Rowntree, Kenneth H. McGill, and Thomas I. Edwards, "Causes of Rejection and the Incidence of Defects among 18 and 19 Year Old Selective Service Registrants," *Journal of the American Medical Association* 123 (September 25, 1943): 181–185, 181.

52. "Press Release: N.Y. State Conference on Social Work (October 22, 1941)," WSP, 3.

53. Sullivan, "Selective Service Psychiatry," 461.

54. Ibid., 453.

55. Sullivan, "Psychiatric Aspect of Morale," 300.

56. Ellen Dwyer, "Psychiatry and Race," 123.

57. Quoted in Yans-McLaughlin, "Science, Democracy, and Ethics," 204.

58. Harry Stack Sullivan, "Schizophrenic Individuals as a Source of Data for Comparative Investigation of Personality," in Sullivan, *Schizophrenia as a Human Process,* 218–232 (originally published in APA, *Proceedings: Second Colloquium on Personality Investigation* [Ann Arbor, MI: UMI, 1930], 43–48), 220.

59. Harry Stack Sullivan, "Socio-psychiatric Research: Its Implication for the Schizophrenia Problem and for Mental Hygiene," in Sullivan, *Schizophrenia as a Human Process* (originally published in *AJP* 87 [1930]: 977–991), 256–270, 266.

60. Historians have shown how such an unexamined conflation of race and sex, as well as the apparent destigmatization of one at the sacrifice of another, has been conspicuous in modern U.S. history. For example, U.S. immigration policies from the 1950s to the 1970s eliminated racially discriminative language, while at the same time, they redefined the category of legitimate citizens based on heterosexuality and marriageability, in effect contributing to homophobia. See Siobhan B. Somerville, "Queer *Loving,*" *GLQ: A Journal of Lesbian and Gay Studies* 11:3 (2005): 335–370.

61. "Proceedings: Selective Service System Seminar for Medical Advisory Board and Army Induction Board Psychiatrists (Washington, DC, January 2–3, 1941)," WSP, 65–66.

62. Menninger, *Psychiatry in a Troubled World,* 277–278; Shephard, *War of Nerves,* 199–200.

63. Sullivan, "Selective Service Psychiatry," 448.

64. Ibid., 450.

65. "Interview with Harry Biele (December 4, 1988)," MSA.

66. Sullivan, "Selective Service Psychiatry," 448–452.

67. Harry Stack Sullivan, "Psychiatry in the Emergency," *MH* 25 (1941): 5–10.

68. Sullivan, "Psychiatric Aspect of Morale," 281–290. Sullivan was asked to discuss Hitler's personality from a psychiatric perspective in the late 1930s and early 1940s. See for example, his brief analysis of Hitler's "disturbed personality" and his "fear of death" as a driving force of Nazi aggression in "Hitler's Terror of Death of Factor in War," *San Francisco News* (September 2, 1939). See also "Doctor Warns Nation of General Paranoia," *Register* (New Haven, CT: June 3, 1940).

69. Sullivan, "Psychiatric Aspect of Morale," 292–293.

70. "Proceedings: The Psychiatrists and the National Emergency (May 5, 1941)," WSP, 23.

71. "Press Release: N.Y. State Conference on Social Work (October 22, 1941)," WSP, 3.

72. Bérubé, *Coming Out under Fire,* 21.

73. "Proceedings: The Psychiatrists and the National Emergency," 7.

74. Indeed, psychiatrists were determined to facilitate communication between local boards and induction centers, not to give up their missions in the face of nonpsychiatric physicians' frustration with psychiatric examiners. The APA recommended that its member psychiatrists send a list of their patients to the state medical officer, so that local examiners could be "precaution[ed]" about dubious individuals. The APA also recommended that social agencies send candidates' personal information to state authorities in New Jersey, New York, and Connecticut. Soon, the Medical Survey Program, a plan to gather personal information from schools and hospitals, was introduced nationwide in 1943. See

"Proceedings: The Psychiatrists and the National Emergency," 53; Shephard, *War of Nerves*, 200.

75. James H. Capshew, *Psychologists on the March: Science, Practice, and Professional Identity in America, 1929–1969* (New York: Cambridge University Press, 1999), 55–56; Ellen Herman, *The Romance of American Psychology* (Berkeley: University of California Press, 1995), chap. 4.

76. Sullivan did not like the term *neuropsychiatry* used officially in the War Department. In 1940, when the National Defense Advisory Council was in the process of organizing its Committee on Neuropsychiatry, Sullivan claimed that neuropsychiatry narrowly focused on disorders of the nervous system and did not deal with "problems in the borderland of the individual and his social setting," as psychiatry did. In his editorial note, he called neuropsychiatry a "product of World-War miscegenation without benefit of scientific legality." See Harry Stack Sullivan, "Editorial Notes: Endocrinoneuropsychiatry," *PSY* 3 (1940): 561–563.

77. Menninger, *Psychiatry in a Troubled World*, 273–274.

78. John W. Appel and Gilbert W. Beebe, "Preventive Psychiatry: An Epidemiologic Approach," *Journal of the American Medical Association* 131 (1946): 1469–1475. See also Paul Wanke, "American Military Psychiatry and Its Role among Ground Forces in World War II," *Journal of Military History* 63 (1999): 127–145. On the increasing emphasis on treatment in 1942 and 1943, see Frank J. Sladen, ed., *Psychiatry and the War* (Springfield, IL: Charles C. Thomas, 1943); Colonel John Boyd Coates Jr., *Preventive Medicine in World War II*, vol. 3: *Personal Health Measures and Immunization* (Washington, DC: Office of the Surgeon General, Department of the Army, 1955), 185–188.

79. Harry Stack Sullivan, "Psychiatry, the Army, and the War," *PSY* 5 (1942): 435–442, 436–437.

80. Ibid., 442.

81. Harry Stack Sullivan, "Therapeutic Aspect of the Psychiatric Consultation with Special Reference to Obsessional and Schizophrenic States (February 8, 1940)," WSP, 50. See also Harry Stack Sullivan, "Some Facts about Psychiatric Therapy and Schizophrenia (February 10, 1940)," WSP, 24.

82. C. C. Fry and E. G. Rostow, *Interim Report OEM cmr. 337* (Washington, DC: National Research Council, April 1, 1945), cited in Menninger, *Psychiatry in a Troubled World*, 227. See also Lewis H. Loeser, "The Sexual Psychopath in the Military Service," *AJP* 102 (July 1945): 92–101.

83. Menninger, *Psychiatry in a Troubled World*, 228–230; Bérubé, *Coming Out under Fire*, 24–25, 264, 270–273; Alfred C. Kinsey, W. B. Pomeroy, and C. E. Martin, *Sexual Behavior in the Human Male* (Philadelphia: W. B. Saunders, 1948); Evelyn Hooker, "The Adjustment of the Male Overt Homosexual," *Journal of Projective Techniques* 11 (1957): 18–31.

84. The process of the desegregation accelerated particularly after 1948, when President Harry Truman set up the Committee on Equality of Treatment and Opportunity in the Armed Services. See *Civil Rights, The White House, and the Justice Department*, vol. 3: *Integration of the Armed Forces*, introduction by Michael R. Belknap (New York: Garland, 1991).

85. John D'Emilio, *Sexual Politics, Sexual Communities: The Making of a Sexual Minority in the United States, 1940–1970* (Chicago: University of Chicago Press, 1983), 48;

John D'Emilio, "Gay Politics and Community in San Francisco since World War II," in *Hidden from History: Reclaiming the Gay and Lesbian Past*, ed. Martin Bauml Duberman, Martha Vicinus, and George Chauncey Jr. (New York: Nal Books, 1989), 456–473, 460; Bernard C. Nalty, *Strength for the Fight: A History of Black Americans in the Military* (New York: The Free Press, 1986); Gary Gerstle, *American Crucible: Race and Nation in the Twentieth Century* (Princeton: Princeton University Press, 2001).

CHAPTER 6   "ONE-MAN" LIBERALISM GOES TO THE WORLD

1. Naoko Shibusawa, *America's Geisha Ally* (Cambridge: Harvard University Press, 2006); Frank Costigliola, "The Nuclear Family: Tropes of Gender and Pathology in the Western Alliance," *Diplomatic History* 21 (Spring 1997): 163–183; Emily S. Rosenberg, "'Foreign Affairs after World War II: Connecting Sexual and International Politics," *Diplomatic History* 18 (Winter 1994): 59–70.

2. Thompson, "The History," 9–10.

3. On Horney's split from the New York Psychoanalytic Society, see Nathan G. Hale Jr., *The Rise and Crisis of Psychoanalysis in the United States: Freud and the Americans, 1917–1985* (New York: Oxford University Press, 1995), 136–145.

4. Douglas Noble, "The History of Washington Psychoanalytic Society and the Washington Psychoanalytic Institute (unpublished, June 26, 1968)," HSP, 29. See also Helen Swick Perry, *Psychiatrist of America: The Life of Harry Stack Sullivan* (Cambridge: Belknap Press of Harvard University Press, 1982), 364.

5. Thompson, "History," 11.

6. Ralph M. Crowley and Maurice R. Green, "Revolution within Psychoanalysis: A History of the William Alanson White Institute (undated)," WAWI.

7. For example, his speech at the Washington Psychoanalytic Society in 1940 suggests his disappointment with the New York group of psychoanalysts. In this speech, he compared psychoanalysis with Christian Science, arguing that "Christian science [*sic*] is a great help to lots of people. . . . If you get a sufficiently bizarre type of confused philosophy, reality is so tainted that it doesn't bother you very much . . . and one very nice way of leading that kind of life . . . is to affiliate yourself with a highly psychoanalytic society, as we have in New York, you see. There are lots of analyzed people running around who associate only with analyzed people." See Harry Stack Sullivan, "Some Facts about Psychiatric Therapy and Schizophrenia (February 10, 1940)," WSP, 36.

8. Jeffrey Potter, *Men, Money, and Magic: The Story of Dorothy Schiff* (New York: Signet Books, 1977), 113. Dorothy Schiff was Sullivan's patient in the 1930s.

9. See, Perry, *Psychiatrist of America*, chap. 35.

10. Ibid.

11. "Cohen, Mabel (interview with Mabel Black Cohen, date unspecified)," HSP.

12. It was well known that Cohen was Sullivan's favorite. She became the new editor of *Psychiatry* after Sullivan's death, because the foundation's board of trustees decided that a new editor *should have been* "closely associated with Dr. Sullivan's . . . teaching and writing, and . . . clinical practice." See Arnold F. Emch, "Editorial Notes: Continuation," *PSY* 12 (1949): 435.

13. "Bruch, Hilde (interview with Hilde Bruch, September 20, 1973)," HSP.

14. See Harry Stack Sullivan, "The Study of Psychiatry," *PSY* 10 (1947): 355–371, in which he described a "dissent member of a seminar" as a "psychiatrist who . . . believes that Freud's original libido theory is an adequate basis for his current clinical thinking." This psychiatrist, Sullivan argued, had to "go away from a session with the feeling that he has been put in the wrong" place (369).

15. "Interview with Ruth Moulton (December 15, 1987)," MSA.

16. Lloyd Frankenberg, "Non-meeting (undated)," HSP.

17. "Hadley, Ernest and Agnes (interview with Agnes Hadley, September 25, 1968)," HSP; "Silverberg, William V. (interview with William V. Silverberg, May 15, 1962)" HSP; Perry, *Psychiatrist of America*, chap. 39; Clifton Read, "Harry Stack Sullivan: A Remembrance (undated)," MSA; "Bourke-White, Margaret (interview with John Vassos and Margaret Bourke-White, September 15, 1964)," HSP.

18. "Blitsten, Dorothy (interview with Dorothy Blitsten, March 17, 1971)," HSP. Ann Bullard, the wife of Dexter Bullard, also remembered that Sullivan "could not stand the color blue." See "File: Bullard, Ann and Dexter (interview with Dexter and Ann Bullard, Chestnut Lodge, February [date unspecified], 1971)," HSP, 8.

19. "Silverberg, William V. (interview with William V. Silverberg, May 15, 1962)," HSP.

20. Frankenberg, "Non-meeting." Throughout his memoir, Frankenberg spelled the name "Jimmy" instead of "Jimmie."

21. Frankenberg, "Non-meeting."

22. All quotes from Frankenberg, "Non-meeting." See also Perry, *Psychiatrist of America*, 339–400. During the time when Sullivan was sick, Jimmie's mother was sick too, and Jimmie was taking care of both. This was an added burden for Jimmie. In a letter to Helen Swick Perry, he wrote, "Don't remember date, as at this time my mother was dying of cancer + I was exhausted, etc., going to see her at the hospital + tending to HSS [Harry Stack Sullivan]." When Jimmie's mother died, he took care of paperwork such as the death certificate. See "Sullivan, James (letter from James Inscoe Sullivan to Helen Swick Perry [undated]; letter from James Inscoe Sullivan to Helen Swick Perry, October 6, 1971)," HSP. All this suggests that Jimmie was in touch with his family, contrary to the image that most of Sullivan's friends had of him as someone who did not have a place to go except Sullivan's.

23. Frankenberg, "Non-meeting."

24. John F. Cuber, "The College Youth Goes to War," *Marriage and Family Living* 5 (Winter 1943): 5–7, 7. See also John F. Cuber, "Readjustment of Veterans," *Marriage and Family Living* 7 (Spring 1945): 28–30.

25. Henry Elkin, "Aggressive and Erotic Tendencies in Army Life," *AJS* 51 (March 1946): 408–413. On postwar Americans' increasing concern about violent masculinity, see, for example, Estelle B. Friedman, "'Uncontrolled Desires': The Response to the Sexual Psychopath, 1920–1960," *Journal of American History* 74 (June 1987): 83–106. On the continuing marginalization of men who were deemed too "feminine" and "soft" in the 1950s, see K. A. Cuordileone, *Manhood and American Political Culture in the Cold War* (New York: Routledge, 2005). On the heightened social concern about sexuality and gender, broadly defined, in the postwar years, see Joanne Meyerowitz, *How Sex Changed: A History of Transsexuality in the United States* (Cambridge: Harvard University Press, 2002).

26. Cuber, "The College Youth," 7.

27. Elkin, "Aggressive and Erotic," 410.

28. Carle C. Zimmerman, "The Social Conscience and the Family," *AJS* 52 (November 1946): 263–268.

29. Lawrence K. Frank, "What Family Do for the Nation," *AJS* 53, no. 6 (1948): 471–473. See also G. Block Chisholm, "Psychological Adjustment of Soldiers to Army and to Civilian Life," *AJP* 101 (November 1944): 300–302.

30. Nadina R. Kavinoky, "Medical Aspects of War Time Marriages," *Marriage and Family Living* 6 (Spring 1944): 25–28.

31. Bernard N. Desenberg, "Home Sex Education and Monogamy," *Marriage and Family Living* 9 (Autumn 1947): 89–92. See also Claude C. Bowman, "Social Factors Opposed to the Extension of Heterosexuality," *AJP* 106 (December 1949): 441–447.

32. Harry Stack Sullivan, *Clinical Studies in Psychiatry* (New York: W. W. Norton, 1956), 157.

33. Ibid., 169.

34. Ibid., 170–177.

35. Ibid., 163–164.

36. Edward A. Strecker, *Their Mothers' Sons* (Philadelphia: Lippincott, 1946), 130–131; Edmund Bergler, *Counterfeit-Sex: Homosexuality, Impotence, Frigidity* (New York: Grune and Strattion, 1958), 193–204.

37. D'Emilio, *Sexual Politics, Sexual Communities,* chap. 3; David K. Johnson, *The Lavender Scare: The Cold War Persecution of Gays and Lesbians in the Federal Government* (Chicago: University of Chicago Press, 2004), 35–36, 75, 113; Margot Canaday, *The Straight State: Sexuality and Citizenship in Twentieth-Century America* (Princeton: Princeton University Press, 2009), 219–221.

38. Harry Stack Sullivan, "Completing Our Mobilization," *PSY* 5 (1942): 263–282, 268–276.

39. Ibid., 281.

40. Ibid., 268.

41. "Proceedings: Round Table on Technical Training of Personnel in the Reestablishment of a Peacetime Society (October 27, 1945)," WSP, 14.

42. Ibid., 16.

43. Gerald N. Grob, *The Mad among Us: A History of the Care of America's Mentally Ill* (New York: Free Press, 1994), 210–221; Hale, *The Rise and Crisis,* 208–209; Jack Pressman, *Last Resort: Psychosurgery and the Limits of Medicine* (New York: Cambridge University Press, 1998), 385; Wade E. Pickren and Stanley F. Schneider, eds., *Psychology and the National Institute for Mental Health: A Historical Analysis of Science, Practice, and Policy* (Washington, DC: APA, 2004).

44. "Proceedings: Round Table," 56–57.

45. Ibid., 60–61.

46. "Panel Discussion: The Reestablishment of Peacetime Society: Responsibilities of Psychiatrists (October 24, 1945)," WSP, 65.

47. Otto Allen Will Jr., "Editorial Notes: The International Mental Health Program," *PSY* 12 (1949): 189–191.

48. Harry Stack Sullivan, "Editorial Note: The Cultural Revolution to End War," *PSY* 9 (1946): 81–87, 83. See also Harry Stack Sullivan, "Your Future and the Newer Psychiatry (an address given at St. John's College, Annapolis, Maryland, in its adult education program, October 31, 1948)," WSP (italics in original).

49. Harry Stack Sullivan, "Editorial Note: For a National Mental Health Council," *PSY* 8 (1945): 235–237.

50. Sullivan, "Cultural Revolution," 86 (italics in original).

51. Harry Stack Sullivan, "Remobilization for Enduring Peace and Social Progress," *PSY* 10 (1947): 239–245, 239; Sullivan, "The Cultural Revolution," 85.

52. Harry Stack Sullivan, "Editorial Note: The Soldier's Return," *PSY* 8 (1945): 111–113, 112.

53. Harry Stack Sullivan, "Mental Health Potentialities of the World Health Organization," *MH* 27 (1948): 27–36, 36 (italics in original).

54. Sullivan, "Remobilization for Enduring Peace," 241.

55. "We, the Undersigned . . . : A Statement by Eight Distinguished Social Scientists on the Causes of Tensions which Makes for War (July 13, 1948)," Louis Wirth papers, Department of Special Collections, University of Chicago. The collection includes the records of the tension project's development between 1948 and 1951.

56. UNESCO, "UNESCO Conference on World Tensions: An International Multidisciplined Group," *PSY* 11 (1948): 231–233, 231.

57. On Benedict's contribution to the Tensions Project, see letters between Klaus Knorr and RFB (from July 9, 1947 to August 5, 1947), Series XVI, Folder 112.14, VC. Her lecture at the seminar on childhood education is in Series XVI, Folder 112.15, VC.

58. Harry Stack Sullivan, "Two International Conferences of Psychiatrists and Social Scientists," *PSY* 11 (1948): 223–229, 225.

59. Ibid., 224.

60. William Alanson White Psychiatric Foundation (WAWPF), "Immediate Retrospects on the I.P.C.," *PSY* 11 (1948): 339–344, 339.

61. A. Querido, "Notes on an Experiment in International Multiprofessional Cooperation," *PSY* 11 (1948): 349–354, 351–352.

62. WAWPF, "Immediate Retrospects," 341.

63. Ibid., 340.

64. Ibid., 344 (italics in original).

65. Ibid., 343.

66. Ibid., 342.

67. Querido, "Notes on an Experiment," 350.

68. Ibid., 351.

69. Ibid., 352.

70. WAWPF, "Immediate Retrospects," 343.

71. Ibid., 343–344.

72. Harry Stack Sullivan, "The School and International Prospect," *PSY* 11 (1948): xvii–xx, xviii.

73. WAWPF, "International Congress on Mental Health, London, August, 1948, Statement by International Preparatory Commission," *PSY* 11 (1948): 235–261, 235. See also 246.

74. Sullivan, "School and International Prospects," xx.

75. Harry Stack Sullivan, "Psychiatry, Education, and the UNESCO 'Tensions Project,'" *PSY* 11 (1948): 371–375, 374.

76. Ruth F. Benedict, "Recognition of Cultural Diversities in the Postwar World," in *An Anthropologist at Work*, ed. Margaret Mead (Boston: Houghton Mifflin, 1959), 439–448, 440.

77. Costigliola, "The Nuclear Family," 165.

78. Frank Costigliola, "'Unceasing Pressure for Penetration': Gender, Pathology, and Emotion in George Kennan's Formation of the Cold War," *Journal of American History* 83.4 (1997): 1309–1339, 1333.

79. Costigliola, "The Nuclear Family," 170.

80. Andrew J. Rotter, "Gender Relations, Foreign Relations: The United States and South Asia, 1947–1964," *Journal of American History* 81 (September 1994): 518–542, 523–525.

81. John W. Dower, *War without Mercy: Race and Power in the Pacific War* (New York: Pantheon Books, 1986); Shibusawa, *America's Geisha Ally*, 22, 131.

82. Petra Goedde, *GIs and Germans: Culture, Gender, and Foreign Relations, 1945–1949* (New Haven: Yale University Press, 2003), chap. 3.

83. Sullivan, "Two International Conferences," 228.

84. Ruth F. Benedict, "Anthropology and the Humanities," in *An Anthropologist at Work*, ed. Margaret Mead (Boston: Houghton Mifflin, 1959), 459–470, 464, 468–469 (italics in original).

85. Johnson, *The Lavender Scare*, 106, 113–114; Canaday, *The Straight State*, 247–248.

INDEX

abuse: history of sexual, 22, 24, 73; of patient, 80–81, 244n. 75; of self, 26, 71
Adler, Alfred, 97
admission: to mental hospital, 17, 19, 23, 67–68, 76, 182, 225n. 18; to the military, 168
adolescence, 27, 30, 106–107, 113, 126
adultery, 26, 100
adulthood, 93, 106–107, 212
African Americans, 86, 104, 109–113, 147, 158, 174–178, 184–185, 218, 235n. 56, 236n. 61. See also race
aggressiveness, 129, 196–197, 205, 207–208, 213, 216, 249n. 69
Alexander, Franz, 242n. 49
Alinder, Gary, 218
Allen, Michael Stuart, 45, 144, 149–152, 219
Allport, Gordon W., 208
alyha, 127–128
American Anthropological Association, 215
American Association of Social Workers, 114
American Council of Education (ACE), 109–110
American Medical Association, 88, 246n. 21
American Psychiatric Association (APA), 92, 94, 114, 159, 161, 163, 181, 217–218, 246n. 21, 249n. 74
American Sociological Society (ASS), 92, 94
anthropology, 114–115, 133, 139, 150, 161, 215–216
Appel, John W., 182
Association of American Medical Colleges, 114
atomic bomb, 206
attendants: characteristics of, 40, 79; at Chestnut Lodge, 192–194; at Sheppard-Pratt, 14–15, 21, 32, 34, 36, 42–43, 67, 78–81, 144, 228n. 71, 242n. 50

bachelorhood, 41, 134, 145–146
Bain, Read, 93, 129
Bare, Richard, 144
Bartemeier, Leo H., 170
Bateson, Gregory, 135, 137

Beebe, Gilbert W., 182
Beers, Clifford B., 89
Benedict, Ruth Fulton: affiliation with Washington School of Psychiatry, 104, 115, 234n. 38; and liberalism, 3, 86; mentioned, 129, 144; and postwar reconstruction, 187, 208, 212–213, 215–217; public image of, 7, 134–135, 145–146; relationship with Ruth Bunzel, 139–140; relationship with Margaret Mead, 6, 123, 134–143; relationship with Natalie Raymond, 136, 138–141; relationship with Edward Sapir, 133–134; as scientist of sexuality, 48, 122–123, 127, 134, 153–154; and World War II, 157, 160, 162; writing on homosexuality, 4–5, 130–131, 139, 141–142
Benedict, Stanley, 135
berdache, 128
Bergler, Edmund, 217
Bieber, Irving, 217
Biele, Harry, 145
bisexuality, 11, 111, 239n. 8
blacks, 27, 109–113, 117, 125, 147–149, 159, 175–178, 184–185, 218, 235n. 56. See also race
Boas, Franz, 91
Boston Psychopathic Hospital, 15
Bradley, A. C., 216
Brazil, 207–208
Bruch, Hilde, 191
Bullard, Ann, 252n. 18
Bullard, Dexter Mean, 145, 169–170, 252n. 18
Bunzel, Ruth, 139
Burgess, Ernest, 94–95, 97–98, 104, 108

Canada, 203, 208
Chapman, Ross McClure, 15–16, 46–47, 80–81, 231n. 61
Chestnut Lodge Hospital, 15, 104, 145, 169, 189, 191–194, 198–199
childhood: of Ruth F. Benedict, 139, 142; scientific theory of, 15, 30, 91, 93, 105, 196; UNESCO seminar on, 207, 211

Chisholm, Brock, 203–204
Civilian Advisory Committee on Selective
  Service (CACSS), 159, 163–164, 166, 168,
  182, 246n. 19
civilization: complexity of, 9; distinction
  between sexes in, 138; and
  homosexuality, 8, 126, 128–129, 131,
  134, 146, 150, 152–153, 171, 196, 241n. 21;
  mentioned, 205–206; and primitivism,
  4–5, 87, 92–93, 109, 116, 122, 134. See also
  primitivism
civil rights movement, 10, 101, 218
class, 38, 98–99, 109, 118, 174, 191, 196
clinical records. See Sheppard and Enoch
  Pratt Hospital; Sullivan, Harry Stack
Cohen, Mabel Black, 191–192, 251n. 12
Cold War, 2, 187, 200, 202, 213
Colloquium on Personality Investigation,
  94–95, 97, 101–104, 108, 171, 241n. 21
Columbia University, 91–92, 129, 139
Committee for Democracy and Intellectual
  Freedom, 162
Committee on Equality of Treatment and
  Opportunity in the Armed Services,
  250n. 84
Committee on Neuropsychiatry, 250n. 76
Committee on Relations with the Social
  Sciences (APA), 92
conservatism, 2, 8, 10
Cornell University, 140
correctional facility, 79, 123–124
Costigliola, Frank, 187
Cressman, Luther, 135
Criteria for the Life History (Dollard), 90, 109
Crowley, Ralph M., 45–46
Cuber, John F., 196, 198, 200, 207
cure : of homosexuality 2, 125; and Native
  American transvestites, 127; of neurosis;
  190; in the "new psychiatry," 31, 151; of
  schizophrenia, 113
Czechoslovakia, 207, 211

Davis, Allison, 104
Davis, Katherine Bemont, 10
de Angulo, Jaime, 141
delinquency, 86, 94, 163
depression, 163
Desenberg, Bernard N., 198, 200
Devereux, George, 127–128, 130, 139–141
diagnosis: as a purpose of staff conference,
  20; of schizophrenia, 28–29, 103, 113; in
  Selective Service screening, 161, 163, 168,
  172; uncertainty of, 29, 88
Dickinson, Robert Latou, 10
discharge: from mental hospital, 15, 17,
  19, 67, 69, 72–73, 75–77, 169; from the
  military, 165, 174, 182, 184
Dollard, John, 3, 87, 90–91, 104, 108–109, 111,
  236n. 61
Dooley, Lucile, 75, 115–116, 190
Dunham, Katherine, 144

effeminacy, 2, 207. See also femininity
Eisenhower, Dwight D., 216

Elgin, William W., 42, 242n. 50
Eliot, Thomas, 92
Elkin, Henry, 196, 198, 200, 207
Elliot, William, 80
Ellis, Havelock, 239n. 8
Ellison, Ralph, 143–144
Ernst, John R., 125
eugenics, 175–176, 239n. 6

"fairy," 24
family: of James Inscoe, 46–47, 252n. 22;
  scientific analysis of, 26, 91, 106, 111,
  115, 124, 172, 196–197, 201, 226n. 38; in
  Sheppard-Pratt clinical records, 19, 28,
  56, 58, 63–64, 71–76, 225n. 18, 225n. 19;
  values, 2; of William V. Silverberg, 132
fatherhood, 22–23, 26, 47–48, 56, 72–73, 133,
  140–141, 212
Federal Bureau of Investigation, 180
feeblemindedness, 180, 248n. 49
fellatio, 23–24, 39, 44, 79
femininity: in behavior, 24, 44; and
  homosexuality, 132, 136, 141, 143;
  imbalance between masculinity and,
  9, 196–197, 202, 205, 213–214; and
  immaturity, 131, 202; integration of
  masculinity and, 200, 206–208, 212–213;
  vs. masculinity, 24, 93, 129, 132–133,
  137, 142, 154, 199. See also effeminacy;
  masculinity
feminism, 93, 124, 127, 129, 133–134, 143
Ferenczi, Sandor, 73, 97, 242n. 49
Fortune, Reo, 135, 137
4F classification, 169, 248n. 49
France, 162, 207, 208, 213
Frank, Lawrence, 3, 95, 104, 145, 187, 197,
  201, 209–211, 233n. 26
Frankenberg, Lloyd, 192–195, 252n. 20
Frazier, E. Franklin, 109, 147, 178
Freud, Sigmund: on homosexuality, 4, 123;
  and psychoanalysis, 8, 15–16, 86, 89, 145,
  195; on sexuality, 26, 108, 226n. 38; and
  the social sciences, 92–94
Freyre, Gilberto, 208
friendship: between Margaret Mead and
  Ruth F. Benedict, 136; between Edward
  Sapir and Ruth F. Benedict, 133–134, 138;
  between Clara Thompson and James
  Inscoe, 47; in children, 106; same-sex, 32,
  98–100, 106, 126, 199, 241n. 21; troubled
  pattern of Sullivan's, 145, 242n. 50
frigidity, 59
Fromm, Erich, 104, 115, 145, 190, 193, 242n.
  49
Fromm-Reichmann, Frieda, 115
Fry, Clements C., 184

Gay, Jan, 48
"gay," use of term, 10–11, 223n. 21
gay culture, 1, 150
gay men: as attendants, 42; healthy,
  31; in the military, 158, 247n. 35; as
  patients, 152; prejudice against, 152; as
  psychiatrists, 3, 5, 13, 41, 104, 132–133, 215

gay rights, 101, 218
gender: equality, 71, 129, 142–143, 155; and homosexuality, 23–24, 130–133, 213; inequality, 5, 60, 127–130, 154; in language, 204, 212–214; mentioned, 2, 4, 10, 21, 52, 77–79, 109, 124, 155, 195, 207; and pathology, 187; and sexuality, 11, 23, 54, 58, 121, 129, 133, 137, 140
Germany, 17, 109, 187, 213–214
Gill, Tom, 115
Great Depression, 2
Groves, Ernest R., 124
Gurvitch, Georges, 208

Hadley, Agnes, 45
Hadley, Ernest E., 45–46, 115
Hamilton, Donald M., 126
Hamilton, Samuel W., 203–204
Harvard University, 91, 93
Healy, William, 95
Hendrick, Ives, 16
Henry, George W., 10, 125, 239n. 8
Henry Phipps Clinic, 15
Hershey, Lewis B., 182, 246n. 19
heteronormativity, 42, 153. See also heterosexism
heterosexism, 41, 177–178, 185. See also heteronormativity
heterosexuality: vs. homosexuality, 4, 122, 153, 168, 173, 217; mentioned, 147, 197, 212; out of balance, 215. See also homosexuality; sexuality
higher education, 62, 65, 75, 169
Hill, Lewis B., 16
Hill, W. W., 127–128, 130
Hitler, Adolf, 180, 249n. 68
Holland, 208
homoeroticism, 24, 30–31, 87, 107–108
homophobia: critique of, 5, 7–9, 21, 33, 48, 82, 86, 98–99, 105–107, 131, 154, 178, 215; disguised, 6; in patients at Sheppard-Pratt, 23, 25; prevalence of, 4, 29, 31, 71, 167, 173, 249n. 60; protection from, 154; and racism, 87, 109–112, 119; and sexism, 123, 129, 141–143
homosexuality: Benedict-Mead discussion of, 135–143; clinical approach to (at Sheppard-Pratt), 21–25, 33–43, 78–82; and cultural sophistication, 131, 144–146, 149–153, 155, 177, 207; and femininity, 24, 132, 141, 143, 154, 188, 196, 199–200; full acceptance of, 87, 126, 168; as health risk; 31–32; vs. heterosexuality, 4, 122, 153, 168, 173, 217; historiography of, 6; as maladjustment to civilization, 93; mentioned, 1, 12, 13–14, 112, 147; post–World War II redefinition of, 188, 196–202, 204, 207, 213–214; and racism, 110–112, 178; and schizophrenia, 28–31, 86, 93; science of, 2–10, 21, 49, 52–53, 71, 83, 118, 121–134, 157–158, 173, 183, 214–218; screening of, 166–174, 184, 248n. 49; and social adjustment, 31; Sullivan-Sapir discussion of, 99–103; Sullivan's writing

on, 43–44, 106–108, 198–200; treatment of, 217. See also heterosexuality; sexuality
"homosexuality," use of term, 10–11
Hooker, Evelyn, 218
Horkheimer, Max, 208
Horney, Karen, 115, 145–146, 189–190, 193, 195, 242n. 49
Hungary, 207
hwame, 127–128
hysteria, 165

idiocy, 54, 201
imbecility, 180, 201
immaturity: and femininity, 132, 200, 202; vs. maturity, 5, 53, 93, 213; in personality, 52, 92–93, 130–131, 163, 213; post–World War II redefinition of, 196, 200–202, 205, 213; psychosexual, 9, 125, 202. See also maturity
immigrants, 17, 64, 104, 179, 249n. 60
immorality, 39, 65
incest, 30, 73
induction (into the army), 159, 164–166, 169, 173–174, 179, 182–183, 246n. 16, 249n. 74. See also induction center
induction center (of U.S. Army), 164, 179, 182, 246n. 16, 249n. 74. See also induction
inhibition: religious, 17; sexual, 13, 48, 107, 111
Inscoe, James (Jimmie): burning Sullivan's letters, 6; conflicting accounts of Sullivan's relationship with, 44–49, 252n. 22; and Sheppard-Pratt, 47, 228n. 71; as Sullivan's partner, 13–14, 80, 99, 118, 133, 135, 141, 143–146, 150, 153–154, 189, 193–195, 242n. 55, 244n. 84
Institute of Ethnic Psychiatry, 116–117
Institute of Human Relations, 95, 108
intelligence: defined by the military, 125, 176, 246n. 16; of the mentally ill, 68, 177; of scientists, 206; social, 201
International Preparatory Commission for the International Congress on Mental Health (IPC), 204, 207–211, 213–215
interpersonal relations, theory of, 3, 90–91, 95–96, 105–108, 110, 114–115, 149, 160, 180, 201
intimacy: heterosexual, 57, 59, 75, 133; interpersonal, 206; same-sex, 31, 78–79, 87, 99–100, 107, 126, 135, 171, 241n. 21
Ireland, 208
Italy, 208

Japan, 98–99, 187, 213–214
Jelliffe, Smith Ely, 92
Jellinek, E. M., 115
Johns Hopkins University, 15, 62, 65
Johnson, Charles S., 3, 86, 109, 112–113, 115, 178
Joint Committee on Psychiatric Education (APA), 114

Kavinoky, Nadina R., 197–198
Kinsey, Alfred C., 10, 48, 218, 228n. 75

Kluckhohn, Florence R., 91, 96
Kolb, Lawrence, 179
Kretschmer, Ernest, 109

Lasswell, Harold, 86, 94, 97–98, 104, 115–116, 233n. 35
Laura Spelman Rockefeller Memorial Foundation, 95, 233n. 26
Layard, J. W., 128
"lesbian," use of term, 10–11, 223n. 21
lesbianism, 2, 124, 134, 135, 138, 142, 247n. 35
Levy, David, 95
Lewis, Oscar, 129–130, 133, 142
liberalism: and conservatism, 2, 8; definition of, 3–4, 86, 158, 217; and homosexuality, 1–3, 5–7, 9, 123, 127, 131; limits of, 86–87, 118, 122, 158–159, 172–173, 181, 204; "one-man," 188; and paternalism, 187; postwar, 218; private, 3, 5–7, 9, 14–15, 32–44, 49, 53, 87, 98, 100–102, 104, 112; public, 3, 5, 9, 15, 53, 88, 102; and race, 178, 185; "us" vs. "others" dichotomy in, 147
life history: and cohort of scientists, 118, 143, 157, 189; mentioned, 26–27, 66, 72, 101, 104, 108, 111, 123; as a method of treatment, 71, 88, 118; as a middle ground between the scientific and the subjective, 70, 74–75, 84–86, 91; in private, 103; as a scientific method, 4, 20, 52, 74, 85–97, 102, 114, 116–117, 121, 215–216. See also subjectivity
Linton, Arthur, 21, 36, 42
local installation board (of U.S. Army), 164, 171, 246n. 21
Lowrey, Lawson G., 95

manliness, 18, 31, 77, 213. See also masculinity
manly-hearted women, 129
marriage: dysfunctional, 27; heterosexual, 2, 19, 26, 40–41, 74–75, 139; mentioned, 136–137; and reproduction, 5, 121, 123, 139, 197; same-sex, 1, 129; scientific concern about, 196–200; sex and, 5, 54, 57–62, 198; "true," 38, 239n. 6
masculinity: vs. femininity, 24, 93, 129, 132–133, 137, 142, 154; and homosexuality, 132–133, 141, 200; imbalance between femininity and, 9, 196–198, 202, 205, 213–214; integration of femininity and, 200, 206–208, 212–213; in the military, 167; modern, 78; traditional, 52, 138; in women, 129, 133. See also femininity; manliness; virility
masturbation: acceptance of, 55–56, 59–60, 111; as common, 53; concern about, 25–26, 54–55; guilt over, 19, 23, 27, 39; and homosexuality, 28; mentioned, 41, 54, 57, 82; mutual, 22, 24–25, 106; stigmatization of, 66, 71
maternity, 136–138, 140, 143. See also motherhood

Mattachine Society, 185
maturity: in appearance, 169, 177; vs. immaturity, 5, 53, 93, 205, 213; and independence, 52, 76–78, 82, 87; and manliness, 31; and marriage, 197–198; and masculinity, 200, 213; of men, 52, 54, 58–65; in post–World War II leadership, 204–205, 210–213; in sexuality, 31, 52, 58, 107–108, 121–123, 173; of women, 59, 132–133, 212. See also immaturity
May, Mark A., 95–96, 108
Mayo, Elton, 93–94
McLean Hospital, 15
Mead, Margaret: on Hiroshima, 206; on homosexuality, 129, 134, 137; and liberalism, 3, 86; and life history, 91; mentioned, 154; and postwar reconstruction, 187, 210–211; public image of, 7; on race, 176–177; relationship with Ruth Fulton Benedict, 6, 123, 134–143; on reproduction, 137–138, 140; as a scientist of sexuality, 5–6, 48; and World War II, 157, 162
Meagher, John F. W., 124–125
medical advisory board (of U.S. Army), 164, 182, 246n. 21
Medical Circular No. 1 (1940), 163–164
Medical Circular No. 1 (revised, 1941), 165, 168, 172, 248n. 49
Medical Survey Program, 249n. 74
medicine. See psychiatry; psychoanalysis
Menninger, Karl A., 115
Menninger, William C., 182, 184
mental hygiene movement, 8, 113, 115–116, 118, 236n. 65
"men-women," 129
Meyer, Adolf, 89–90, 232n. 8
middle class, 16, 145, 190. See also class
modernity, 4, 7, 10, 49, 52, 58, 85–86, 93–94, 117, 121
Mohave Indians, 127–128, 139
morale, 1, 161–162, 171, 180–181, 185
morality, 14, 23–27, 37, 51, 74–75, 136, 157, 183, 196–197, 200, 206. See also immorality
Moreno, J. L., 176
moronity, 201
motherhood, 26, 59, 72–73, 105, 124, 136–138, 140, 147, 169, 199–200
Moulton, Ruth, 192
Mullahy, Patrick, 149, 243n. 63

nadle, 127
Naess, Arne, 208
National Association for the Advancement of Colored People (NAACP), 184
National Committee for Mental Hygiene (NCMH), 89, 159, 163
National Defense Advisory Council, 250n. 76
National Institute of Mental Health, 114, 203
National Mental Health Act (1946), 203

Native Americans, 7, 98–100, 116–117, 126–130, 223n. 18, 241n. 21
neurosis, 26, 93, 109, 114, 145, 190, 195
new psychiatry, *See* psychiatry
New York Psychoanalytic Society, 189, 251n. 3
Noble, Douglas, 115
North Piegan Indians, 129
Norway, 207

objectivity: critique of, 4, 94, 114; as a masculine trait, 207; scientific, 6, 49, 91; vs. subjectivity, 4, 6, 91. *See also* subjectivity
occupational therapy, 15, 66–67, 71, 76, 225n. 18, 226n. 20
Office of War Information, 162
Ogburn, William, 92
orgasm, 58–59

Painter, Thomas, 48, 228n. 75
paranoia, 29, 125, 151, 163, 167
Park, Robert E., 86, 92, 95, 104
parole, 15, 17, 72–73
Parsons, Elsie Clews, 128–130, 133, 142, 240n. 14
participant observation, 91, 95–96, 101–102, 110, 114, 117, 215
Partridge, George E., 16, 38
paternalism, 112, 154, 187–188, 194–195, 210
patients. *See* Sheppard and Enoch Pratt Hospital; Sullivan, Harry Stack
Patterns of Culture (Benedict), 131, 139, 141
Paul, Randolph, 115
"Peeping Tom," 248n. 49
Perry, Helen Swick, 45, 144, 147–151, 153, 252n. 22
personality development, theory of, 3, 31, 104–106, 109, 116, 169, 205, 212
Personal Psychopathology (Sullivan), 87, 105–108, 111, 113, 117
petting, 25, 57–58
Pima Indians, 128
Plant, James S., 95, 97–98
Pope, Ray, 193–194
Porter, William C., 171, 173, 246n. 19
Powdermaker, Hortense, 108–109, 111, 117, 235n. 51
Pratt, Enoch, 15
preadolescence, 106, 113, 199
premarital sex, 54, 57–60, 66, 238n. 3
prepsychotic personality, 165
primitivism: and African Americans, 112; and civilization, 5, 87, 92–93, 109, 116, 122; and femininity, 143; and homophile attitude, 4, 37–38, 100, 122, 128; and homosexuality, 7, 126–129, 131, 134, 142; as human nature, 86, 94; and lack of social maladjustment, 93; in masculinity, 196–197; and schizophrenia, 109, 116, 132; as underdeveloped personality, 92–93; white scientists' approach to, 117. *See also* civilization

prison, 79, 179
privacy, 6, 103, 169
prostitution, 23, 25, 45, 196
psychiatric screening, *See* homosexuality; Selective Service System
psychiatry: biological, 88–89; centralization of, 202–203; impact of World War II on, 158–159, 161, 164–165, 172, 181–183; mentioned, 2, 103, 133, 167, 208; the new, 15, 20, 31, 82, 88–90, 95–96, 113–114, 161, 165, 167, 183; reform of, 88–90, 92–93, 96–98, 113–115, 118; social, 95–97, 98, 104; Sullivan's place in, 13, 144, 189–192. *See also* psychoanalysis
Psychiatry (journal), 104, 115–116, 211, 234n. 39
psychoanalysis: culture of, 145, 242n. 50, 251n. 7; and psychiatry, 8, 13–16, 89–90, 92, 115, 143, 152, 217; schisms in, 189–190, 195; at Sheppard-Pratt, 15–17, 66–68, 73–75; and the social sciences, 83, 90–93, 97, 104, 108, 114–115, 160–161; theory of, 86; during World War II, 168, 180. *See also* Freud, Sigmund; psychiatry
psychopathic personality, 28, 163, 248n. 45. *See also* racism
psychotic personality, 174, 248n. 49

"queer," use of term, 11
queerness, 7, 166, 168–170

race: assumed differences of, 126, 147, 162, 176, 178, 212; as barrier, 110, 113, 185; consciousness, 147; discrimination and, 147, 155, 158, 174–178, 180, 249n. 60; discussed at Sheppard-Pratt, 29, 74; human, 126, 132; scientific analysis of, 109–113, 155, 174, 177–178, 212. *See also* African Americans; blacks; Native Americans; whites
racism, 5, 87, 109, 112–113, 119, 147, 153, 155, 158, 175–178, 184–185, 212, 215. *See also* race
Raymond, Natalie, 136, 138–142
Read, Clifton, 81, 146–148, 150, 154, 175, 193
recovery: high rate of (at Sheppard-Pratt), 132; from homosexuality, 36; hope for, 113; of James Inscoe from an assumed mental illness, 7; and manliness, 77; sign for, 30; social, 72–73, 169
regionalism, 51, 64–65, 109
rehabilitation, 174
relativism, 3, 85, 127, 172, 212
religion, 17, 28, 51, 56–57, 74, 180
reproduction, 5, 121, 123, 132, 137–138, 140–141, 197
Richmond, Winfred V., 124, 132
Rioch, David McKenzie, 194
Rioch, Janet McKenzie, 180, 192
Robbins, Bernard, 36, 78–80
Roosevelt, Franklin Delano, 159, 163
Rosanoff, Aaron, 125
Rostow, Edna G., 184
Rowland, Howard, 115
Russia, 17, 64

same-sex marriage. *See* marriage

Sapir, Edward: as friend of Sullivan and James Inscoe, 99, 146; on homosexuality, 98–100, 133, 241n. 24; and liberalism, 3, 86; mentioned, 119, 123, 144; relationship with Ruth Fulton Benedict, 133–135, 138; Sullivan's collaboration with, 45, 91, 94–96, 98–104, 108, 115–116, 171, 189

Sapir, Jean, 45, 108, 138, 146, 153

Sapir, Philip, 144, 242n. 55

Schiff, Dorothy, 144

schizophrenia: definition of, 13, 25, 28–31, 109; and "generating" mothers, 200; and homosexuality, 20, 28–31, 81–82, 86, 93, 98–99, 123–125, 132, 151–152, 167–171, 181; and neurosis, 145; patients diagnosed with, 13–14, 17, 20, 29, 43, 63–64, 103, 171; rarity in primitive society, 116; Sullivan's expertise in, 13–14, 48, 113; treatability of, 28, 113, 117; treatment of, 14, 80–82

Schwartz, Morris S., 104

Selective Service System, 159–161, 169, 182, 189; screening, 8, 112, 158–185, 192, 195, 204, 246n. 16, 246n. 17, 247n. 31, 248n. 49. *See also* the Civilian Advisory Committee on Selective Service

Selective Training and Service Act (1940), 159

self-awareness: and homosexuals, 130; as male quality, 17; as modern quality, 66, 73, 87; same-sex, 32, 98–100, 126, 136, 199, 241n. 21, 247n. 35; significance of (in treatment), 51, 65, 71–72, 75, 77; and women, 83

Selling, Lowell S., 125, 132

Sex and Temperament in Three Primitive Societies (Mead), 129, 137, 141

sexism, 5, 130, 133, 155, 202, 215

sexuality: abnormal, 1, 4, 102; female, 26–27, 57–60, 212; gender and, 140, 143, 155; homosexuality as a high-risk, 41; homosexuality as the most apt, 122; human, 2–3, 30, 44, 48; immature, 198; male, 18, 52, 54–55, 60, 197, 202, 205; mature, 31; mentioned, 7, 10–14, 21, 25, 42, 86, 101, 103, 106, 121, 135–137, 167, 214; 1920s' exploration of, 58; 1920s' freedom of, 2, 57–58; normal, 3; of "others," 86–87, 122, 126, 130–131; as part of person as a whole, 217; politics of, 8; and queerness, 166; in science, 108, 111–112; secular vs. religious approach to, 56. *See also* heterosexuality; homosexuality; lesbianism; transvestism

sexual minority, 1–11, 42, 122–125, 130–133, 152–155, 159, 171–173, 185, 189, 198, 215–218, 244n. 75. *See also* homosexuality

"sexual minority," use of term, 11, 223n. 21

sexual psychopaths, 248n. 49

Shaw, Clifford, 94

Sheppard, Moses, 15

Sheppard and Enoch Pratt Hospital (Sheppard-Pratt): Ross M. Chapman at, 47, 80–81; characteristics of (as hospital),

13, 15–21, 78; clinical culture of, 21, 24–25, 60–63, 65–66, 77–78, 80–84, 86, 93–94, 98; clinical practice at, 28–32, 36, 87, 89–90, 96, 99–102, 117, 132, 151–152, 225n. 18, 225n. 19, 226n. 20; clinical records at, 13–14, 18–21, 47, 85, 225n. 7, 226n. 21, 226n. 22, 227n. 62; James Inscoe at, 47, 228n. 71; and liberalism, 14, 18; mentioned, 108, 112–113, 130, 147–148; patients at, 13–18, 21–29, 32–45, 49–60, 63–65, 67–77, 79, 103, 107, 110–111, 126, 145, 171; as sex-segregated institution, 79–80, 126; Sullivan's departure from, 49, 53, 79, 87, 118, 123, 145

Shibusawa, Naoko, 187

Silverberg, William V., 16, 132–133, 145, 190, 193, 241n. 20, 242n. 49

Singleton, Anne (pseud. Ruth Fulton Benedict), 135

Socarides, Charles, 217

Social Science Research Council, 95, 104, 109, 233n. 26

social work, 15, 56, 114, 207

sociology, 29, 90, 114–115, 197, 208

sodomy, 27, 166

Soviet Union (USSR), 116, 187, 213

Stanton, Alfred H., 104

Stekel, Wilhelm, 97

stenographer, 20. *See also* typist

Stephens, Gordon, 212

Stevenson, George H., 181

Stieglitz, Edward, 194

Stonewall (riot), 102, 218

subjectivity: debate over, 92, 95; in history of science, 5, 10; of homosexuals, 7, 80–82, 102–104, 154–155, 207, 215; in life history, 87, 90, 103; of the mentally ill, 52–53, 61, 65, 88, 94, 144, 152; mentioned, 118, 135, 157, 207, 218; vs. objectivity, 4, 6, 91; of "others," 189, 206, 211; in private, 103–104, 132, 144, 152, 214–215; and science, 6–7, 14, 19–20, 37–38, 44, 48–49, 70, 74, 151; in science, 82, 85, 90, 95, 102, 108, 123, 147, 215; science's declining engagement with, 117–118, 189, 215–218; of scientists, 5, 19, 53, 80–82, 88, 94, 96, 102–104, 108, 111–112, 122–123, 133, 151–153, 178, 204, 211, 215; in scientists' careers, 44, 117; sexual, 5, 119, 144, 148, 215; of youths, 60. *See also* objectivity

Sullivan, Harry Stack (Harry): at Chestnut Lodge Hospital, 104, 145, 189, 191–193, 198–200; and demise of psychiatric screening system, 180–183; departure from Sheppard-Pratt, 49, 53, 79, 87, 118, 123, 145; expertise in schizophrenia, 13–14, 48, 113; and female patients, 17, 69; in historiography, 5–7; IPC participants' critique of, 209–211; and liberalism, 3–4, 14–15, 87–88, 118–119, 188–189; and making of psychiatric screening system, 158–160, 163–164, 168; on masturbation, 55–56, 71; on medical education, 97–98, 114–115; on mental hygiene movement,

115–116, 118; 1930s patients of, 148–150; as physician at Sheppard-Pratt, 20–21; place in psychiatry and psychoanalysis, 13, 144–145, 189–192; place in social sciences, 87, 91, 94–95, 108–109; protectiveness of patients, 22–23, 72–73, 181; as psychiatric interviewer, 68–70; public vs. private approaches to homosexuality, 4–5, 8–9, 13–15, 41–42, 44, 52–53, 82–83, 98–103, 107–108, 122–123, 144, 152–157, 167–168, 172–173, 214–215, 218; relationship with James Inscoe, 13–14, 44–49, 80, 99, 118, 133, 135, 141, 143–146, 150, 153–154, 189, 193–195, 242n. 55, 244n. 84, 252n. 22; on race, 109–113, 147, 175–178; students of, 150–152; and UNESCO, 211–212; on "us" vs. "others," 200–201, 204–207; writing on homosexuality, 43–44, 106–108, 198–200
Sweden, 208
Switzerland, 208
Szalai, Alexander, 208

Taylor, Harold C., 108–109
Thom, Douglas A., 167, 169
Thomas, William I., 91–92
Thompson, Clara M., 46–47, 115, 144–146, 168, 180, 190, 194, 242n. 49
transvestism, 127, 140, 149, 239n. 8
trauma, 23, 32
typist, 20, 67. See also stenographer

United Kingdom, 162, 207–208
United Nations, 201
United Nations Educational, Scientific, and Cultural Organization (UNESCO), 9, 185, 188, 193, 202, 204, 207–208, 211–212, 214–216; UNESCO Seminar on Childhood Education, 207, 211; UNESCO Tensions Project, 212
United States Army, 158, 171, 196. See also Selective Service System
United States Bureau of the Census, 88
United States Public Health Service, 179, 203
University of Chicago, 91–93, 104, 108, 124

Vassos, John, 147–148, 193
Veteran's Administration, 203
Vietnam War, 185
virility, 4, 25, 138, 154, 196–197, 207, 213. See also manliness; masculinity

War Department, 159, 180, 182, 250n. 76
Washington-Baltimore Psychoanalytic Society, 115, 242n. 49, 251n. 7
Washington School of Psychiatry, 104, 113–114, 189–190, 194, 244n. 74
Weininger, Benjamin, 151
White, William Alanson, 94, 114–115, 237n. 80
whites, 27, 110–113, 117–119, 147, 158–159, 174–178, 185, 235n. 56, 236n. 60. See also race
Will, Otto Allen, 150–151
William Alanson White Institute of Psychiatry, 190. See also William Alanson White Psychiatric Foundation
William Alanson White Psychiatric Foundation, 116, 144, 182, 190, 203
Williams, Frankwood E., 114
Wolbarst, Abraham L., 126
womanliness, 77. See also manliness
working class, 145. See also class
World Federation for Mental Health (WFMH), 188, 193, 202, 204, 207, 211
World Health Organization (WHO), 188, 193, 202–204
World War I, 27, 159
World War II, 2, 8–9, 155, 157, 185, 200

Yale University, 91, 95, 104, 108–109, 116–117
Young, Kimball, 91–92
youth: African American, 109; education of, 73, 121; homosexual experience in, 22, 121; and immaturity, 92; maladjustment of, 116, 126, 198; mass screening of, 183; mentioned, 136; 1920s' culture of, 25–27, 51–52, 57, 60, 238n. 3; seduction of, 171; white, 175

Zilboorg, Gregory, 97, 245n. 7
Zimmerman, Carle C., 197, 201

ABOUT THE AUTHOR

NAOKO WAKE grew up in Japan as a child of a marine scientist and a yoga teacher. After completing her BA and MA at Kyoto University, she went to America's heartland, to attend Indiana University, Bloomington, where she received her PhD in 2005. She is currently a faculty member in the History, Philosophy, and Sociology of Science Program at Lyman Briggs College, Michigan State University, in East Lansing, where she teaches courses on the history of sexuality, gender, medicine, illness, and literature.